Targeted Intraoperative Radiotherapy in Oncology

Mohammed Keshtgar • Katharine Pigott
Frederik Wenz
Editors

Targeted Intraoperative Radiotherapy in Oncology

Springer

Editors
Mohammed Keshtgar
Division of Surgery
and Interventional Sciences
Department of Breast Surgery
University College London Medical
School; Royal Free London NHS
Foundation Trust
Hampstead
UK

Katharine Pigott
Department of Clinical Oncology
Royal Free London Foundation
NHS Trust
London
UK

Frederik Wenz
Department of Radiation Oncology
University Medical Center Mannheim
University of Heidelberg
Mannheim
Germany

ISBN 978-3-662-50925-8 ISBN 978-3-642-39821-6 (eBook)
DOI 10.1007/978-3-642-39821-6
Springer Heidelberg New York Dordrecht London

Printed on acid-free paper

Springer is part of Springer Science+Business Media (www.springer.com)

Foreword

Targeted intraoperative radiotherapy was developed more than a decade ago so that radiation was applied during operation targeted to the peri-tumoral tissues. The technique was designed at University College London for breast cancer and has through a randomized controlled trial disseminated all over the world. The targeted intraoperative radiotherapy in oncology is the first reference textbook in this field, edited by the pioneers of this technology. A panel of multidisciplinary experts who have been involved with the TARGIT technology for many years contributed to this book. It covers the scientific background of this technology, including radiobiology, mechanism of action and radiation safety aspects. It also provides a well-illustrated practical guidance to clinicians from various disciplines involved in management in cancer. It comprehensively covers the quality assurance and commissioning of the equipments and also provides detailed information on how to use the system in the operating room. The book also provides the latest updates on the results of randomised controlled trials and all the literatures related to this technology. The quality of life and health economics and cosmesis is also covered, along with training requirements to introduce this innovative technology into the health care system. Although the emphasis has been on breast cancer, applications in other cancers including rectal, brain, head and neck and cervical cancers as well as its use in bone metastasis is discussed. We congratulate the editorial team with an excellent review on this topic, which will alter the management of patients with many solid tumors, especially breast cancer, in the coming years.

Cornelis J.H. van de Velde
Department of Surgery
President European CanCer Organization (ECCO)
Brussels, Belgium

David Azria
Coordonnateur du pôle de Radiothérapie Oncologique
Président de la CME
ICM
Montpellier, France

Preface

Over the past few decades, the major change in the management of early breast cancer has been the shift towards less invasive approaches. These include breast conservation surgery and sentinel lymph node biopsy. Postoperative radiotherapy is regarded as an essential adjunct to BCS and cannot be safely omitted. There is overwhelming evidence that this approach decreases the risk of local recurrence and improves survival. The aim of radiotherapy is to selectively kill any residual tumour cells without damaging normal cells.

It is important to remember that whole breast radiotherapy is not without risks. Although treatment regimens have become safer with careful planning using computed tomography and treatment delivery using tangential fields, healthy tissues such as the heart, ribs and lungs do receive a small but significant dose of radiation.

Although the recurrence rate in breast cancer is low, the results of many clinical trials and observational studies have demonstrated that around 90 % of local recurrences after BCS occur within the same quadrant of the breast that harboured the primary tumour (index quadrant). This observation raises the question of whether whole breast radiotherapy is necessary in all patients and whether radiotherapy to the index quadrant of the breast alone would be sufficient. This has led to growing interest in accelerated partial breast irradiation (APBI), which aims to decrease the volume of breast treated and increase the daily fraction size of radiation.

A Photon Radiosurgery System (PRS) was first introduced at the London Royal Free Hospital in 1995 to assess its role in the treatment of solitary brain metastases. The tip of the probe was placed into the tumour, using standard stereotactic techniques, allowing for the delivery of a prescribed therapeutic radiation dose directly into the centre of the metastasis. Subsequently, the system was trialed for the first time in treatment of primary breast cancer at the University College London after the design and development of polymer applicators of various diameters to insert into the tumour cavity after resection.

In March 2000, an international, phase 3 randomised controlled trial in early breast cancer was launched as a non-inferiority trial and enrolled over 3,400 patients from 33 centres in eleven countries. The trial results indicate that the TARGIT technique using Intrabeam™ is safe and the efficacy falls within the pre-specified non-inferiority margin of 2.5 % for local recurrence as compared to external beam radiotherapy. Subsequently this technique was used for other solid tumours which is at various stages of development.

TARGIT Academy was subsequently established in 2010 to ensure appropriate introduction of this new technology into routine clinical practice. The focus of the Academy is on quality assurance and high standards in clinical education and training. It runs regular training courses in London and Mannheim and offers high-quality hands-on training and provides a networking platform which enables interaction and cooperation between surgeons, radiation oncologists, medical physicists and the extended multidisciplinary team.

This book is prepared by a panel of multidisciplinary experts who have been involved with the TARGIT technology from the outset. The purpose of this book is to provide a practical guide to clinicians from various disciplines who treat cancer patients. Although the emphasis is on breast cancer, however we have included the experience in brain tumours, rectal cancer and spinal metastases. We have presented case histories to enhance the learning points. We hope that you find this book a useful adjunct to your day-to-day practice.

Hampstead, UK — Mohammed Keshtgar
London, UK — Katharine Pigott
Mannheim, Germany — Frederik Wenz

Contents

Contributors

Maha Abdel Hadi Department of Surgery, University of Dammam, Dammam, Saudi Arabia

Yasser Abo-Madyan Department of Radiation Oncology, University Medical Center Mannheim, University of Heidelberg, Mannheim, Germany

Department of Clinical Oncology and Nuclear Medicine (NEMROCK), Faculty of Medicine, Cairo University, Cairo, Egypt

Michael Alvarado Division of Surgical Oncology, Department of Surgery, University of California, San Francisco, CA, USA

Kenneth Geving Andersen Section for Surgical Pathophysiology, 7621, Rigshospitalet, Copenhagen University, Copenhagen, Denmark

Department of Breast Surgery, Rigshospitalet, Copenhagen University, Copenhagen, Denmark

Gustavo Baldassarre Division of Experimental Oncology, CRO-IRCCS, National Cancer Institute, Aviano, Italy

Barbara Belletti Division of Experimental Oncology, CRO-IRCCS, National Cancer Institute, Aviano, Italy

Frederic Bludau Department of Orthopaedic and Trauma Surgery, University Medical Centre Mannheim, University of Heidelberg, Mannheim, Germany

Chris Brew-Graves Division of Surgery and Intervention Science, Department of Surgery, University College London, London, UK

Sven Clausen Department of Radiation Oncology, University Medical Center Mannheim, University of Heidelberg, Mannheim, Germany

David J. Eaton Department of Radiotherapy, Royal Free London NHS Foundation Trust, Hampstead, London, UK

Michael Ehmann Department of Radiation Oncology, University Medical Center Mannheim, University of Heidelberg, Mannheim, Germany

Sam Eljamel Centre for Neurosciences, Ninewells Hospital and Medical School, Dundee, Scotland, UK

Henrik Flyger Department of Breast Surgery, Herlev Hospital, Copenhagen University, Herlev, Denmark

Regina Gonzalez Department of Radiotherapy, Guy's and St Thomas' Hospitals, London, UK

Carsten Herskind Department of Radiation Oncology, University Medical Center Mannheim, University of Heidelberg, Mannheim, Germany

Mohammed Keshtgar Division of Surgery and Interventional Sciences, Department of Breast Surgery, Royal Free London Foundation Trust, University College London, Hampstead, UK

Samuele Massarut Breast Surgery Unit, CRO-IRCCS, National Cancer Institute, Aviano, Italy

Mario Mileto Breast Surgery Unit, CRO-IRCCS, National Cancer Institute, Aviano, Italy

Stephen Morris Division of Surgical Oncology, Department of Surgery, University of California, San Francisco, CA, USA

Katia Pasciuti Department of Radiotherapy, Royal Free London Foundation Trust, Hampstead, London, UK

Katharine Pigott Department of Radiation Oncology, Royal Free London Foundation Trust, Hampstead, UK

Wojciech P. Polkowski Department of Surgical Oncology, Medical University of Lublin, Lublin, Poland

Tina Reis Department of Radiation Oncology, University Medical Center Mannheim, University of Heidelberg, Mannheim, Germany

Claire Reynolds Department of Radiotherapy, Royal Free London Foundation Trust, London, UK

Frank Schneider Department of Radiation Oncology, University Medical Center Mannheim, University of Heidelberg, Mannheim, Germany

Magda Skórzewska Department of Surgical Oncology, Medical University of Lublin, Lublin, Poland

Elena Sperk Department of Radiation Oncology, University Medical Center Mannheim, University of Heidelberg, Mannheim, Germany

Klaus Wasser Institute of Clinical Radiology and Nuclear Medicine, University Medical Center Mannheim, University of Heidelberg, Mannheim, Germany

Grit Welzel Department of Radiation Oncology, University Medical Center Mannheim, University of Heidelberg, Mannheim, Germany

Frederik Wenz Department of Radiation Oncology, University Medical Center Mannheim, University of Heidelberg, Mannheim, Germany

Norman R. Williams Clinical Trials Group, Division of Surgery and Interventional Science, Faculty of Medical Sciences, University College London, London, UK

Targeted Intraoperative Radiotherapy: Concept and Review of Evidence in Breast Cancer

1

Mohammed Keshtgar and Frederik Wenz

1.1 Introduction

The development of the classic radical mastectomy in the latter part of the nineteenth century is credited to William S. Halsted, of the Johns Hopkins Hospital, Baltimore (1898) (Halstead 1894). In 1922 Geoffrey Keynes, surgeon at St. Bartholomew's Hospital, London, began experimenting with the use of radium enclosed in hollow platinum needles in the treatment of advanced breast cancer. Following on from his experience with advanced disease, he took the courageous leap of faith and started treating women with early breast cancer with local excision (lumpectomy) and radium needles inserted into the unaffected quadrants of the breast and the axillary plus supraclavicular lymphatic fields (Keynes 1937).

M. Keshtgar, BSc, FRCSI, FRCS (Gen), PhD (✉)
Division of Surgery and Interventional Sciences,
Department of Breast Surgery, University College
London Medical School, Royal Free London
Foundation NHS Trust, Pond Street,
Hampstead, London NW3 2QG, UK
e-mail: m.keshtgar@ucl.ac.uk

F. Wenz
Department of Radiation Oncology,
University Medical Center Mannheim,
University of Heidelberg,
Theodor-Kutzer-Ufer 1-3,
D-68167 Mannheim, Germany
e-mail: frederik.wenz@medma.uni-heidelberg.de,
frederik.wenz@umm.de, http://www.umm.de

Over the past few decades, the major change in the surgical management of early breast cancer has been the shift towards minimally invasive approaches. These include breast conservation surgery (BCS) and sentinel lymph node (SLN) biopsy. BCS was introduced to reduce the physical and psychological consequences of removing the whole breast.

Postoperative radiotherapy to the whole breast with boost to the tumour bed is regarded as an essential adjunct to BCS and cannot be safely omitted. There is overwhelming evidence that this approach decreases the risk of local recurrence and improves survival (Fisher et al. 1991). The aim of radiotherapy is to selectively kill any residual tumour cells without damaging normal cells. This is achieved by generating free radicals, which cause single- or double-stranded breaks in the cell's DNA. Considering that tumour cells have less ability to repair DNA damage than normal cells and are more frequently in the radiosensitive part of the cell cycle, they are most vulnerable to the effects of radiation therapy.

It is important to remember that whole breast radiotherapy is not without risk. Although treatment regimens have become safer with careful planning using computed tomography and treatment delivery using tangential fields, healthy tissues such as the heart, ribs and lungs do receive a small but significant dose of radiation.

Other issues with whole breast radiotherapy include the time constraint of between 3 and 7 weeks of daily visits to hospital, which is a great inconvenience for patients. The radiotherapy

M. Keshtgar et al. (eds.), *Targeted Intraoperative Radiotherapy in Oncology*,
DOI 10.1007/978-3-642-39821-6_1, © Springer-Verlag Berlin Heidelberg 2014

equipment is expensive to purchase and run, and requires installation in a shielded building. Moreover, geographic miss (delivery of radiotherapy to a wrong site) is possible during boost radiotherapy, especially following oncoplastic breast procedures where the incision is some distance from the original site of tumour in the majority of cases. Cosmesis can also be impaired by the short- or long-term radiotoxicity. Finally, the resultant delay in radiotherapy in order to accommodate chemotherapy might compromise local control (Bowden et al. 2006). A delay of more than 6 weeks has been shown to significantly increase the risk of recurrence at 5 years (Punglia et al. 2010).

1.2 The Case for Change

The results of many clinical trials and observational studies have demonstrated that around 90 % of local recurrences after BCS occur within the same quadrant of the breast that harboured the primary tumour (index quadrant). This observation raises the question of whether whole breast radiotherapy is necessary and whether radiotherapy to the index quadrant of the breast alone would be sufficient for the management of breast cancer patients (Bartelink et al. 2007; Veronesi et al. 1993; Clark et al. 1992).

This has led to growing interest in accelerated partial breast irradiation (APBI), which aims to decrease the volume of breast treated and increase the daily fraction size of radiation. Several APBI techniques are available, including linac-based intensity-modulated radiotherapy, multicatheter interstitial brachytherapy, balloon-based APBI using the MammoSite™ brachytherapy applicator (Hologic, Inc., MA, USA), a newly developed modified form of balloon-based brachytherapy called Xoft Axxent Electronic Brachytherapy™ (Xoft, Inc., CA, USA), intraoperative radiotherapy using a mobile linear accelerator in the operating theatre (http://www.intraopmedical.com/) and the novel technique of targeted intraoperative radiotherapy (IORT) using INTRABEAM® (Carl Zeiss Surgical, Oberkochen, Germany).

1.3 Targeted Intraoperative Radiotherapy (TARGIT)

1.3.1 INTRABEAM

INTRABEAM is a mobile, miniature X-ray generator powered by a 12-V supply. Accelerated electrons strike a gold target at the tip of a 10-cm-long drift tube with a diameter of 3 mm, resulting in the emission of low-energy X-rays (50 kV) in an isotropic dose distribution around the tip. The irradiated tissue is kept at a fixed, known distance from the source by spherical applicators to ensure a more uniform dose distribution. The tip of the electron drift tube sits precisely at the epicentre of a spherical polymer applicator, the size of which is chosen to fit the cavity after the breast cancer has been excised. Using this method, the walls of the tumour cavity are irradiated to a biologically effective dose (20 Gy to the tissue in contact with the applicator) that rapidly attenuates over a distance of a few centimetres. As a result, surrounding healthy tissue is spared and the device can be used in an unmodified operating theatre (Fig. 1.1).

The mechanism of action of this approach is described in detail later in this textbook. In brief, a study of the impact of wound fluid after BCS for breast cancer showed that wound fluid (taken from the drain over the first 24 h after BCS without TARGIT) stimulated proliferation, migration

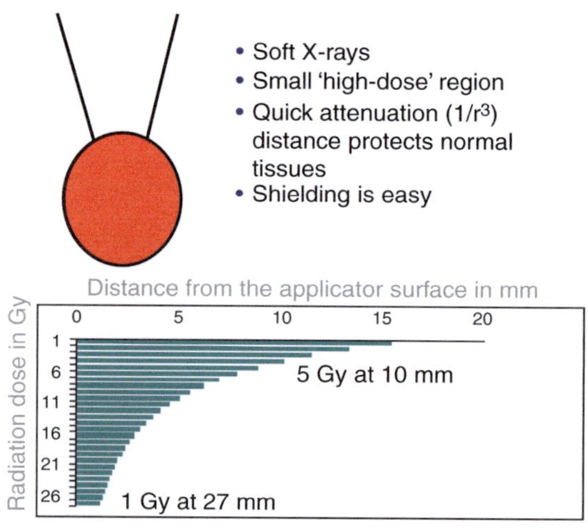

Fig. 1.1 Rapid attenuation of the radiation dose as the distance increases

and invasion of breast cancer cell lines; however, the stimulatory effect almost completely disappeared when fluids from TARGIT-treated patients were used. This was attributed to an alteration in the molecular composition and biological activity of the wound fluid (Belletti et al. 2008). The other possible explanation is the timeliness of this approach, with delivery of radiotherapy soon after the primary tumour has been excised.

1.3.2 Historical Perspective

A Photon Radiosurgery System (PRS) was introduced at The Royal Free Hospital in 1995 to assess its role in the treatment of solitary brain metastases. The tip of the probe was placed into the tumour, using standard stereotactic techniques, allowing for the delivery of a prescribed therapeutic radiation dose directly into the centre of the metastasis. A dose of 10–20 Gy was prescribed to the margin of the treatment volume defined as the volume seen on CT scan with a 2 mm margin. Between April 1995 and April 1997 eleven patients with cerebral metastases were treated with the PRS. Ten patients were treated successfully with no morbidity and good local tumour control at the treated site at their time of death from systemic disease. One patient developed a hemiplegia postoperatively and died 35 days later from widespread systemic disease and treatment complications. This system offered the combined advantages of treatment at the same sitting as the confirmatory biopsy. On the whole it was well tolerated and provided good local tumour control (Porter et al. 1998).

Subsequently, the system was trialed for the first time in treatment of primary breast cancer at the University College London after the design and development of polymer applicators of various diameters to insert into the tumour cavity after resection (Vaidya et al. 1999).

1.3.3 TARGIT Randomised Controlled Trial

In March 2000, an international, phase 3 randomised controlled trial was launched as a non-inferiority trial and over the years enrolled patients from 33 centres in ten countries. It compared outcomes in patients aged 45 years or older with invasive ductal carcinoma undergoing BCS followed by either whole breast external beam radiotherapy (EBRT) over several weeks or a risk-adaptive approach using single-dose TARGIT. Under the risk-adaptive approach, if the final pathology report demonstrated unpredicted prespecified adverse features, then EBRT was to be added to TARGIT afterwards, omitting boost radiation. The primary outcome measure in this study was local recurrence, with several secondary outcome measures including toxicity, survival, cosmesis, quality of life and health economics.

Randomisation to the TARGIT or the EBRT arm was done either before lumpectomy (pre-pathology) or after lumpectomy (post-pathology). Among the patients allocated to receive TARGIT, those in the pre-pathology group received it immediately after surgical excision under the same anaesthesia, while those in the post-pathology group received it as a subsequent procedure.

The original recruitment goal of 2,232 (powered to test non-inferiority; hazard ratio: <1.25) was reached in early 2010 (Vaidya et al. 2010); 1,113 patients were randomly allocated to TARGIT and 1,119 to EBRT. Fourteen percent of the TARGIT group with poor prognostic factors also received EBRT in a risk-adaptive approach, with omission of boost radiotherapy to the tumour bed, as stated above. At 4 years, there were six local recurrences in the TARGIT group and five in the EBRT group. The Kaplan-Meier estimate of local recurrence in the conserved breast at 4 years was 1.20 % (95 % CI 0.53–2.71) after TARGIT compared with 0.95 % (0.39–2.31) in the EBRT group; the difference between the groups was not statistically significant. The frequency of any complications and major toxicity was similar in the two groups and grade 3 radiation-induced toxicity was lower in the TARGIT group; however, seromas needing more than three aspirations were more common in the TARGIT group. There was no difference in wound breakdown.

The early results of this study therefore provided level 1 evidence that the single dose of radiotherapy delivered at the time of surgery

Table 1.1 Updated summary of the results of the TARGIT-A trial

	Events		
	5-year cumulative risk (95 % CI)		
	TARGIT	EBRT	HR (95 % CI)
Ipsilateral breast recurrence (IBR)	23	11	
	3.3 % (2.1–5.1)	1.3 % (0.7–2.5)	2.07 (1.01–4.25)
All recurrences (ipsilateral and contralateral breast, axillary and distant)	69	48	
	8.2 % (6.3–10.6)	5.7 % (4.1–7.8)	1.44 (0.99–2.08)
Mortality	37	51	
	3.9 % (2.7–5.8)	5.3 % (3.9–7.3)	0.70 (0.46–1.07)

using the TARGIT technique is safe and that for selected patients with early breast cancer it can be considered as an alternative to EBRT delivered over several weeks.

Recruitment to the TARGIT trial continued after the *Lancet* publication, primarily to allow completion of sub-protocols; the final recruitment goal of 3,451 women was achieved in June 2012 and the trial then closed to recruitment.

The updated results were presented at the San Antonio Breast Cancer Symposium (Vaidya et al. 2012) (Table 1.1): 1,721 patients were randomly allocated to receive TARGIT and 1,730 to receive EBRT. 1,010 patients had a minimum of 4 years of follow-up and 611 patients had a minimum of 5 years of follow-up. Primary events (local recurrence) had increased from 13 to 34 since the *Lancet* publication.

For the primary outcome of ipsilateral breast recurrence (IBR), the absolute difference at 5 years was 2.0 %, which was higher with TARGIT and reached the conventional levels of statistical significance ($p=0.042$), but was within the pre-specified non-inferiority margin; in the pre-pathology arm the absolute difference in 5-year IBR was 1 % and in the post-pathology arm it was higher, at 3.7 %.

For the secondary outcome, there was a non-significant trend towards improved overall survival with TARGIT [HR=0.70 (0.46–1.07)] due to fewer non-breast cancer deaths [17 vs. 35, HR 0.47 (0.26–0.84)]. Cardiovascular deaths were 1 vs. 10 and deaths from cancers other than breast were 7 vs. 16.

The results indicate that the risk-adapted approach using single-dose TARGIT had a slightly higher local recurrence rate than EBRT for the primary endpoint of IBR, but was within the preset non-inferiority boundary, with the pre-pathology group performing better than the post-pathology stratum. In addition there was a trend towards improved overall survival in the TARGIT arm due to fewer non-breast cancer deaths. However, longer follow-up is needed to consolidate these findings.

A pilot of the cosmesis subprotocol in 118 patients indicated a superior cosmetic outcome in the first year for those receiving TARGIT (Keshtgar et al. 2013). Results from a pilot patient preference study of 58 patients confirmed that 54 (93 %) of the subjects would undergo TARGIT if it offered equivalent or some added risk compared with EBRT (Alvarado et al. 2010).

1.3.4 TARGIT as a Boost

The safety and tolerability of the TARGIT technique was initially established in a phase II study (Vaidya et al. 2011). In this study, 299 patients (with 300 cancers) underwent BCS and received a single 20 Gy dose of radiotherapy during surgery. In these patients, IORT replaced the boost radiation and all patients subsequently received standard whole breast EBRT. The treatment was well tolerated by all patients, and with median follow-up of 60.5 months (range 10–120 months), the 5-year Kaplan Meier estimate for ipsilateral recurrence was reported at 1.74 % (standard error 0.77). This is one of the lowest recurrence rates reported in the literature and we believe that this approach of using IORT as a boost at the time of surgery for the primary breast cancer in high-risk patients is superior to the current conventional practice. To test this hypothesis, a randomised trial (TARGIT-Boost) has been designed which has commenced. In this trial, patients with high-risk breast cancer who are suitable for BCS will be randomised to receive IORT as a boost radiation versus standard EBRT.

1.3.5 TARGIT in Exceptional Circumstances

A study of use of the TARGIT technique in 80 patients with exceptional circumstances who could not receive standard EBRT has also been published recently (Keshtgar et al. 2011). This group included patients with previously irradiated breasts, scleroderma, systemic lupus erythematosus, motor neuron disease, Parkinson's disease, ankylosing spondylitis, morbid obesity and cardiovascular or severe respiratory disease. After a median follow-up of 38 months, only two local recurrences had been observed, which is an annual local recurrence rate of 0.75 % (95 % confidence interval, 0.09–2.70 %).

In summary, the evidence is mounting that TARGIT should replace whole breast EBRT in selected patients with early breast cancer. The technique is relatively easy to use and does not require shielding of the operating theatre, and healthy tissues are largely protected. Furthermore, TARGIT is suitable for developing countries – an unusual example where a new health technology is more affordable than the existing standard and can optimise treatment and reduce the number of unnecessary mastectomies.

These results heavily influenced the outcome of the recent St Gallen consensus in 2011. In response to the question, "Should partial breast irradiation, including IORT, be applied in selected patients including the elderly?" 87 % of experts who were present voted 'yes'.

1.4 Concluding Remarks

The management of breast cancer has undergone evolutionary changes over the years, from radical mastectomy to BCS and from radical axillary dissection to targeted SLN biopsy. The early results from the TARGIT trial provide level 1 evidence that IORT is safe and can be offered in a single fraction to a selected group of patients with early breast cancer.

We are entering a new era of personalised care in breast cancer management using risk-adaptive approaches. Based on current evidence and until national bodies such as NICE issue guidance on its use, we propose that TARGIT can be safely offered as a single fraction in elderly and selected women with early breast cancer and in compelling special circumstances where EBRT is not feasible or possible. For the other patient groups there is still an opportunity to enter them into clinical trials (Fig. 1.2).

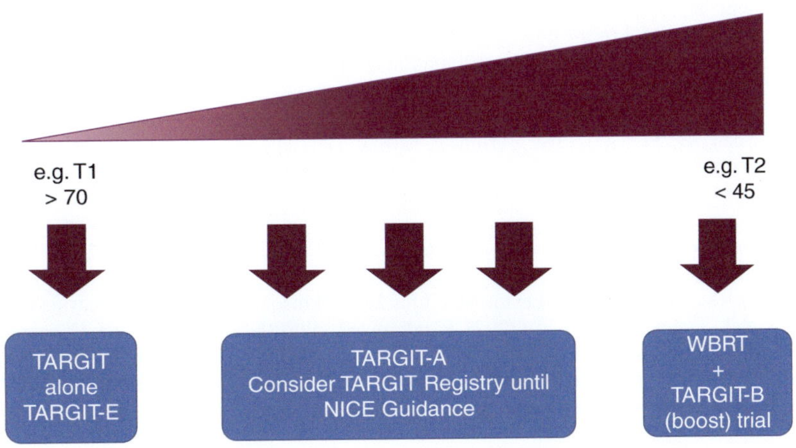

Fig. 1.2 Working towards personalised care in breast cancer using a risk-adaptive approach

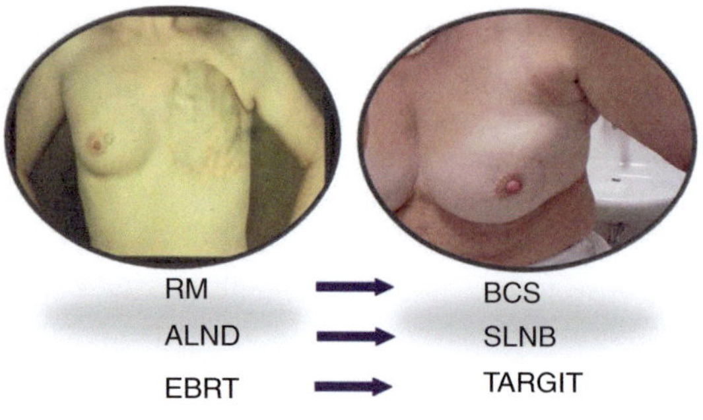

Fig. 1.3 Historical milestones in the loco-regional treatment of breast cancer : from radical mastectomy (*RM*) to breast conserving surgery (*BCS*), from axillary lymph node dissection (*ALND*) to sentinel node biopsy (*SLNB*) and a recent move from radical external beam radiotherapy (*EBRT*) to a targeted intra-operative radiotherapy (*TARGIT*)

The quest for optimal treatment for early breast cancer has come a long way in the past 100 years and we are set for the next revolution in the management of breast cancer, moving from radical whole breast radiotherapy to a targeted partial breast irradiation (Fig. 1.3). Let's watch this space….

References

Alvarado M, Connolly JS, Oboite M, Park C, Esserman L (2010) Patient preference in breast cancer radiotherapy. J Clin Oncol 28(Suppl):e11005

Bartelink H, Horiot JC, Poortmans PM, Struikmans H, Van den Bgaert W, Fourquet A et al (2007) Impact of a higher radiation dose on local control and survival in breast-conserving therapy of early breast cancer: 10-year results of the randomized boost versus no boost EORTC 22881–10882 trial. J Clin Oncol 25:3259–3265

Belletti B, Vaidya JS, D'Andrea S, Entschladen F, Roncadin M, Lovat F et al (2008) Targeted intraoperative radiotherapy impairs the stimulation of breast cancer cell proliferation and invasion caused by surgical wounding. Clin Cancer Res 14:1325–1332

Bowden SJ, Fernando IN, Burton A (2006) Delaying radiotherapy for the delivery of adjuvant chemotherapy in the combined modality treatment of early breast cancer: is it disadvantageous and could combined treatment be the answer? Clin Oncol (R Coll Radiol) 18:247–256

Clark RM, McCulloch PB, Levine MN, Lipa M, Wilkinson RH, Mahoney LJ et al (1992) Randomized clinical trial to assess the effectiveness of breast irradiation following lumpectomy and axillary dissection for node-negative breast cancer. J Natl Cancer Inst 84:683–689

Fisher B, Anderson S, Fisher ER, Redmond C, Wickerham DL, Wolmark N et al (1991) Significance of ipsilateral breast tumour recurrence after lumpectomy. Lancet 338:327–331

Halstead WS (1894) The results of operations for cure of the cancer of breast performed at the Johns Hopkins Hospital from June 1889 to January 1894. Ann Surg 20:497–555

Keshtgar M, Williams NR, Corica T, Hedges R, Saunders C, Joseph D (2010) Early evidence of better cosmetic outcome after intraoperative radiotherapy compared with external beam radiotherapy for early breast cancer: objective assessment of patients from a randomised controlled trial. Ann Surg Oncol 17(Suppl 1):S13

Keshtgar MR, Vaidya JS, Tobias JS, Wenz F, Joseph D, Stacey C et al (2011) Targeted intraoperative radiotherapy for breast cancer in patients in whom external beam radiation is not possible. Int J Radiat Oncol Biol Phys 80:31–38

Keshtgar MR, Williams NR, Bulsara M, Saunders C, Flyger H, Cardoso JS et al (2013) Objective assessment of cosmetic outcome after targeted intraoperative radiotherapy in breast cancer: results from a randomised controlled trial. Breast Cancer Res Treat 140(3):519–525

Keynes G (1937) The place of radium in the treatment of cancer of the breast. Ann Surg 106:619–630

Porter DG, Bradford R, Cosgrove GR, Black P, Arbitt E (1998) CT-directed stereotactic photon radiosurgery system in the management of cerebral metastases – a multi-centre prospective evaluation [Abstract]. Br J Neurosurg 11:478

Punglia RS, Saito AM, Neville BA, Earle CC, Weeks JC (2010) Impact of interval from breast conserving surgery to radiotherapy on local recurrence in older women with breast cancer: retrospective cohort analysis. BMJ 340:c845

Vaidya JS, Baum M, Tobias JS, Houghton J (1999) Targeted Intraoperative Radiotherapy (TARGIT)-trial protocol. Lancet http://www.thelancet.com/protocol-reviews/99PRT-47

Vaidya JS, Joseph DJ, Tobias JS, Bulsara M, Wenz F, Saunders C et al (2010) Targeted intraoperative radiotherapy versus whole breast radiotherapy for breast cancer (TARGIT-A trial): an international, prospective, randomised, non-inferiority phase 3 trial. Lancet 376:91–102

Vaidya JS, Baum M, Tobias JS, Wenz F, Massarut S, Keshtgar M et al (2011) Long-term results of targeted intraoperative radiotherapy (Targit) boost during breast-conserving surgery. Int J Radiat Oncol Biol Phys 81:1091–1097

Vaidya JS, Wenz F, Bulsara M, Joseph D, Tobias JS, Keshtgar M et al (2012) Targeted intraoperative radiotherapy for early breast cancer: TARGIT-A trial – updated analysis of local recurrence and first analysis of survival. Cancer Res 72(24 Suppl):S4–2

Veronesi U, Luini A, Del Vecchio M, Greco M, Galimberti V, Merson M et al (1993) Radiotherapy after breast-preserving surgery in women with localized cancer of the breast. N Engl J Med 328:1587–1591

Mechanism of Action of TARGIT

2

Gustavo Baldassarre, Barbara Belletti, Mario Mileto, and Samuele Massarut

2.1 Introduction

The X-ray generator INTRABEAM delivers a highly localised dose of low-energy photons (50 kV) to the tumour bed immediately after wide local excision for early breast cancer. This modality differs from conventional external beam fractionated radiotherapy (EBRT) in several respects. First, the highly localised radiation field is characterised by a non-uniform dose distribution. In fact, the dose delivered to the cavity with INTRABEAM abruptly decreases in a manner proportional to the cube of the distance from the applicator. In contrast, EBRT delivers the same dose to the whole breast. A second important aspect to be taken into account is that intraoperative radiotherapy (IORT) distributes the total dose in a single fraction during surgery, thereby avoiding geographical miss and unwanted delay in RT application. A third important difference is that low-energy photons have an increased relative biological effect (RBE) compared with high-energy photons. Finally, the typical duration of the application (from 30 to 50 min), results in sublethal damage to the irradiated tissue. Since residual proliferating cancer cells are much less able to repair sublethal DNA damage in comparison with normal epithelial cells, the long treatment time of IORT with INTRABEAM is likely to result in a better therapeutic index.

From a biological point of view, IORT with the INTRABEAM technique offers a unique opportunity to study the immediate effect of radiotherapy on human tissues in vivo.

G. Baldassarre, MD (✉) • B. Belletti
Division of Experimental Oncology, CRO-IRCCS, National Cancer Institute, Via F. Gallini 2, 33081 Aviano, Italy
e-mail: gbaldassarre@cro.it

M. Mileto • S. Massarut, MD
Breast Surgery Unit, CRO-IRCCS, National Cancer Institute, Via F. Gallini 2, 33081 Aviano, Italy
e-mail: smassarut@cro.it

2.2 Tumour Killing

Several studies have addressed the ability of the INTRABEAM system to kill normal and/or tumour-derived cell lines in vitro. One of the most accurate studies demonstrated that low-energy X-rays are able to effectively kill both normal rodent and glioblastoma cell lines with a high linear energy transfer (LET) (Astor et al. 2000).

The LET describes the rate at which a type of radiation deposits energy as it passes through tissue. Higher levels of deposited energy cause more cells to be killed by a given dose of radiation therapy. X-rays, gamma rays and electrons are known as low-LET radiation while neutrons, heavy ions and pions are classified as high-LET radiation.

Radiobiologically, the high RBE values demonstrated by the low-energy X-rays are similar to those obtained for high-LET radiation and may prove extremely important in treating solid

M. Keshtgar et al. (eds.), *Targeted Intraoperative Radiotherapy in Oncology*,
DOI 10.1007/978-3-642-39821-6_2, © Springer-Verlag Berlin Heidelberg 2014

tumour types with different radiosensitivity. In fact, high-LET radiations provide a significant increase in the dose delivered to the tumour compared with clinically used low-LET radiations (Astor et al. 2000).

Importantly, the experimentally evaluated RBE for INTRABEAM is very similar to that theoretically calculated (Brenner et al. 1999), and both convey that RBE increases as the radiation dose from the applicator decreases.

2.3 Modifications of the Tumour Micro-environment

Taking advantage of the opportunity to study the immediate effect of radiotherapy on human tissues in vivo, we recently demonstrated that TARGIT treatment acts also by modifying the local post-surgery micro-environment (Belletti et al. 2008).

This biological evidence could at least in part explain the preferential localisation of breast cancer recurrences in the index quadrant within the tumour bed. Since the advent of IORT, the most common explanation for this observation has been the presence of "residual" tumour cells in the postoperative milieu. However, several studies have suggested that this cannot be the only explanation. Although residual tumour cells may still be present even when meticulous care is taken to ensure that excision margins are microscopically free of tumour, it is difficult to explain why radiotherapy reduces the risk of recurrence by the same proportional extent no matter how wide the excision margin.

Interestingly, the possible deleterious effects of surgical wounding have been speculated for a long time and have been demonstrated in mice (Demicheli et al. 2001; Fisher et al. 1989; Tsuchida et al. 2003). Moreover, experimental and clinical observations suggest that the extent of surgery may represent a variable that enhances tumour burden (Tsuchida et al. 2003; Tagliabue et al. 2006). This effect has been previously related to growth factor produced by stromal cells during the wound healing process (Tagliabue et al. 2003; Coussens and Werb 2002).

Accordingly, wound axillary fluids harvested from breast cancer patients have been proved to stimulate HER2-positive breast carcinoma cell growth in 2D assay, an effect that could be only partially abrogated by impairing HER-2 signal transduction (Tagliabue et al. 2003). This observation implies that several growth factors and cytokines secreted in the wound fluids participate in the stimulation of breast carcinoma. We confirmed and expanded this observation by demonstrating that wound fluids collected from the breasts of breast cancer patients not only stimulated 2D proliferation but also enhanced breast cancer cell growth in a 3D model system that more closely resembled the in vivo situation (Fig. 2.1).

We have also demonstrated that wound fluids act as chemo-attractants for breast carcinoma cells, which again provides a possible explanation as to why local recurrences peak between 2 and 3 years after primary surgery at the site of surgery (Baum et al. 2005). Indeed, we have provided the first formal demonstration that wound fluids harvested from breast cancer patients who have undergone wide local tumour excision stimulate breast cancer cell motility, invasion and growth in three-dimensional contexts (Belletti et al. 2008). Thus, the wound fluid may stimulate the growth of any residual tumour cells and/or attract breast cancer cells at the site of surgery, suggesting an additional molecular and biological explanation for the high local recurrence rate of breast cancer.

We can therefore speculate that surgical excision of the cancer is certainly beneficial but the act of surgery may have harmful effects (Demicheli et al. 2001; Baum et al. 2005) and we should strive to understand and reduce these. We have demonstrated that TARGIT almost completely abrogates the stimulatory effects of surgical wound fluid on cancer cells in vitro (Fig. 2.2), suggesting that it may confer more benefits than those expected from the tumoricidal effect of radiotherapy.

Importantly, our observations are in line with the clinical evidence demonstrating that TARGIT is able to control local recurrences as well as EBRT when used alone in selected

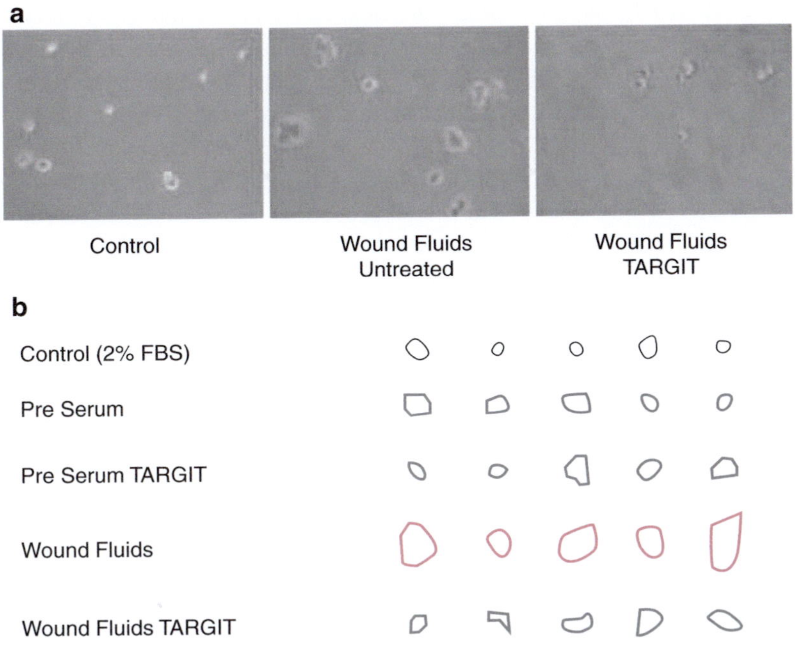

Fig. 2.1 TARGIT impairs the proliferative activity of wound fluids from breast cancer patients. This figure shows the colony formation assay. In (**a**), MCF-7 breast cancer cells were included in a 3D Matrigel matrix and incubated in medium supplemented with 2 % FBS (control) or wound fluids from untreated or TARGIT-treated breast cancer patients as indicated. Only wound fluids from untreated patients were able to stimulate MCF-7 cell growth in 3D matrix. (**b**) Depicts the areas of representative colonies formed by MCF-7 cells in the presence of the indicated stimuli (all used at 2 % concentration). The larger size of colonies formed in the presence of wound fluids from untreated patients is evident. *Pre Serum* indicates the serum collected from untreated or TARGIT-treated women the day before surgery

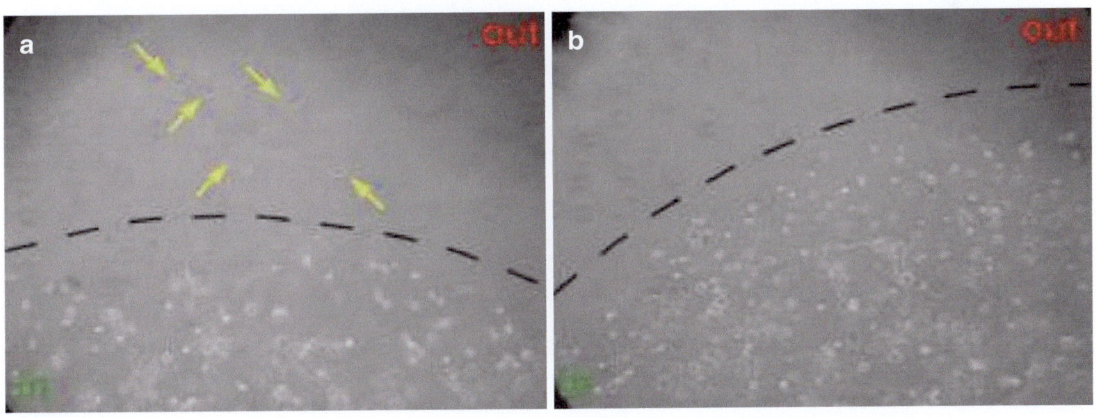

Fig. 2.2 TARGIT decreases the chemo-attractant activity of wound fluids from breast cancer patients. This figure shows an evasion assay. MDA-MB-231 highly metastatic breast cancer cells were included in a 3D Matrigel matrix and incubated in medium supplemented with 5 % wound fluids from untreated (**a**) or TARGIT-treated (**b**) breast cancer patients. Only cells incubated with wound fluids from untreated patients were able to evade the matrix (*yellow arrows*) in response to chemo-attractant stimuli

patients (Vaidya et al. 2010), but also results in better local control compared with that obtained with the EBRT boost when used as a tumour bed boost in unselected breast cancer patients (Vaidya et al. 2011).

The latter clinical observation suggests that the beneficial effect of TARGIT could have contributed in achieving such a low rate of recurrence not only through better cell killing (probably the main mechanism of action) but also by modifying the wound micro-environment, making it less favourable for cancer cell growth and invasion. Of course, while our studies do not provide proof for the superiority of IORT, they do provide a biological rationale for that possibility. As a corollary we can also speculate that the effects of radiotherapy may be completely different when radiation is applied to a wounded tissue as compared with application to an already repaired breast, as in the case of EBRT in breast cancer therapy. To prove this hypothesis we generated two different mouse models of breast radiotherapy (Fig. 2.3) that indeed confirmed our speculation (manuscript in preparation).

From a biochemical point of view, we demonstrated by a proteomic analysis on 174 known cytokines that TARGIT is able to modify in vivo in humans the levels of several factors involved in

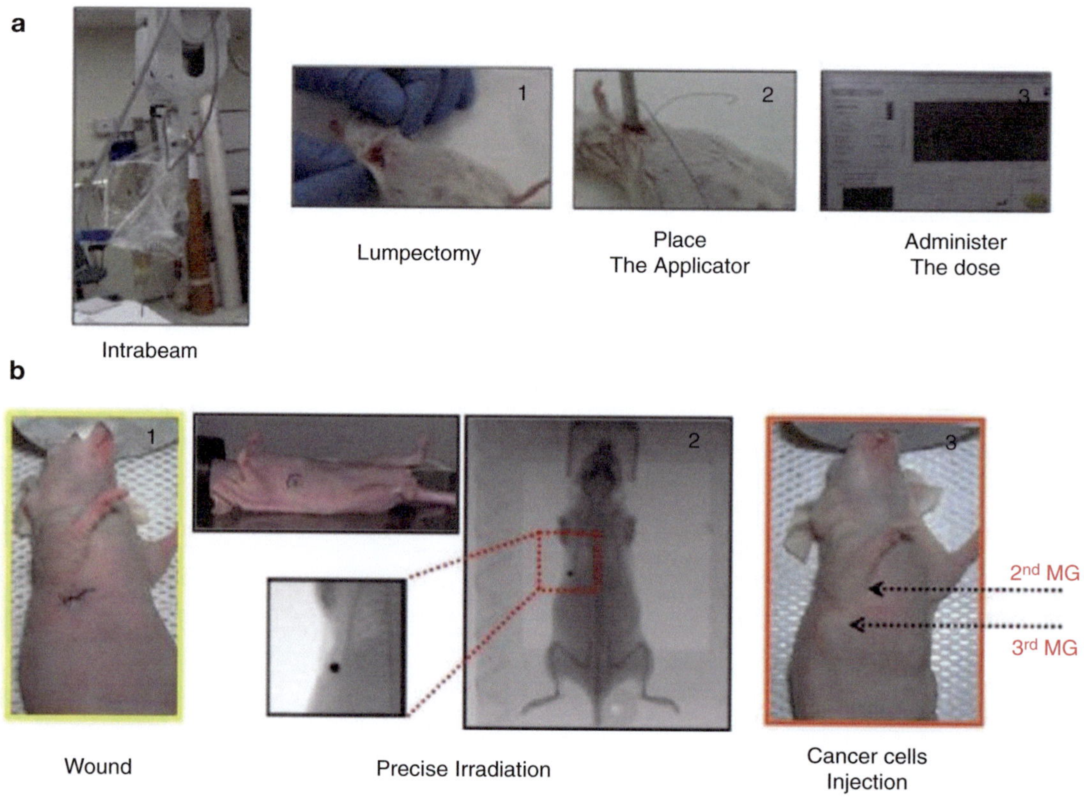

Fig. 2.3 Mouse models of TARGIT and precise irradiation. In (**a**) the *INTRABEAM apparatus* applied to the mouse breast irradiation is shown. Briefly, after anaesthesia, female SV129 mice underwent lumpectomy and then the INTRABEAM applicator was placed in the wounded tissue. Delivered doses (up to 8 Gy at 2 mm) could be delivered with two different applicators in order to vary the time of exposure. Wounded and irradiated tissues could be studied after different time points from irradiation to gain new insights into the biology of the irradiated wounded tissues. In (**b**) the *precise irradiator* was used as a model of wounded and undamaged breast. Briefly, the second mammary gland of nude female mice was wounded or not (*1*) and then the irradiation of both second and third mammary glands was performed using an area as small as 2×2 mm^2 (*2*). Breast cancer cells were then injected in the third mammary gland (*3*) and tumour growth followed over time. In this manner it was possible to identify the specific effects of radiation on the wound-induced growth of breast cancer cells in vivo

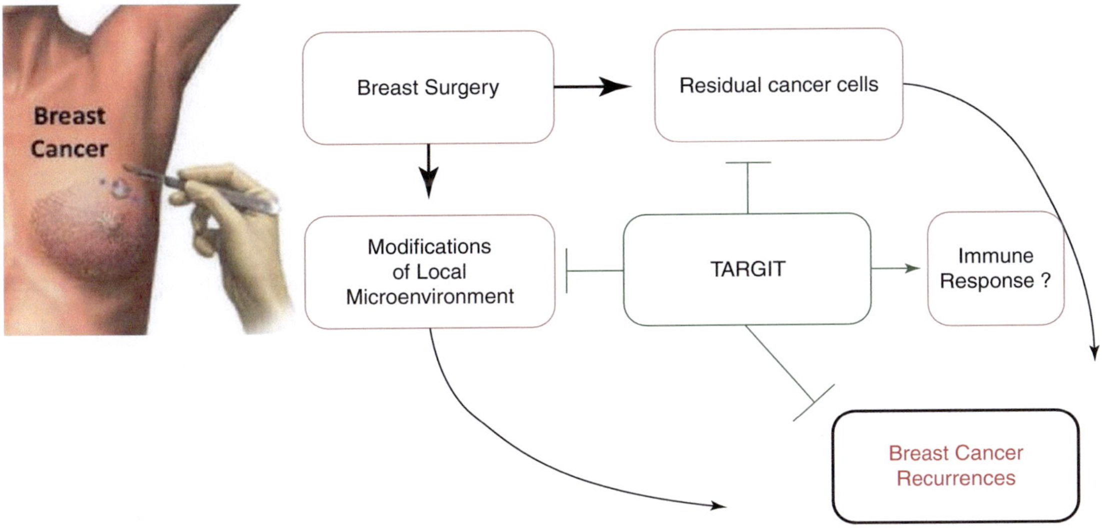

Fig. 2.4 TARGIT mechanisms of action. After lumpectomy for breast cancer, the wound response along with the presence of residual cancer cells in the local micro-environment may stimulate local and/or distant recurrences of the disease. TARGIT may function not only by killing residual tumour cells with the high RBE of low-energy photons but also by modifying the post-surgery tumour bed and possibly by impinging on the immune response via the modulation of specific cytokines. With these combined actions, TARGIT successfully prevents recurrence formation after wide local excision of early breast cancer

the control of cell growth motility and metastasis formation, such as IL-6, IL-8, HGF, UPA, leptin and RANTES (Belletti et al. 2008). Moreover, in accordance with previous observations on the effects of radiotherapy on modification of cytokine expression in humans and animal models (Yamazaki et al. 2005; Jones et al. 1999; Büttner et al. 1997), we observed a specific increase in IL-5 and IL-4 following TARGIT that could also reflect a different immune response in the local micro-environment. Indeed, the modification of immune response by radiotherapy has recently been proposed (Formenti and Demaria 2008; Formenti and Demaria 2009).

In conclusion, we propose that perioperative treatments such as TARGIT could reduce tumour recurrence by beneficially altering the tumour micro-environment, in addition to the conventionally known tumoricidal effect (Fig. 2.4).

These findings may also stimulate research into the development of novel perioperative local and systemic treatments especially directed at compensating for the harmful consequences of surgery and wound healing.

2.4 Highlights

- The isotropic non-uniform dose distribution obtained with INTRABEAMallows delivery of high doses to the tumour bed and spares normal tissues.
- The high RBE of low-energy photons effectively kills cancer cells.
- TARGIT treatment modifies the local post-surgery micro-environment, making it less conducive to cancer cell growth.
- TARGIT treatment alters cytokine production induced by the act of surgery that is necessary for the proper wound healing response and is known to participate in tumour growth and spread.
- Mouse models of TARGIT shed new light on the complex relationship between wound response and radiotherapy in breast cancer.

Acknowledgements We wish to thank all our collaborators for their scientific and highly professional contributions. This work was supported in part by grants from the Italian Association for Cancer Research (AIRC IG 10459 to B.B.), from Regione Friuli Venezia Giulia (to G.B.) and from CRO Intramural Grant (to G.B. and S.M.).

References

Astor MB, Hilaris BS, Gruerio A, Varricchione T, Smith D (2000) Preclinical studies with the photon radiosurgery system (PRS). Int J Radiat Oncol Biol Phys 47: 809–813

Baum M, Demicheli R, Hrushesky W, Retsky M (2005) Does surgery unfavourably perturb the "natural history" of early breast cancer by accelerating the appearance of distant metastases? Eur J Cancer 41:508–515

Belletti B, Vaidya JS, D'Andrea S, Entschladen F, Roncadin M, Lovat F et al (2008) Targeted intraoperative radiotherapy impairs the stimulation of breast cancer cell proliferation and invasion caused by surgical wounding. Clin Cancer Res 14:1325–1332

Brenner DJ, Leu C-S, Beatty JF, Shefer RE (1999) Clinical relative biological effectiveness of low energy x-rays emitted by miniature x-ray devices. Phys Med Biol 44:323–333

Büttner C, Skupin A, Reimann T, Rieber EP, Unteregger G, Geyer P, Frank KH (1997) Local production of interleukin-4 during radiation-induced pneumonitis and pulmonary fibrosis in rats: macrophages as a prominent source of interleukin-4. Am J Respir Cell Mol Biol 17:315–325

Coussens LM, Werb Z (2002) Inflammation and cancer. Nature 420:860–867

Demicheli R, Valagussa P, Bonadonna G (2001) Does surgery modify growth kinetics of breast cancer micrometastases? Br J Cancer 85:490–492

Fisher B, Gunduz N, Coyle J, Rudock C, Saffer E (1989) Presence of a growth-stimulating factor in serum following primary tumor removal in mice. Cancer Res 49:1996–2001

Formenti SC, Demaria S (2008) Local control by radiotherapy: is that all there is? Breast Cancer Res 10:215

Formenti SC, Demaria S (2009) Systemic effects of local radiotherapy. Lancet Oncol 10:718–726

Jones BM, Kwok CC, Kung AW (1999) Effect of radioactive iodine therapy on cytokine production in Graves' disease: transient increases in interleukin-4 (IL-4), IL-6, IL-10, and tumor necrosis factor-alpha, with longer term increases in interferon-gamma production. J Clin Endocrinol Metab 84:4106–4110

Tagliabue E, Agresti R, Carcangiu ML, Ghirelli C, Morelli D, Campiglio M et al (2003) Role of HER2 in wound-induced breast carcinoma proliferation. Lancet 362:527–533

Tagliabue E, Agresti R, Casalini P, Mariani L, Carcangiu ML, Balsari A et al (2006) Linking survival of HER2-positive breast carcinoma patients with surgical invasiveness. Eur J Cancer 42:1057–1061

Tsuchida Y, Sawada S, Yoshioka I, Ohashi Y, Matsuo M, Harimaya Y et al (2003) Increased surgical stress promotes tumor metastasis. Surgery 133:547–555

Vaidya JS, Joseph DJ, Tobias JS, Bulsara M, Wenz F, Saunders C et al (2010) Targeted intraoperative radiotherapy versus whole breast radiotherapy for breast cancer (TARGIT-A trial): an international, prospective, randomised, non-inferiority phase 3 trial. Lancet 376:91–102

Vaidya JS, Baum M, Tobias JS, Wenz F, Massarut S, Keshtgar M et al (2011) Long-term results of targeted intraoperative radiotherapy (Targit) boost during breast-conserving surgery. Int J Radiat Oncol Biol Phys 81:1091–1097

Yamazaki H, Inoue T, Tanaka E, Isohashi F, Koizumi M, Shuo X et al (2005) Pelvic irradiation-induced eosinophilia is correlated to prognosis of cervical cancer patients and transient elevation of serum interleukin 5 level. Radiat Med 23:317–321

3 How to Use the INTRABEAM System

Regina Gonzalez and Claire Reynolds

3.1 Introduction

Mobile radiotherapy systems offer a versatility desirable for certain cancer treatments where the patient requires some form of surgical intervention. These systems can be taken into operating rooms and used to irradiate the tumour or tumour bed as part of a surgical procedure. Mobile techniques include brachytherapy treatments using sealed sources (i.e. HDR), electron units (Mobetron, Novac-7) and photon units (INTRABEAM®).

Most of these mobile units still present major radiation shielding requirements, and they are therefore usually confined to dedicated operating rooms. The miniature X-ray source INTRABEAM has been proven to meet minimal radiation shielding requirements thanks to the rapid dose fall-off in soft tissue at this energy range, approximately $1/r^3$ ($1/r^2$ due to the inverse square law, and $1/r$ due to attenuation in tissue). This will be covered in the chapter "Radiation Protection".

This chapter describes the routine use of this relatively new X-ray INTRABEAM® PRS500 equipment, further details can be found in (Carl Zeiss Surgical 2007; Biggs and Thomson 1996). The system provides a means for minimally invasive, highly focussed treatment of selected lesions as well as for the intraoperative radiation therapy of a tumour bed anywhere in the body.

3.2 Components

The INTRABEAM system has several subassemblies. The system configuration used during performance verification checks and treatment is described next.

3.2.1 Main System Components

3.2.1.1 X-ray Tube (XRS) with Internal Radiation Monitor (IRM)

Electrons are emitted by thermoionic emission when the filament contained in the cathode (electron gun) is heated. These electrons are then accelerated by anodes along different accelerating sections from 50 to 0 V, in 10-kV increments. The effective emitted radiation energy is approximately 20 keV. Following this acceleration, the electrons enter a 10 cm long, 3.2 mm diameter probe. The first part of this probe, the snout or mounting collar, contains deflecting coils that steer the electron beam down the evacuated drift tube towards a thin (approx. 1 μm) concave gold target at the hemispherical tip of the probe. Part of the energy produced from the interaction of the electrons

R. Gonzalez (✉)
Department of Radiotherapy,
Guy's and St Thomas' Hospitals, London, UK
e-mail: regina.gonzalez@gstt.nhs.uk

C. Reynolds
Department of Radiotherapy,
Royal Free London Foundation Trust,
Pond Street, Hampstead, London NW3 2QG, UK
e-mail: clairehourihane@nhs.net

M. Keshtgar et al. (eds.), *Targeted Intraoperative Radiotherapy in Oncology*,
DOI 10.1007/978-3-642-39821-6_3, © Springer-Verlag Berlin Heidelberg 2014

with the target material is converted into radiation in the form of characteristic and bremsstrahlung radiation. These X-rays are generated in a nearly spherical distribution centred at the tip of the probe. The radiation that passes back along the path of the electron beam is detected by the IRM. The signal from the IRM is calibrated to the dose rate before the probe is placed in the patient for treatment. The integrated IRM output is used during treatment as a direct measure of treatment dose to the patient. The total exposure is then controlled by the accumulated counts monitored by the IRM as well as by a timer which serves as a backup.

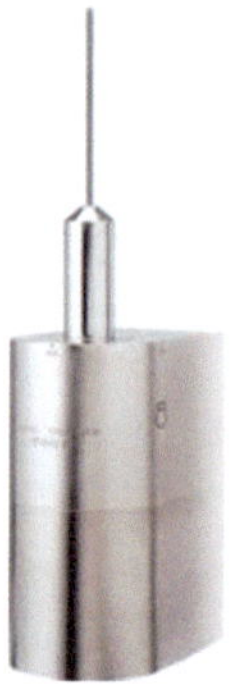

3.2.1.2 Control Console

The XRS is powered by this component. The control console receives instructions from the user terminal to perform QC and treatment tasks. It executes them, monitors them and displays current data during the process. The XRS provides the control console with feedback signals regarding the operational status of the variables relating to X-ray production, interlock status, etc. It sends raw data back to the user terminal, which are then transformed into QC and treatment records. The XRS is connected to the control console via a low-voltage (12-V) cable. An air pressure sensor located within the control console is used to correct output measurements.

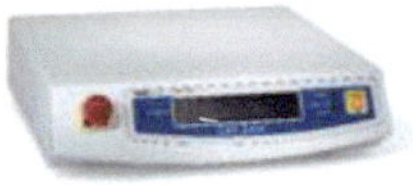

3.2.1.3 User Terminal and INTRABEAM Software

This is the primary interface between the user and the INTRABEAM system. The user is able to set up the control console to perform the main functions of the system: pre-treatment verification, treatment planning, logging of all procedure variables and events, and saving and printing of treatment and performance data. The integrated user terminal has been designed for easy transport and safe use in theatres.

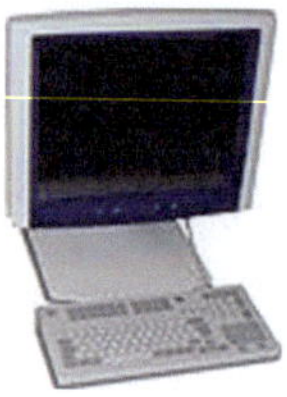

3.2.2 Verification Components

The INTRABEAM is supplied with a range of shielded accessories used during the pre-treatment procedure.

3.2.2.1 Photodiode Array (PDA)

This is used to determine the optimum voltage from the deflection coils in the *X* and *Y* directions and isotropy settings of the XRS prior to treatment. It contains five diodes placed on the four side faces and the top face of a cube, such that all are equidistant from the centre of radiation of the XRS probe. When the probe is inserted into the PDA, the axis markings on the side of the PDA housing must be aligned with the matching axis marking on the XRS housing. Signals from the PDA will be displayed on the user terminal measuring the distribution (isotropy) of X-rays emitted from the tip of the probe.

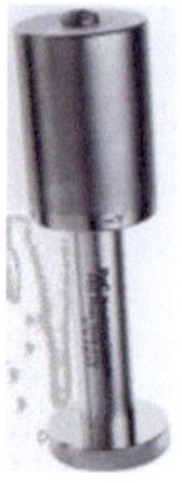

3.2.2.2 Probe Adjuster/Ion Chamber Holder (PAICH)

The PAICH (Fig. 3.1) has two primary functions: (1) to maintain straightness of the XRS probe and (2) to provide a means of accurate positioning of an ionisation chamber in relation to the probe tip. It is essential for the XRS probe to be straight in order to maintain an isotropic radiation output. The "runout" (deviation from perpendicular) of the probe is determined using the probe adjuster. Probe straightness is measured optically to 0.1 mm by a method in which the probe intercepts a portion of a light beam from an LED across one edge of the tip of the tube. The light beam is detected as it strikes an opposing photodiode. As the PAICH is rotated around the probe, any mechanical deviation of the tube from the axis of rotation will be represented by a change in the light detected.

3.2.2.3 Electrometer and Ion Chamber (IC)

A shielded IC (type PTW 23342 for very low radiation therapy energies) parallel plane chamber is used to verify the output of the XRS and to calibrate the IRM readings. The electrometer (PTW Unidos E) measures and displays the current generated by the IC. The customised shield serves not only to provide radiation safety but also to reproducibly position the chamber inside the PAICH with respect to the tip of the probe whenever taking output measurements.

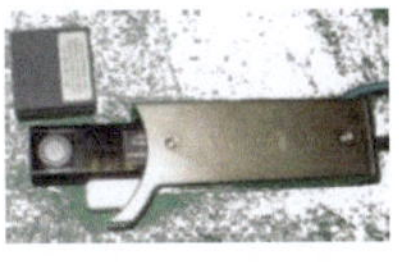

3.2.2.4 External Radiation Monitor (ERM)

Older INTRABEAM systems (i.e. PRS 400) utilised a radiation detector external to the XRS, measuring the radiation exiting the patient. The ERM used detectors with the purpose of independently monitoring the constancy of the radiation emitted by the XRS and during the course of treatment, thus providing a further backup to the timer for controlling dose delivery and end of treatment. New systems do not include this external monitor.

3.2.3 Other Components

3.2.3.1 Applicators

Spherical applicators, ranging from 1.5 to 5 cm in 0.5-cm increments, fill the entire cavity left after tumour excision. The XRS probe is located in the centre of the applicator, and thus the tumour bed. The material of the applicator is medical-grade acrylic and it can be steam sterilised up to 100 times. For smaller applicators, aluminium is inserted around the cavity where the tip of the probe will be present (Fig. 3.2). This is to remove lower energy characteristic line from the radiation spectrum due to the presence of components at the probe tip other than the gold target material. For larger applicators, the thickness of the material will be sufficient to harden the beam. The aluminium will also reduce the higher signal that would otherwise be obtained from radiation passing back through the probe as these photons go through less material with decreasing applicator diameter.

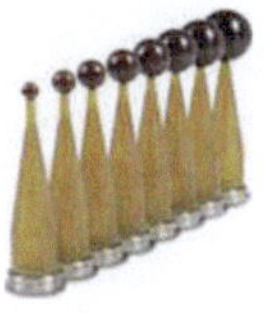

The treatment time for each applicator is worked out using the "transfer function" for the relevant applicator and PDD data of the bare probe as given in the calibration files.

3.2.3.2 Stand

The stand allows positioning of the XRS with 6 degrees of freedom. Electromagnetic clutches lock the radiation source in the treatment position. The stand requires careful balance setup for weight compensation.

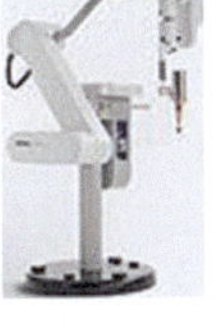

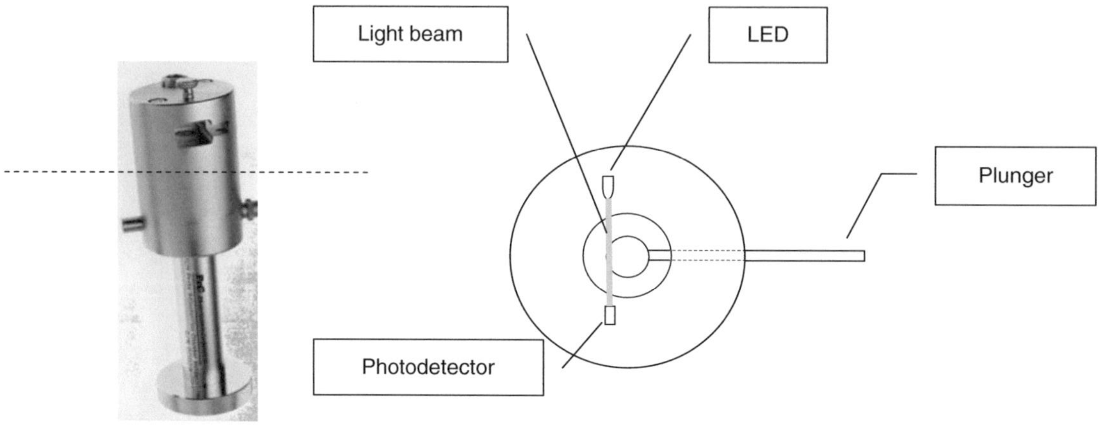

Fig. 3.1 Top view diagram of PAICH cross-section

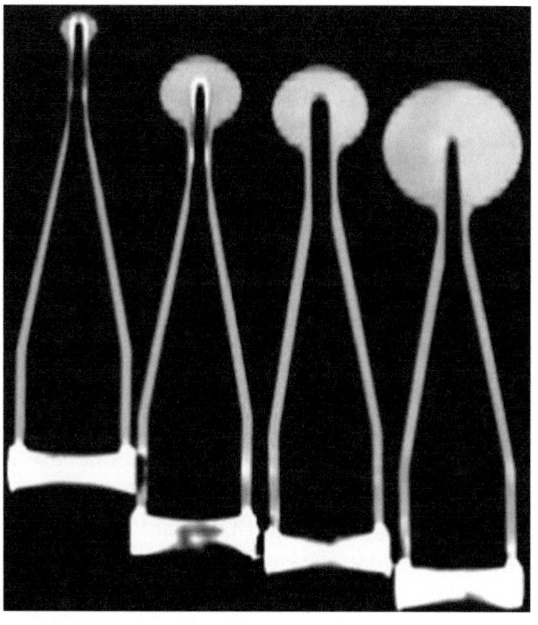

Fig. 3.2 CT image showing cross-sections of 1.5, 3.0, 3.5 and 5.0 cm diameter applicators, illustrating the aluminium inserted in the two smallest applicators

3.2.3.3 Interlock System and Safety Features

The whole system features various interlock mechanisms to avoid unintended radiation emission and loss or incorrect data transmission. Radiation emission is audio and visually indicated on the X-ray source and user interface. Further safety systems such as a theatre door switch can be added to an external interlock switch on the INTRABEAM control console. The count rate is constantly monitored by the IRM and its ratio with the planned treatment time is checked via the control console. Any deviation from tolerance will stop any emission of radiation. The system also features an optical interlock able to detect whether the appropriate verification device has been correctly attached to the X-ray source, whether the source has been mounted correctly onto the floor stand and whether an applicator has been correctly attached to the floor stand. The INTRABEAM PRS500, and older versions, is not capable of detecting the applicator size. For this reason, it is recommendable to independently verify such parameters once the surgeon has attached it to the stand. Finally, the software follows a series of verification steps such that only when they have been correctly completed by trained and authorised staff will emission of radiation be allowed.

3.2.3.4 Ancillary Components

Ancillary components include *connectors* that will provide signal feedback and low-voltage power between different components; *V&X block guides* for the safety coupling between the XRS and pre-treatment components; and a *protector sheath* to cover the XRS probe while not in use or out of its carrying tray.

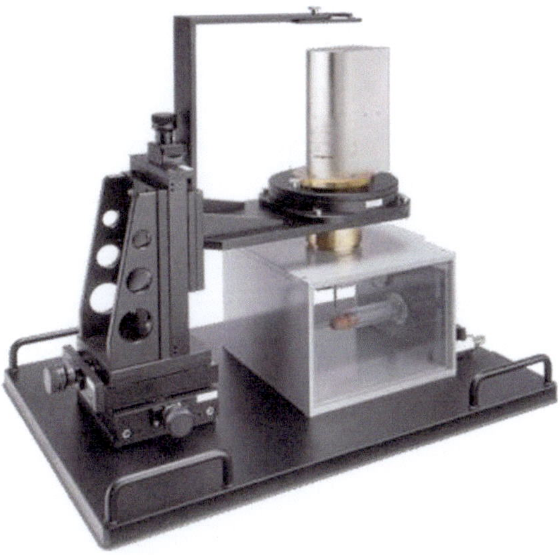

Fig. 3.3 Zeiss water phantom

3.3 Calibration of the System

The dosimetry check of the INTRABEAM is predefined by the manufacturer, Zeiss, with calibration files linked to the XRS serial number provided on a CD to be loaded onto the user interface. Calibration of the XRS to quantify the depth dose rate characteristics (PDDs) of its X-ray emission must be performed annually. These PDDs and other checks such as output measurements are carried out at the Carl Zeiss manufacturing plant using their own water phantom (simliar to the commercially available model shown in Fig. 3.3).

The purpose of any commissioning study by the hospital's radiotherapy department will be to develop and implement a method to independently verify the internal dosimetry of the system vs. quoted data: dosimetric determination of the PDDs (with bare probe and with applicators), absolute dose, isotropy and long-term stability of the XRS. These independent verification tests will be explained in the chapter "Quality Assurance and Commissioning". Here, we will only cover the sequential procedures designed to verify the correct operation of the INTRABEAM system prior to patient treatment.

These checks, specifically dose calibration and probe straightness, are vital to ensure accuracy of dose delivery. This is because, since the electrons are made to drift along a thin tube of 3 mm outside diameter and 2 mm inside diameter, any bending of more than 0.1 mm in the tube will reflect the electrons back and will reduce the output dose rate per minute.

3.3.1 Treatment Verification Tests

When logging in the user terminal, the software will display the "System Quality Assurance" tab by default. Once the XRS in use has been selected, the following optional and mandatory tests are performed prior to treatment:

3.3.1.1 Probe Adjuster (Optional Test, PAICH Tool)

The probe adjuster is used to verify and, if necessary, adjust the straightness of the XRS probe to ensure proper alignment of the electron beam with the mechanical centre of the probe (Fig. 3.4). This test will be performed if the isotropy verification test has been unsuccessful and/or the XRS probe is suspected to be bent. Insert the XRS into the PAICH and connect both to the control console. The two bar graphs on the right side of the window display the current deviation of the XRS probe as the PAICH is rotated 360°, with the second graph indicating the same deviation at a different sensitivity setting. As the PAICH is rotated, the deviation bar moves. The runout must not exceed the specified tolerance (0.10 mm). This is calculated according to the formula below, where the maximum and minimum deviations are the values of the high and the low cursor associated with each bar.

$$\text{Runout (mm)} = \text{maximum deviation (mm)} - \text{minimum deviation (mm)}$$

If the probe needs adjusting, press "Zero" before rotating the PAICH around the probe to where the deviation bar is at its maximum. At this point, depress the plunger and then release it. After releasing the plunger, the bars should be closer to the centre of the graph.

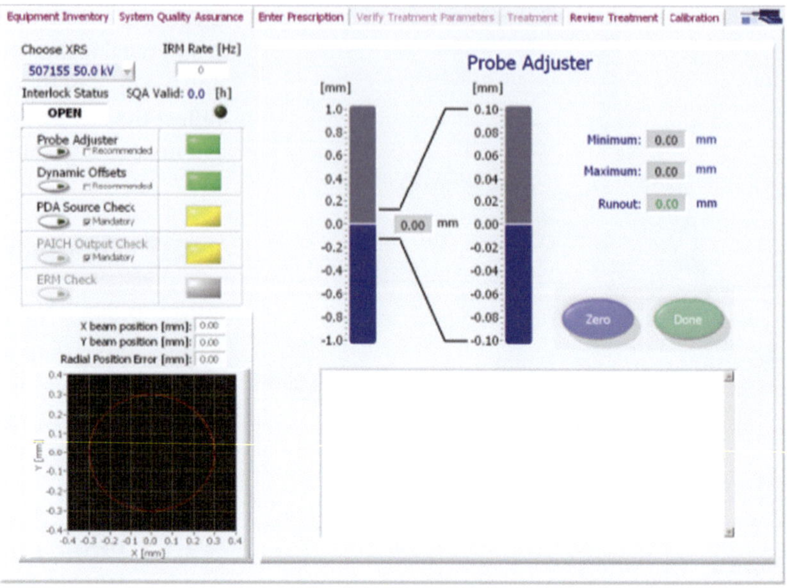

Fig. 3.4 Probe adjuster window

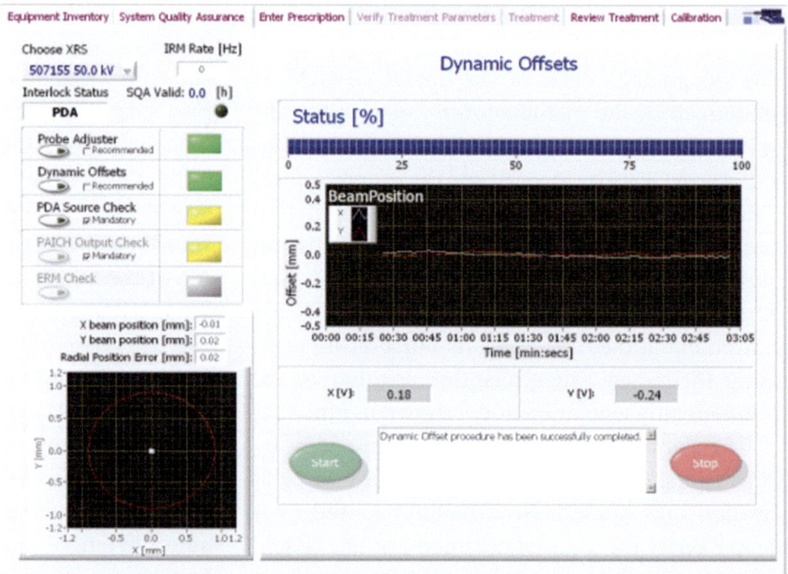

Fig. 3.5 Dynamic offsets window

3.3.1.2 Dynamic Offsets (Optional Test, PDA Tool)

This test must be run after centring the XRS probe. It verifies the stability as well as the beam position over a period of time at the deflector coil voltages set for optimum output (electron beam centred on the target). With the XRS probe inserted into the PDA, align the +X and +Y markings on both the XRS and the PDA. Both the XRS and the PDA must be connected to the control console. Once the process has been started, it will run automatically and last a few minutes. During this time, the main beam position graph should show both coordinate signals (X and Y) to be approximately flat with no fluctuation greater than ±0.1 mm around 0 (beam centre) (Fig. 3.5). The graph at the bottom left corner will provide the same information radially.

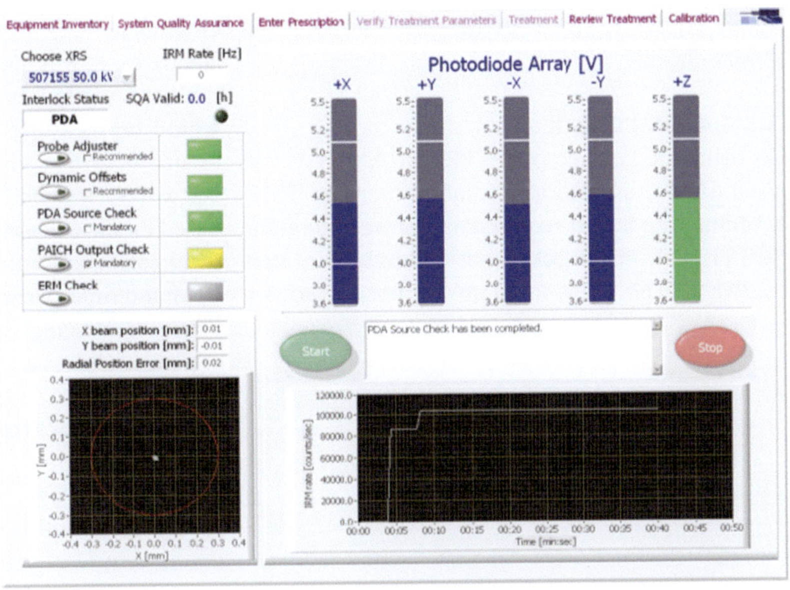

Fig. 3.6 PDA source check window

3.3.1.3 PDA Source Check (Mandatory Test, PDA Tool)

This test is used to verify the XRS probe's spherical emission pattern. With the XRS probe inserted into the PDA, align the +X and +Y markings on both the XRS and the PDA. Both the XRS and the PDA must be connected to the control console. Once the process has been started, it will run automatically and last a few minutes. The test begins by measuring the dark counts from the IRM over a 30-s period, ensuring they are less than a predefined maximum value. X-ray emission is shut off during this portion of the test. The system then turns on X-rays. During this time, the bar graph "Photodiode Array [V]" will display the signals obtained from the four lateral sensors with respect to the one in the Z position (Fig. 3.6). If the beam is nearly isotropic, the height of the first four bars should follow closely the one displayed by Z. The XRS isotropy should fall within the specified tolerance provided the probe is straight and the deflector coils are set for optimum output. If this is the case, the IRM count rate [Hz] information obtained during this test will be used in the treatment administration. The IRM rate will be compared with the corresponding IRM at the time of the last calibration.

PAICH Output Check (Mandatory Test, PAICH Tool) (Fig. 3.7)

This procedure checks the amount of radiation being generated by the XRS, in air, against an expected value in the Z-axis. With the XRS inserted into the PAICH, insert the shielded IC into the PAICH slot and connect it to the electrometer UNIDOS E. The slot is positioned such that the front chamber window is symmetrically located 1 cm from the tip of the source, perpendicular to its axis. The settings of the electrometer should be "Current" and "Low pA". Any setting changes to the electrometer will require ending the INTRABEAM software application. Both the XRS and the PAICH must be connected to the control console. "Zero" the electrometer prior to commencing the test. Once the test has been started, it will run automatically and last a few minutes. The final dosimeter reading obtained will be the average of readings obtained during a period of time. The final output shown is temperature and pressure corrected. The corrected output will be compared to the corresponding output at the time of the last calibration.

After all mandatory checks have been carried out successfully, they will be valid for 36 h. Once treatment has been started, it needs to be delivered within 90 min to avoid having to repeat the mandatory checks.

3.3.1.4 ERM Check

As mentioned earlier, old INTRABEAM systems used to have an external radiation monitor. This monitor is no longer required; therefore, although still present, this check is not highlighted in the software. The ERM used to be positioned as close as possible to the patient (i.e. on the gantry stand) as it was dependent on the intensity of radiation exiting from the patient. Its count rate would be measured during the first 30 s of the treatment. This count rate would be used to project a total number of counts for the treatment based on the calculated treatment time, setting an extra safety control to terminate the beam if the IRM and timer were to fall outside of the bounds during treatment.

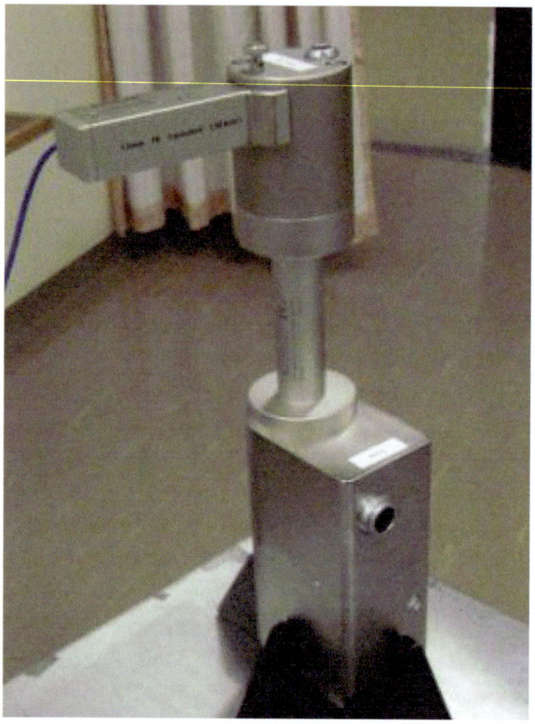

Fig. 3.7 Output check set up

3.3.2 Calibration Tests

What follows next is a series of tests that allow further non-routine pre-treatment calibration of the system (e.g. yearly calibrations, compliance with department's QA programme or after repair).

3.3.2.1 Time/Date

This procedure synchronises the date and time between the user terminal and the control console (Fig. 3.8). The latter adopts the date and time from the former.

3.3.2.2 Deflection Calibration (PDA Tool) (Fig. 3.9)

It is recommended that this test is performed at least once a year (i.e. after a new calibration file has been imported as a result of recalibration). This procedure determines the sensitivity of the beam deflecting coils. The procedure will show the Z signal (voltage reading) change with the

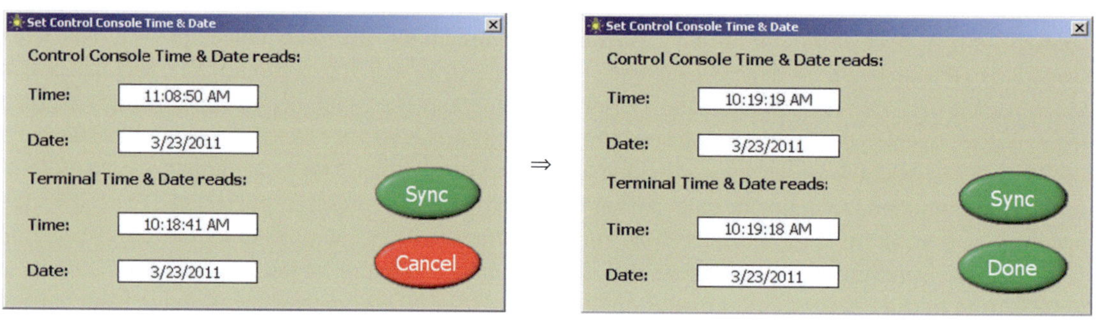

Fig. 3.8 Date/Time synchronisation

change in electron beam direction as the applied voltage in the coils (X and Y) changes. The end result will indicate the alignment of the electron beam with respect to the physical centre of the XRS probe (optimum output for a given set of deflecting voltages). Once the process has been started it will run automatically and take around 20 min to complete.

3.3.2.3 IRM Linearity (PDA Tool) (Fig. 3.10)

It is recommended that this test is performed at least once a year (i.e. after a new calibration file has been imported as a result of recalibration). This procedure will test the response of the IRM by determining the linear correlation between the individual beam currents and the associated count

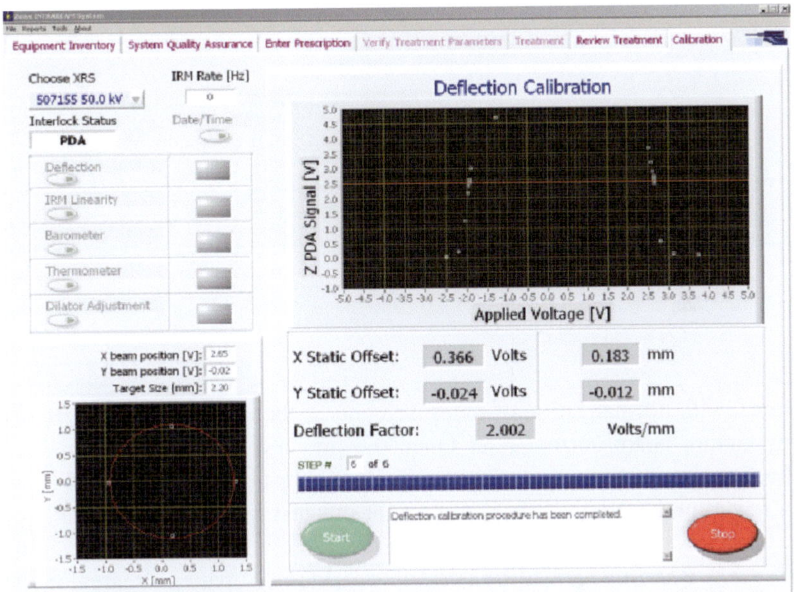

Fig. 3.9 Deflection calibration window

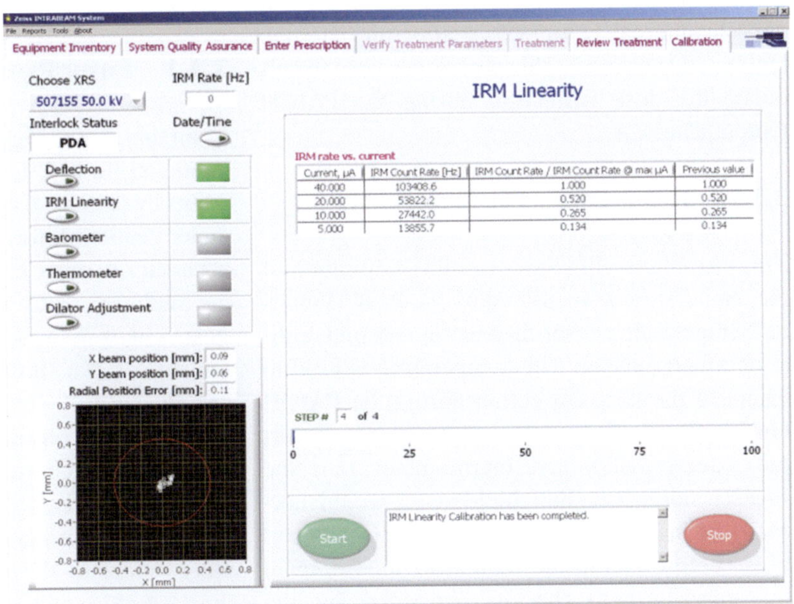

Fig. 3.10 IRM linearity window

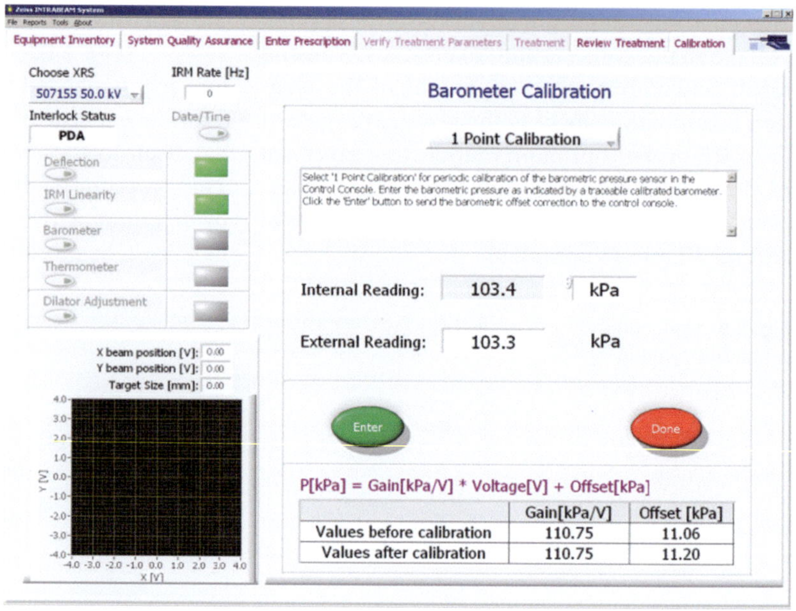

Fig. 3.11 Barometer calibration window

rates, with normalisation of measurements at the maximum beam current rate. Once the process has been started it will run automatically and last a few minutes. No tolerances are set for this test.

3.3.2.4 Barometer Calibration (Fig. 3.11)

This procedure will allow (1 point) calibration of the air pressure as measured by the control console internal barometer against an external, calibrated barometer. This pressure is used to calculate the dose correction during the PAICH Output Check.

3.3.2.5 Thermometer Calibration (Fig. 3.12)

This procedure will allow (1 point) calibration of the temperature as measured by the PAICH internal temperature sensor against an external, calibrated thermometer. This temperature is used to calculate the dose correction during the PAICH Output Check. To proceed with this test, insert the external calibrated thermometer into the PAICH slot where the shielded IC would normally be inserted. Leave the thermometer to stabilise before taking the final reading. Compare this reading with the one provided by the INTRABEAM system.

3.4 Patient Treatment Menu

Only when all relevant verification tests have been successfully performed will the system allow the input, verification and delivery of the patient treatment. What follows next is a step by step guide to the software menu for treatment.

3.4.1 Enter Prescription

From this menu (Fig. 3.13) you may initiate a new treatment (or call up the details of previous treatments by ticking "Continue with previous patient" under "Patient Information"). Under this tab, it is necessary to enter certain information chosen for the treatment: XRS, applicator type and size. The treatment # increments automatically. Enter the Patient ID (i.e. hospital number) and click on "More" to fill in patient-related information: name, date of birth, sex and treatment site with exact location coordinates. Once the prescription and treatment depth (mm from surface of applicator) have been entered, the system will automatically calculate the treatment time (h:m:s) and dose rate at depth (Gy/min). This calculation is described in Appendix A. A depth dose graph

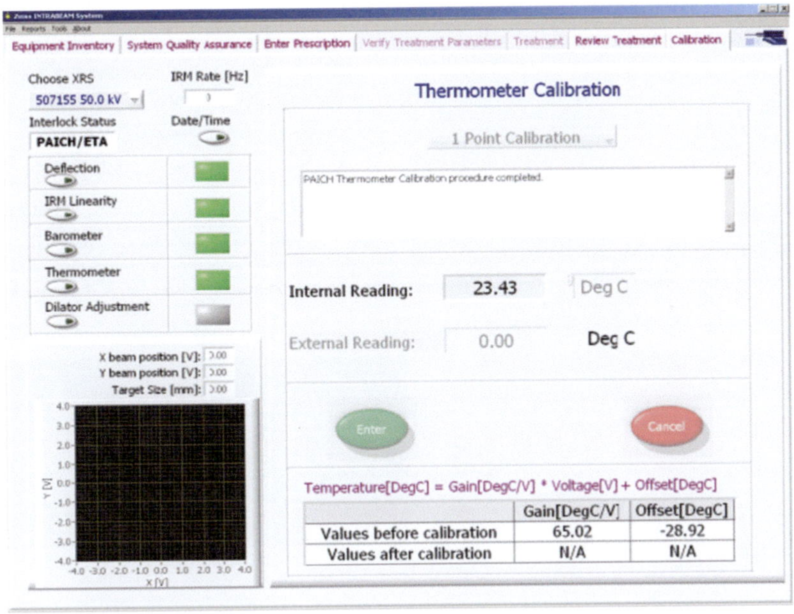

Fig. 3.12 Thermometer calibration window

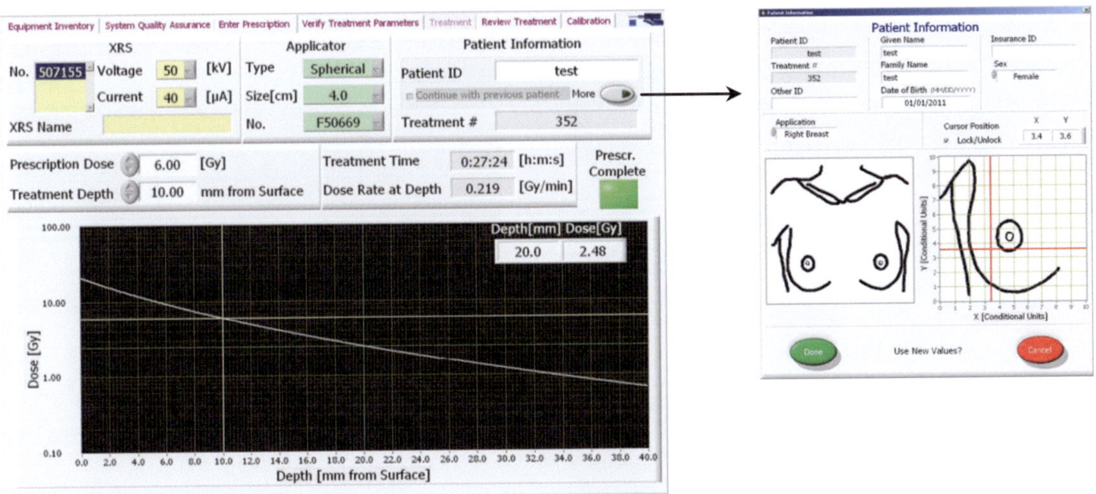

Fig. 3.13 Enter treatment window

relevant to the chosen parameters will be displayed at the bottom of the window.

3.4.2 Verify Treatment Parameters

Under this tab (Fig. 3.14), an independent operator/physician must verify all the parameters entered under the "Enter Prescription" tab. No editing can be done here, so any correction will have to be made by going back to the previous "Enter Prescription" tab. A verification password needs to be entered before moving on to the "Treatment" tab.

3.4.3 Treatment

At this point, the system verifies that all interlocks are satisfied, including correct insertion of the applicator into the XRS, in order to verify

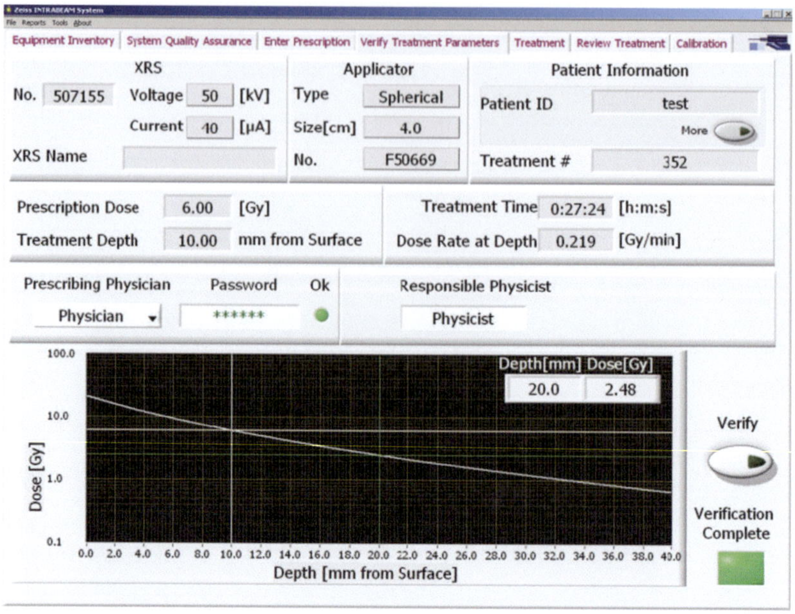

Fig. 3.14 Verify treatment prescription window

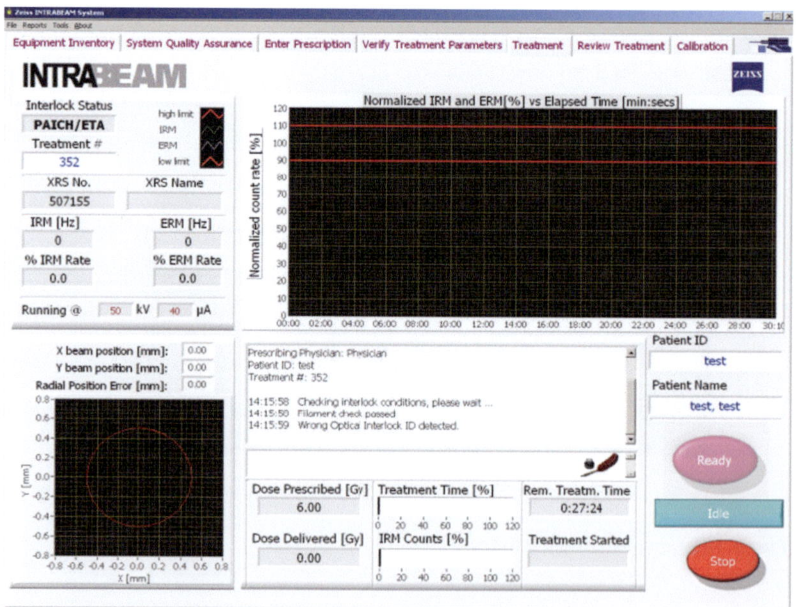

Fig. 3.15 Treatment window

that it is safe to proceed. Once these checks have been completed, the software will enable X-ray production. During this time a graph will display the normalised IRM (%), confirming beam stability over the whole treatment time (Fig. 3.15). There are various mechanisms to control the production of radiation. Some of them are controlled by hardware and some by software:

3.4.3.1 Hardware

The IRM and treatment timer counters each contain a setpoint register (IRM limit and run time respectively) and a cumulative counts register. Prior to the start of treatment, the setpoint registers are loaded with the end point values obtained from the verification tests and the chosen treatment parameters, whereas the cumulative count registers are initialised to zero. The IRM counters will count the pulses from the IRM monitor, incrementing at a rate based on its input signal (IRM input pulses), and will continually compare the accumulated counts with the count limit. The timer count register will also increment at a rate based on the input coming from a clock oscillator. When the limit has been reached, a signal sent to the control console causes X-ray production to terminate, resulting in a normal end of treatment.

3.4.3.2 Software

During radiation the control console measures the IRM count rate and elapsed treatment time. If the IRM count rate deviates by more than a certain percentage from the expected rate, the software will pause the X-rays. Under normal operating conditions, the end of treatment will be controlled by the IRM reaching its setpoint value. If the IRM falls out of bounds during treatment, the system will pause. Should the operator elect to continue treating, the treatment timer will be used as the end of treatment controller.

The "Pause" button may be used at any time during the treatment to suspend radiation. X-rays will not be generated, but the system will remain armed and will continue with the treatment when the "Ready" button is pressed again. If the treatment needs to be aborted, the "Stop" button is pressed instead. This option does not allow resumption of the treatment. Under these circumstances, the rest of the treatment can only be delivered by inserting the remainder of the dose from the "Enter Prescription" tab and following the subsequent treatment tabs as described above. Troubleshooting of power failures and other potential interlock conditions is described further in Appendix B.

3.4.4 Review Treatment

This tab provides a means to review, save on a pdf file or print the final treatment delivered.

3.5 Miscellaneous

3.5.1 Equipment Inventory

This tab lists all the equipment (XRSs, QA instruments and applicators) associated with the system as well as other relevant information (Fig. 3.16). Thus, when receiving a replacement XRS (e.g. due to calibration of your main XRS), this new XRS will have to be registered in the system via the Equipment Inventory and its calibration files loaded in the relevant folder.

3.5.2 Applicator Sterilisation Monitor

The number of sterilisations that an applicator has undertaken after use during treatment is registered under the "Equipment Inventory" tab (Fig. 3.17). However, there will be occasions, e.g. when the surgeon is checking the most suitable applicator size for use in the patient, when the "discarded" applicator will not be registered as it will not have been entered under the "Treatment" tab. As the tested applicator will equally require sterilisation, the software provides a way to manually keep count of the number of sterilisations for these "test" applicators. In the main window menu, go to "Tools\Applicator Sterilization". Select the "tested" applicator and move it from the left to the right panel. Under the "Equipment Inventory" tab the sterilisation counts on the "tested" applicator will be incremented.

Appendices

Appendix A: Treatment Calculation Time

Depth Dose Curve in Water

During production or recalibration, Zeiss determines the depth dose curve of a given XRS in a specially designed water phantom that allows the mounting and positioning of the XRS without the stand, as well as the insertion of the ion chamber (IC) inside a purpose-made holder within the

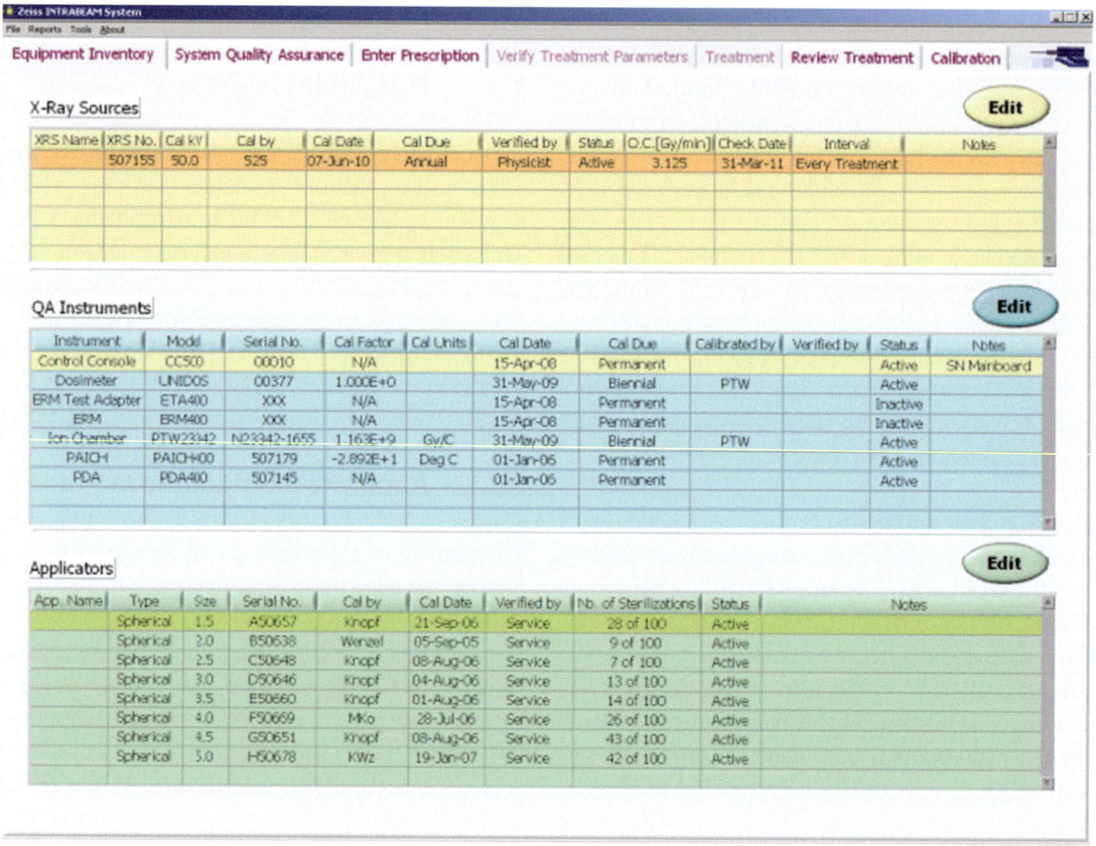

Fig. 3.16 Equipment inventory window

Fig. 3.17 Applicator sterilisation monitor window

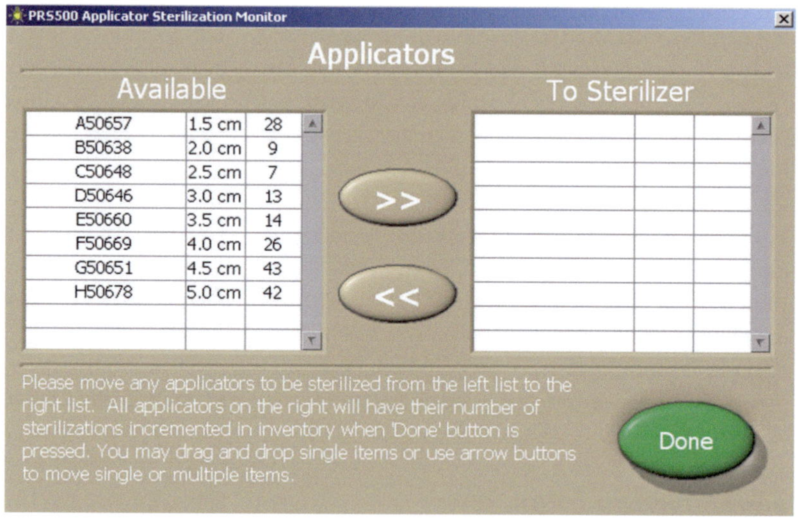

phantom. The current obtained from the IC measured at different depths (z) will allow calculation of the depth dose curve from the following equation:

$$D_{w,z}\left[Gy/\min\right]=IC_{TP,z}\left[nC/s\right]\times N_s\left[R/C\right]\times k_q\times f\left[Gy/R\right]\times 60\left[s/\min\right]$$

where $D_{w,z}$ = absorbed dose to water at depth z; $IC_{TP,z}$ = ion chamber current reading in water phantom at depth z, temperature and pressure corrected; N_s = calibration factor for the ion chamber used during the water phantom measurements taken from the PTW calibration certificate;

f = conversion factor from roentgens to grays with a value of 8.81 mGy/R, as extracted from ICRU Report 17; and k_q = beam quality correction factor – this takes the value of 1 for beam qualities in the (PTW) T30 to T50 range (accelerating voltage of 30 to 50 kV with effective energies of approx. 17–20 kV).

A fit function of the depth dose curve is generated mathematically to account for the impossibility of measuring directly on the surface of the XRS tip.

Similarly, depth dose curves are obtained with applicator, for each of the clinical applicators. The ratio between the depth curves with and without applicator provides the transfer function (Y_z) for each applicator. Again, a fit function of these depth dose curves will be generated to account for the impossibility of directly measuring from the surface of the applicator.

Both calibration files, bare probe depth dose curve and applicator transfer functions, will be loaded onto the user terminal. The information is securely linked via the serial numbers of XRS and each individual applicator.

Original PAICH Output and IRM

Baseline values for dose rates and IRM rates are also loaded onto the system via calibration files obtained from measurements taken with the Zeiss factory PAICH and IC.

Thus, the original PAICH output at factory will be given as:

$$D_{original}\left[Gy/\min\right] = IC_{TP}\left(PAICH_{factory}\right)\left[nC/s\right] \times N_{k,factory}\left[Gy/C\right] \times k_q \times 60\left[s/\min\right]$$

where IC_{TP} = ion chamber current reading inside the PAICH, temperature and pressure corrected; $N_{k,factory}$ = calibration factor for the ion chamber used during the $PAICH_{factory}$ measurements and taken from its PTW Air Kerma calibration certificate; and k_q = beam quality correction factor as above.

Customer's PAICH Output and IRM

The PAICH output measurement performed during the pre-treatment quality control determines the output of the XRS before the actual treatment session:

$$D_{customer}\left[Gy/\min\right] = IC_{TP}\left(PAICH_{customer}\right)\left[nC/s\right] \times N_{k,customer}\left[Gy/C\right] \times k_q \times 60\left[s/\min\right]$$

where $N_{k,customer}$ = calibration factor for the ion chamber used during the $PAICH_{customer}$ measurements taken from its PTW Air Kerma calibration certificate.

The software will compare the PAICH output value calculated during pre-treatment QA with that given in the stored calibration file. The software will not permit delivery of treatment when the deviation revealed by the comparison exceeds 10 %. If the deviation is between 5 and 10 %, the software will require the customer to acknowledge a warning message.

The actual absolute dose output in water (depth dose curve to be used for treatment) is calculated from the fitted depth dose curve in water and the factory and customer's PAICH outputs:

$$D_{w,z(treat,bareXRS)}\left[Gy/\min\right] = D_{w,z}\left[Gy/\min\right] \times \frac{D_{customer}}{D_{factory}}$$

Finally, the total depth dose curve for the XRS plus applicator chosen will be:

$$D_{w,z(treat)}\left[Gy/\min\right] = D_{w,z(treat,bareXRS)}\left[Gy/\min\right] \times Y_z$$

The calculated treatment time given by the INTRABEAM for a prescribed dose $D_{w,z}$ (Gy) will be:

$$\text{Calculated Treatment Time}\left[\min\right] = \frac{D_{w,z}\left[Gy\right]}{D_{w,z(treat)}\left[Gy/\min\right]} \quad \text{or,}$$

$$\text{Calculated Treatment Time}\left[s\right] = \frac{D_{w,z}\left[Gy\right]}{D_{w,z(treat)}\left[Gy/\min\right]} \times 60\left[s/\min\right]$$

This time and the actual IRM rate [count/s] measured during the pre-treatment QA procedure are used to calculate the total number of IRM counts that correspond to the treatment dose prescribed, $D_{w,z}$ [Gy].

$$\text{Total Counts [counts]} = I_{actual}\ [counts/s] \times \text{Treatment Time [s]}$$

where I_{actual} = IRM rate during pre-treatment QA procedure.

The actual treatment time, i.e. time during which radiation is being emitted, may increase or decrease depending on whether the dose rate of the XRS changes during treatment. The radiation will stop once the total IRM counts have been reached. However, if the calculated counts are not reached during 110 % of the calculated treatment time, then the system will stop the treatment. The delivered dose, up until the system stops the radiation, is recorded at all times.

Appendix B: Troubleshooting

The following flowcharts aim to provide a quick guide to the essential steps to follow when a problem or interlock with the INTRABEAM system is encountered. Any problem beyond the common faults/interlocks given here will require consultation with the manufacturer before an attempt is made to resolve it.

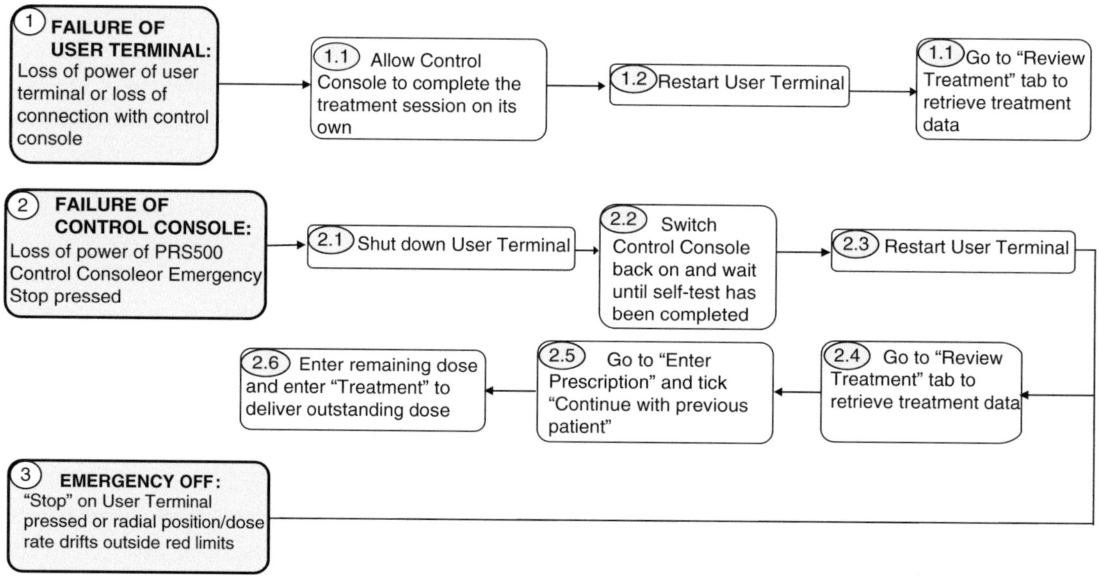

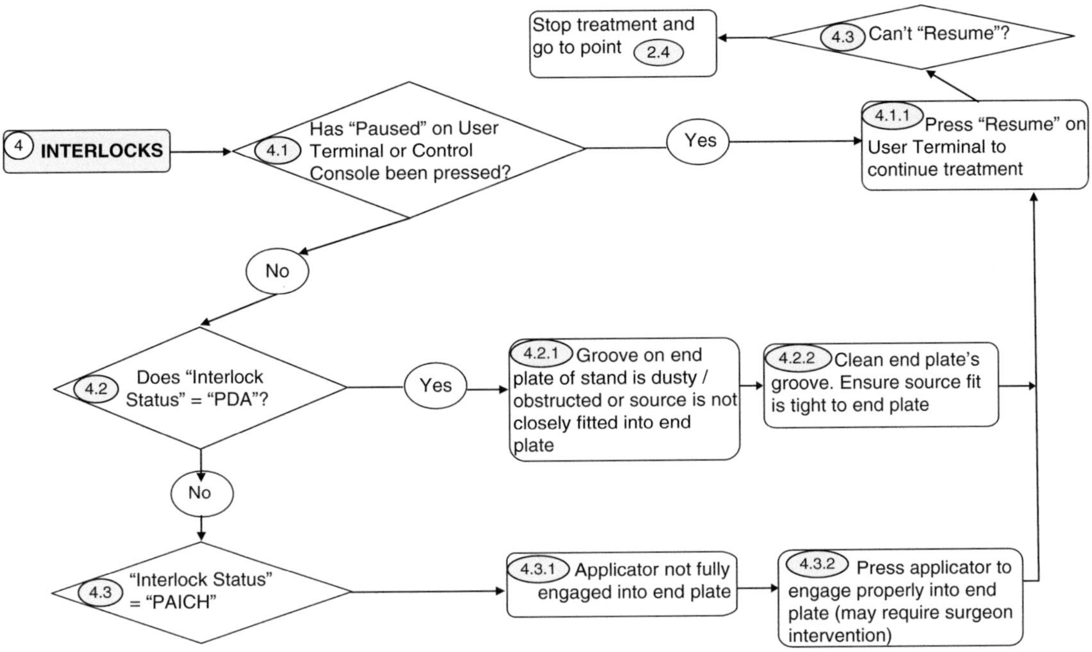

References

Carl Zeiss Surgical (2007) INTRABEAM® system PRS 500 with XRS 4. Carl Zeiss Surgical, Oberkochen

Biggs DS, Thomson ES (1996) Radiation properties of a miniature X-ray device for radiosurgery. Br J Radiol 69:544–547

Quality Assurance and Commissioning

4

Frank Schneider, Sven Clausen
and David J. Eaton

4.1 Dosimetry

The X-ray source (XRS 4) of the INTRABEAM® system accelerates electrons with a maximum voltage of 50 kV. These are steered down a 10-cm-long drift tube (probe) to strike a thin gold target at the end, and generate bremsstrahlung photon radiation in an approximately isotropic distribution (Wenz and Kraus-Tiefenbacher 2011). The probe tip consists of beryllium, transparent to X-rays above an energy of 10 keV, coated with nickel and titanium nitride, to give a durable and biocompatible surface. All of these materials will affect the characteristic spectrum of the source, to give an effective energy of approximately 20 kV for the probe only (Beatty et al. 1996; Dinsmore et al. 1996). With a spherical breast applicator attached, the beam will be hardened due to the additional material in the path of the radiation, which preferentially absorbs lower energy photons. The applicators are made from a biocompatible polyetherimide material (Ultem®), with an additional aluminium layer inside the smaller sizes (≤3.0 cm diameter) to give similar levels of hardening and shield the shaft from excess leakage.

4.1.1 Factory Calibration

Before delivery of a new system and as part of the annual service, the XRS 4 is calibrated in the factory by the vendor. Dose rate as a function of depth is measured using a soft X-ray ionisation chamber in a water tank, similar to the one described below. During production, depth doses are measured for the user probe only, and for a standard factory probe with each of the user applicators added. These values form the basis of the calibration files supplied with the unit. Each year the depth dose for the probe only is updated and a new calibration file is returned along with the source.

Ionisation chamber readings are corrected to standard temperature and pressure and converted to dose using an exposure calibration factor for the chamber and a Roentgen to Gray conversion factor. For 50 kV, a beam quality of 0.6 mm Al (half value layer) or an effective energy of 20 kV is used for these coefficients, corresponding to the probe at 1 cm depth in water. Dose values for the probe are fitted to a triple exponential function based on the Lambert-Beer absorption law, to enable extrapolation to the surface (Fig. 4.1). Dose fall-off away from the surface is approximately inversely proportional to distance cubed. Applicator dose values are converted into a transfer function, which is fitted to a double exponential best fit curve. For a certain depth:

F. Schneider (✉) • S. Clausen
Department of Radiation Oncology, University Medical Center Mannheim, University of Heidelberg, D-68167 Mannheim, Germany
e-mail: frank.schneider@umm.de; sven.clausen@umm.de

D.J. Eaton
Department of Radiotherapy, Royal Free London NHS Foundation Trust, Pond Street, Hampstead, London NW3 2QG, UK
e-mail: davideaton@nhs.net

M. Keshtgar et al. (eds.), *Targeted Intraoperative Radiotherapy in Oncology*,
DOI 10.1007/978-3-642-39821-6_4, © Springer-Verlag Berlin Heidelberg 2014

$$\text{Dose rate (probe and applicator)} = \text{Dose rate (probe alone)} \times \text{Transfer function (applicator)} \quad (1)$$

Baseline readings are also acquired during factory calibration for the IRM feedback monitor and output measured using the PAICH attachment. These are supplied with the calibration file and are used for comparison with PDA and PAICH checks performed before each treatment. Any small differences in the daily output are used to adjust the planned treatment time:

$$\text{Planned treatment time} = \frac{\text{Prescription dose}}{\text{Dose rate (probe and applicator)} \times \text{Daily output difference}} \quad (2)$$

Every 2 years, the user chamber and electrometer are returned to a standards laboratory to update the calibration factors for these instruments, and a new certificate is provided to the user. The air kerma factor from this certificate is then updated on the system at the same time as the replacement calibration file is installed.

During production, the isotropy of the applicators is measured using the water tank and values tabulated for each applicator size by removing the anisotropy due to the factory standard source:

$$\text{Isotropy (applicator)} = \text{Isotropy (probe and applicator)} - \text{Isotropy (probe alone)} \quad (3)$$

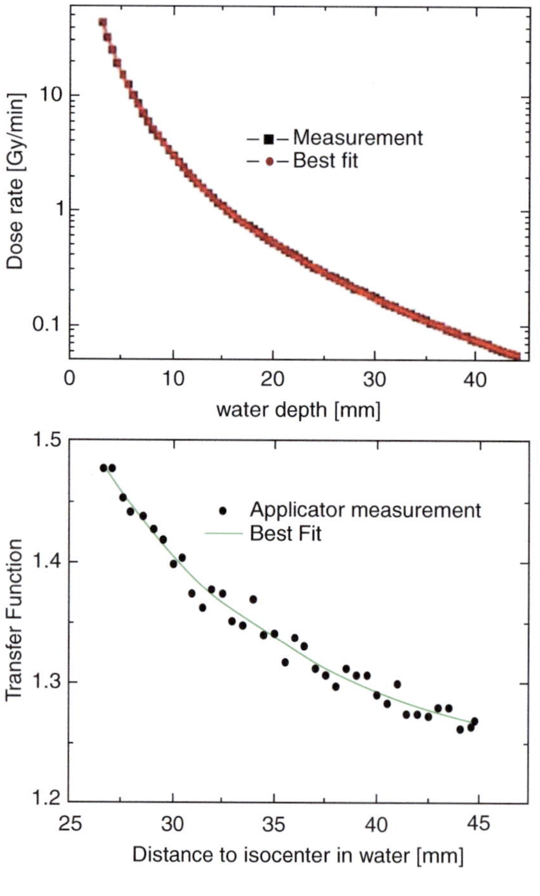

Fig. 4.1 Measurements of depth dose for probe only and applicator, with best fit lines overlaid

Further details on all these procedures can be found in Carl Zeiss Meditec AG (2011).

4.2 Commissioning

The extent of measurements undertaken for a commissioning process will depend on the local requirements, national regulations and personal interest. The minimum which has to be done before using the INTRABEAM system clinically is to perform the internal quality assurance tests defined by the system itself and to designate the radiation protection areas, which are described in more detail in the Chap. 5. In some countries it is necessary to verify the system using an independent method. In that case, some of the following approaches can be used. Further details on this topic can be found in a recent review article (Eaton 2012).

4.3 Independent Quality Assurance

4.3.1 Water Phantom

Zeiss offers a special water phantom (dimensions: 58×40×52 cm) to independently measure depth dose curves and isotropy of the XRS 4 in the local centre. The phantom consists of a water tank, filled with 6 l of water, and two cavities for placing a soft X-ray ionisation chamber (PTW type 23342) below or beside the XRS 4 (Fig. 4.2). A stepping mechanism allows a linear movement of the XRS 4 in three directions with positional accuracy of ±0.1 mm. Using the chamber cavity below the XRS 4 allows measurement of dose rates at different depths to confirm the calibration file of the system. To determine the isotropy, the XRS 4 can be rotated in steps of 45° around the vertical axis of the probe. Using the chamber cavity to the side of the XRS 4, dose rate measurements can be recorded at different source angles. All measurements can be done with and without an applicator. These measurements can be used to independently verify the calibration data, measured by the vendor.

Solid water-equivalent phantom materials may also be used to measure output at different depths (Härtl et al. 2009). Care must be taken, however, that the material is water-equivalent at low kilovoltage energies. The major source of error in these measurements will be positioning of the source and detector. An appropriate code of practice should be used to convert chamber readings into dose. The ionisation chamber should be linked to a national standard laboratory by direct calibration or local intercomparison against a secondary standard instrument. Intercomparison may be performed using the INTRABEAM system or a superficial unit of similar beam quality. Beam quality may be determined by measuring the half value layer, with the source collimated to approximate narrow beam geometry (Eaton and Duck 2010).

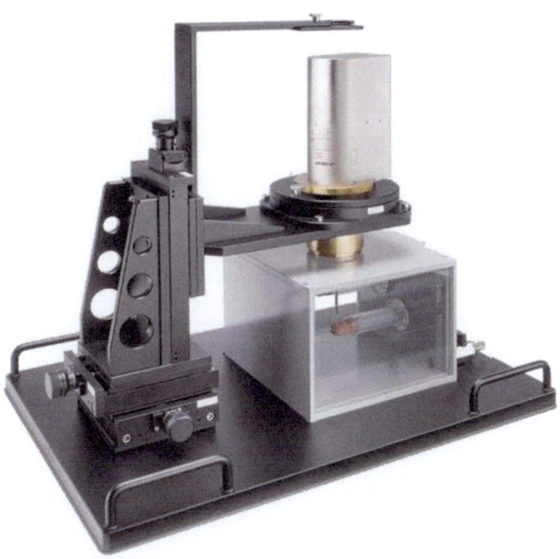

Fig. 4.2 Water phantom to measure depth doses and isotropy

4.3.2 Film Measurement

An alternative approach to measure depth dose curves and isotropy of the XRS 4 with high spatial resolution is film dosimetry using radiochromic films, such as Gafchromic® films (ISP, New Jersey, USA). These are made by laminating an active layer between two polyester layers. Some advantages of these films are water resistance, tissue equivalence, wide detectable dose range, low energy dependence and the possibility of handling them in room light (Schneider et al. 2009a).

Gafchromic films have been used to determine the depth doses and spatial dose distributions of the INTRABEAM system, as shown in Fig. 4.3 (Schneider et al. 2009b). To analyse the isotropy, an applicator or probe shape was cut out from the film and the film was then placed around an applicator or the bare probe. This setup was sandwiched between two halves of solid water blocks, and irradiated. Afterwards it was scanned and evaluated according to standard local protocols.

The verification of the depth dose curve is more difficult because the film has to be calibrated from pixel values (grey values) into dose. This can be done by irradiating a film along an extension of the axis of the probe. A profile on the scanned film along this axis gives a curve

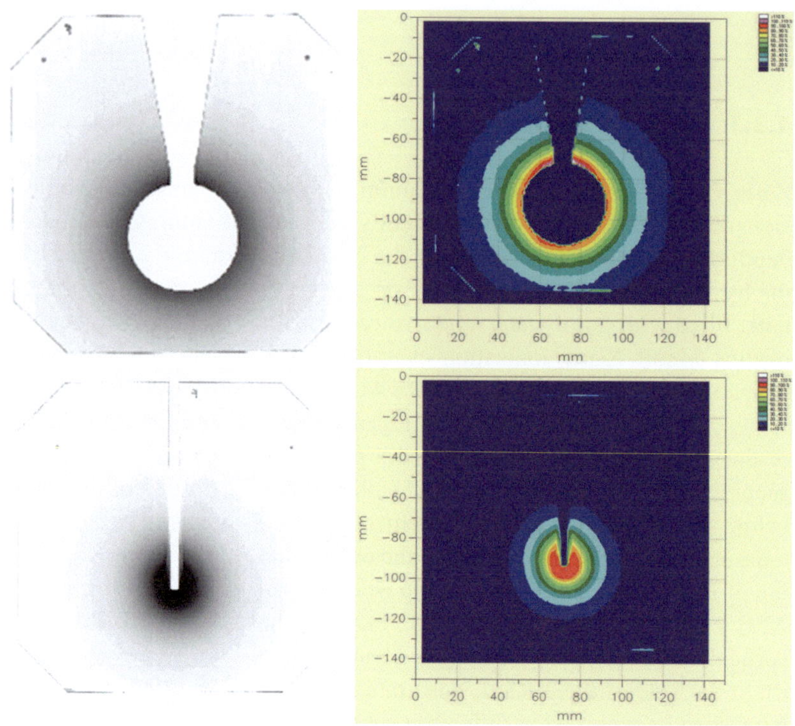

Fig. 4.3 Evaluation of isotropy using Gafchromic films

representing grey values as a function of depth. An exponential function can be fitted to that curve in Mathematica or Mathlab. In a second step the depth dose curve, which is calculated by the INTRABEAM terminal, can be fitted using another exponential function. Finally these two functions can be correlated to obtain an assignment of grey values to dose (Schneider et al. 2009b). However, in this approach some extra knowledge is needed to keep the compound error of the film-scanner system as low as possible (Schneider et al. 2009a; Andres et al. 2010).

4.3.3 TLD Measurement

Thermoluminescent dosimeters (TLDs) are small, portable, tissue equivalent and independent of dose rate or temperature, making them a useful addition to more accurate measurements with an ionisation chamber. Energy and dose dependence (supralinearity) necessitate calibration in a similar beam quality and dose level, but this can potentially be performed using a superficial therapy X-ray unit instead of the INTRABEAM system (Eaton and Duck 2010). Common clinical uses of TLDs in radiotherapy include checking the dose in vivo to normal tissues such as the eyes, and they have been also been used with INTRABEAM to measure skin doses during breast intraoperative radiotherapy (Eaton et al. 2012; Fogg et al. 2010).

TLDs have been used to measure depth doses for the XRS 4 alone (Hakim et al. 1997; Soares et al. 2006), but may be less practical for this purpose than other methods using an ionisation chamber or film. However, they can be used as a quick and simple method to verify isotropy as described in the following example.

Five packets of TLD rods (LiF) were prepared by heat sealing four TLD rods (LiF) in plastic envelopes. These were then taped to the surface of one of the larger applicators (to minimise positional uncertainties), in the five orthogonal positions of the diodes in the PDA attachment (±*X*, ±*Y*, +*Z*). The source was mounted on the support stand and the applicator attached, then the end of the applicator was submerged in water to give

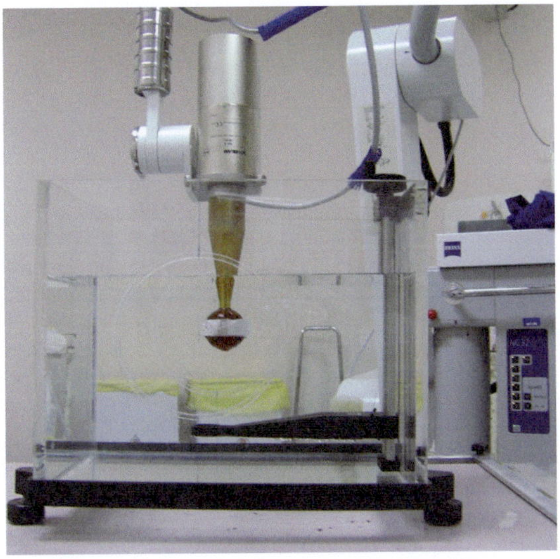

Fig. 4.4 TLD measurement setup for verification of isotropy

Table 4.1 TLD isotropy results after return of x-ray source from factory calibration in 2011, using a 4.5 cm diameter applicator

Direction	Mean packet reading (nC)	Relative difference from mean lateral plane value (%)	Relative difference from forward value (+Z) (%)
+*Z*	21,659	(+5.4)	–
−*X*	20,204	−1.7	−6.7
+*X*	20,484	−0.3	−5.4
−*Y*	21,149	+2.9	−2.4
+*Y*	20,340	−1.0	−6.1

full scatter conditions (Fig. 4.4). The TLDs were irradiated for 5–10 min, then read out according to standard local protocols. No calibration or supralinearity correction was applied since the doses were relative and expected to be similar to each other.

The mean reading from each packet was compared to the forward (+*Z*) and mean lateral plane values as shown in Table 4.1. The standard deviation of lateral readings (*X*, *Y*) was 1.9 % and the difference between the mean lateral plane value and the forward direction (*Z*) was −5.2 %. The manufacturer-quoted anisotropy for this applicator is −8.3 to +0.4 % relative to the forward direction, so these values are acceptable.

4.4 Monte Carlo Simulation

Geant4 is a Monte Carlo open source toolkit developed at CERN. For medical use, a low-energy package can be included to get more precise physical processes in the low-keV energy range needed for intraoperative radiation therapy (Gallina et al. 2002). The code was verified for medical applications in external and internal radiotherapy (Carrier et al. 2004; Milhoretto et al. 2010). In order to simulate the XRS 4, the geometry had to be implemented with a sub-millimetre accuracy and materials had to be defined by their elemental compositions (Yanch and Harte 1996).

This has been done by defining a particle source of electrons with a mean energy of 50 keV and a Gaussian energy spread with a full width at half maximum of 5 keV (Clausen et al. 2012). Using those geometries and parameters, a phase space file was written during a simulation, which included every particle (electron, photon, positron) emitted by the XRS 4. That file was then used to perform further simulations much faster, which could be used to confirm the isotropy and the depth dose in a relative way (Nwankwo et al. 2013).

References

Andres C, del Castillo A, Tortosa R, Alonso D, Barquero R (2010) A comprehensive study of the Gafchromic EBT2 radiochromic film. A comparison with EBT. Med Phys 37:6271–6278

Beatty J, Biggs PJ, Gall K, Okunieff P, Pardo FS, Harte KJ et al (1996) A new miniature x-ray device for interstitial radiosurgery: dosimetry. Med Phys 23:53–62

Carl Zeiss Meditec AG (2011) INTRABEAM® dosimetry. Carl Zeiss Meditec AG, Oberkochen

Carrier JF, Archambault L, Beaulieu L, Roy R (2004) Validation of GEANT4, an object-oriented Monte Carlo toolkit, for simulations in medical physics. Med Phys 31:484–492

Clausen S, Schneider F, Jahnke L, Fleckenstein J, Hesser J, Wenz F (2012) A Monte Carlo based dose calculation method for intravaginal TARGIT brachytherapy using the INTRABEAM system with a cylindrical applicator. Z Med Phys 22:197–204

Dinsmore M, Harte KJ, Sliski AP, Smith DO, Nomikos PM, Dalterio MJ et al (1996) A new miniature x-ray source for interstitial radiosurgery: device description. Med Phys 23:45–52

Eaton DJ (2012) Quality assurance and independent dosimetry for an intraoperative x-ray device. Med Phys 39:6908–6920

Eaton DJ, Duck S (2010) Dosimetry measurements with an intra-operative x-ray device. Phys Med Biol 55:N359–N369

Eaton DJ, Best B, Brew-Graves C, Duck S, Ghaus T, Gonzalez R et al (2012) In vivo dosimetry for single fraction targeted intraoperative radiotherapy (TARGIT) for breast cancer. Int J Radiat Oncol Biol Phys 82:e809–e814

Fogg P, Das KR, Kron T, Fox C, Chua B, Hagekyriakou J (2010) Thermoluminescence dosimetry for skin dose assessment during intraoperative radiotherapy for early breast cancer. Australas Phys Eng Sci Med 33:211–214

Gallina P, Francescon P, Cavedon C, Casamassima F, Mungai R, Perrini P et al (2002) Stereotactic interstitial radiosurgery with a miniature X-ray device in the minimally invasive treatment of selected tumors in the thalamus and the basal ganglia. Stereotact Funct Neurosurg 79:202–213

Hakim R, Zervas NT, Hakim F, Butler WE, Beatty J, Yanch JC et al (1997) Initial characterization of the dosimetry and radiology of a device for administering interstitial stereotactic radiosurgery. Neurosurgery 40:510–516, discussion 516–517

Härtl PM, Dobler B, Kölbl O, Treutwein M (2009) Practical dosimetry and constancy check at introduction of intraoperative radiotherapy with Intrabeam® (Zeiss). Z Med Phys 19:288–293

Milhoretto E, Schelin HR, Setti JA, Denyak V, Paschuk SA, Evseev IG et al (2010) GEANT4 simulations for low energy proton computerized tomography. Appl Radiat Isot 68:951–953

Nwankwo O, Clausen S, Schneider F, Wenz F (2013) A virtual source model of a kilo-voltage radiotherapy device. Phys Med Biol 58:2363–2375

Schneider F, Polednik M, Wolff D, Steil V, Delana A, Wenz F, Menegotti L (2009a) Optimization of the Gafchromic EBT protocol for IMRT QA. Z Med Phys 19:29–37

Schneider F, Fuchs H, Lorenz F, Steil V, Ziglio F, Kraus-Tiefenbacher U et al (2009b) A novel device for intravaginal electronic brachytherapy. Int J Radiat Oncol Biol Phys 74:1298–1305

Soares C, Drupieski C, Wingert B, Pritchett G, Pagonis V, O'Brien M et al (2006) Absorbed dose measurements of a handheld 50 kVP X-ray source in water with thermoluminescence dosemeters. Radiat Prot Dosimetry 120:78–82

Wenz F, Kraus-Tiefenbacher U (2011) Physical and technical aspects. Intraoperative radiotherapy for breast cancer, 1st edn. UNI-MED Verlag AG, Bremen

Yanch J, Harte KJ (1996) Monte Carlo simulation of a miniature, radiosurgery x-ray tube using the ITS 3.0 coupled electron-photon transport code. Med Phys 23:1551–1558

5 Radiation Protection

David J. Eaton and Frank Schneider

5.1 Advantages of the INTRABEAM System

Brachytherapy[1] is a form of radiation therapy that uses small radioactive sources placed a short distance from the treatment area. The steep dose gradient with these sources allows a high dose to be delivered to the target while sparing the surrounding normal tissue.

Soon after the discovery of radioactive materials over a 100 years ago, needles of radium-226 were used for therapeutic purposes. Caesium-137 was also used but more recently iridium-192 has been the material of choice due to a shorter half-life, lower energy (Table 5.1) and high specific activity. This final property has allowed very small but high-activity sources to be fabricated and stored on a coiled wire loop in a shielded container, known as high dose rate (HDR) systems. By connecting an applicator inserted into the patient to this wire, the source can be automatically driven into position, known as remote afterloading. Operator doses are greatly reduced using these systems; however, the source is always "on", there is a risk of contamination, and the activity decays with time, so the source needs replacing every few months to maintain treatment times at a practical length.

Intraoperative radiotherapy has many benefits, as described in previous chapters, and can be performed using electron linear accelerators (linacs, e.g. *Mobetron*, IntraOp Medical Inc and *Liac*, Sordina SpA) operating at megavoltage energies. More recent designs of these units are self-shielding with beam stoppers, but there may still be limitations to the number of procedures that can be performed (Daves and Mills 2001; Soriani et al. 2010).

The INTRABEAM system operates at a peak voltage of 50 kV, so has a much lower energy than

Table 5.1 Representative energies of different brachytherapy sources

Radiation source	Energy
Radium-226	830 keV
Caesium-137	662 keV
Iridium-192	380 keV
Electron linacs	4–12 MeV
INTRABEAM	50 kV

Values are the average energy of the radionuclides (Khan 2003), or the nominal energy of the X-ray sources. X-ray systems are often described in terms of their peak accelerating voltage (e.g. 50 kV), although only a few electrons will possess the corresponding maximum energy (50 keV) and the effective energy of the beam spectrum will be lower (e.g. 20-30 keV for the INTRABEAM)

[1] From the Greek word 'brachy' meaning short or close.

D.J. Eaton (✉)
Department of Radiotherapy, Royal Free London NHS Foundation Trust, Pond Street, Hampstead, London NW3 2QG, UK
e-mail: davideaton@nhs.net

F. Schneider
Department of Radiation Oncology, University Medical Center Mannheim, University of Heidelberg, D-68167 Mannheim, Germany
e-mail: frank.schneider@umm.de, http://www.umm.de

M. Keshtgar et al. (eds.), *Targeted Intraoperative Radiotherapy in Oncology*,
DOI 10.1007/978-3-642-39821-6_5,

afterloading brachytherapy or electron linac approaches. This greatly simplifies the shielding requirements, yet maintains the benefits of short range delivery with rapid attenuation of dose, an electronic source that can be readily switched on and off, and the efficiency of treatment during surgery. These combined features have led to the title of "electronic brachytherapy" (Park et al. 2010). Caution is still advised, since the unshielded dose rate from the source can reach 1 Gy/min, much higher than a diagnostic X-ray source with which theatre staff may be familiar. However, shielding requirements are practical and straightforward, as will be described in this chapter.

5.2 Legislation

Hazards associated with higher doses of radiation have led to strict legal requirements, which will be specific to each country. Most of Europe derives its laws from the European Union directives, given in Table 5.2. There will also usually be a national license or authorisation to use radiation, which must be obtained before beginning to use any material or equipment.

In the UK, safety of staff and members of the public is covered by the Ionising Radiation Regulations (1999) of the Health and Safety at Work Act (1974). These define the role of a Radiation Protection Adviser, who is the qualified radiation expert for the organisation, and a Radiation Protection Supervisor, who supervises compliance with the specific procedures relating to the safety of the radiation technique (the Local Rules). Safety of the patient is covered by the Ionising Radiation (Medical Exposure) Regulations (2000), which require any radiation exposure to be justified by a defined practitioner (usually a radiation oncologist) and delivered by defined operators. Both the staff operating the INTRABEAM system and the surgeon who positions the applicator are considered to be operators and should be named in the local procedures.

In the USA, the system is still considered to be an emerging technology and although it has received Food and Drugs Administration clearance, it is not currently covered by Nuclear Regulatory Commission regulations. The specific requirements of each state will also vary. Guidelines have been produced by the American Association of Physicists in Medicine (AAPM, Thomadsen et al. 2009), which are summarised in Table 5.3.

Table 5.2 Summary of legal requirements in Europe

Directive 96/29/Euratom
Consultation with Qualified (radiation) Expert:
Controlled area definition and working instructions
Prior critical examination and acceptance
Regular checking and calibration
Dose monitoring and training
Directive 97/43/Euratom
Justification, optimisation and limitation of exposures
Medical Physics Expert closely involved in radiotherapeutic practices

Table 5.3 Summary of legal requirements in the USA

AAPM guidelines
The services of an Authorised Medical Physicist shall be required in facilities using electronic brachytherapy units:
Dosimetry and treatment calculations
Calibration validation and quality assurance
Shielding and area designation
Dose monitoring and training
Physically present during treatments

All of these documents describe the close involvement of experts in radiation physics, who should be consulted with regard to both commissioning a new service and ongoing clinical support.

5.3 Basics of Radiation Protection

The philosophical basis underlying radiation safety is to keep doses to staff (and others not undergoing treatment) as low as reasonably practicable (ALARP).[2]

[2] Or alternatively as low as reasonably achievable (ALARA).

Table 5.4 Sources of annual (background) radiation doses to the UK population

Annual UK effective dose – 2,700 μSv
Cosmic rays (11 %)
Radon gas (48 %)
Ground or buildings (13 %)
Internal (food, e.g. bananas, brazil nuts) (9 %)
Medical procedures (19 %)

Data from Health Protection Agency

Table 5.5 Typical radiation doses

	Dose (μSv)
Chest X-ray	20
Return flight from UK to Australia	200
CT scan	2,000–10,000
Annual occupational limit for radiation workers	20,000
Acute radiation sickness	>1,000,000

Data from Health Protection Agency

Four general principles can be used to achieve this:

- Time
- Distance
- Shielding
- Contamination

Radiation exposure is directly proportional to time, but follows an inverse square dependence on distance. For example, if the distance is doubled, the exposure is reduced by a factor of 4. Therefore distance can have a large impact on doses received. As mentioned earlier, less shielding is required for lower energy X-rays.

Because the INTRABEAM system is an electronic X-ray source, there is no issue of contamination, since the radiation exposure only occurs when the beam is on. If any intervention for the patient is required, the radiation can be switched off (paused) and poses no further hazard during this time.

Radiation dose may be measured using a number of different units. The most fundamental is the Gray (Gy), which is commonly used to describe the amount of radiation given therapeutically, since it corresponds to the energy deposited per unit mass and can be readily measured. However, effective doses to individuals for protection considerations are quoted in Sieverts (Sv), which take account of the relative biological effect of different types of radiation and different sensitivities of different tissues in the body. Typical values are thousandths (mSv) or millionths (μSv) of this unit, and the latter will be used for all subsequent quoted values, since many detectors read in this scale.

Although current models for risk from radiation equate any dose with some risk, it is important to consider small exposures in context. Every individual receives some exposure to ionising radiation from natural background sources, listed in Table 5.4, as well as any medical exposures. Some comparative doses for common activities, legislative limits and adverse effects are given in Table 5.5.

5.4 Prospective Dose Survey

A major component of the prior risk assessment of an operating theatre to be used for IORT is to simulate a treatment and measure the effective doses in various locations. These readings can then be used to estimate the expected doses to operators and other staff or members of the public not involved in the procedure. Specific measures for designation of controlled areas and shielding requirements are based on these assessments, in order to keep doses below legislative limits. Reference data can be used to estimate the effect of shielding by certain materials, such as concrete or plasterboard in the floors and walls, but it is important to perform an actual survey in the theatre to be used, to take account of specific geometry and construction (Eaton et al. 2011). Dosimeters reading directly in μSv, such as that shown in Fig. 5.1, can be used to measure prospective doses, as well as doses during the first few clinical treatments and at regular intervals thereafter, to confirm the sufficiency of the measures implemented. Two examples of this process are described in the following sections.

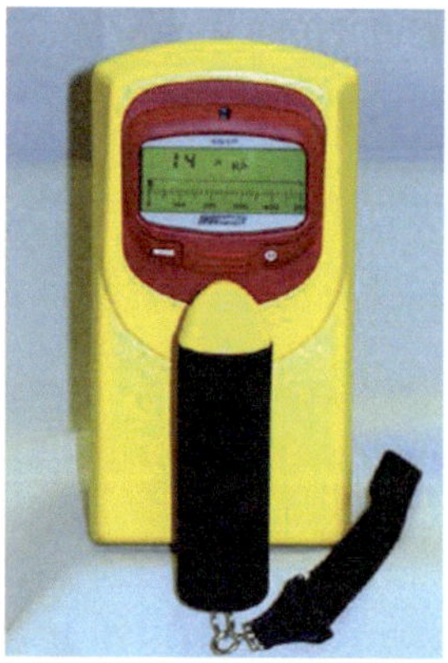

Fig. 5.1 Example of an environmental dosimeter

5.4.1 Example 1: London, UK

A prospective survey was performed as shown in Fig. 5.2. UK guidelines for the designation of controlled and supervised areas are an instantaneous dose rate of greater than 2,000 and 7.5 μSv/h, respectively, or a time-averaged dose rate (TADR, over 8 h) of 7.5 or 2.5 μSv/h, respectively (Institute of Physics and Engineering in Medicine 2002). Following these criteria, the main theatre was designated a controlled area. The two side rooms (anaesthetic and scrub) could have been designated as supervised areas based on the TADR for two patients per day. However, it was only possible to lock the outer doors, so it was decided to designate all three rooms as controlled for simplicity. Access hatches and the areas just outside the side doors into the corridor from the theatre were designated as supervised to limit use and reduce loitering during the procedure.

Further shielding measures are shown in Fig. 5.3. The large screen for staff was constructed from a decommissioned simulator control room window and thick lead sheets in the wooden surround. Due to the low energy of the radiation, only 0.25 mm or more of lead equivalent is required. Above this level, radiation scattered around the screen dominates primary transmission. Lead aprons could also be used, and are readily available, but do not provide

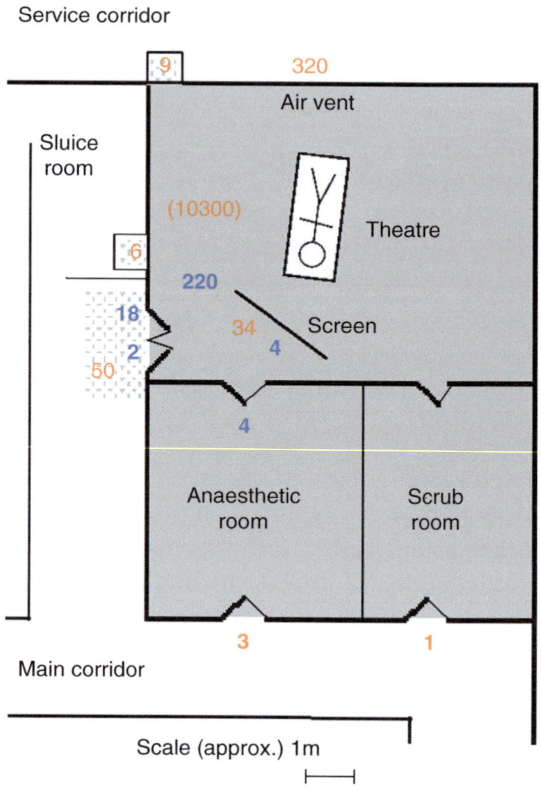

Fig. 5.2 Dose rates (in μSv/h) measured around theatre for the unshielded source and applicator (*orange*), and simulated treatment (*blue*) using bolus around applicator to model attenuation by the patient and tungsten-rubber shielding sheets over the surface, as shown in Fig. 5.3. Controlled areas are shown in *dark grey* and supervised areas in *hatched grey* (Figure modified from Eaton et al. 2011)

whole body protection and may be cumbersome to wear. No permanent modification of the theatre was required, but a second small screen was constructed to cover an air vent at the rear, which connected to a service corridor. Tungsten-rubber shielding sheets are provided by the manufacturer to reduce external dose rates by placing them over the treatment area. They each provide 0.1 mm lead equivalent attenuation (50 kV), or approximately 95 % reduction.

With these measures in place, the measured doses from the first 20 patient treatments were acceptable (Fig. 5.4). Further details of all these measurements and the justification for

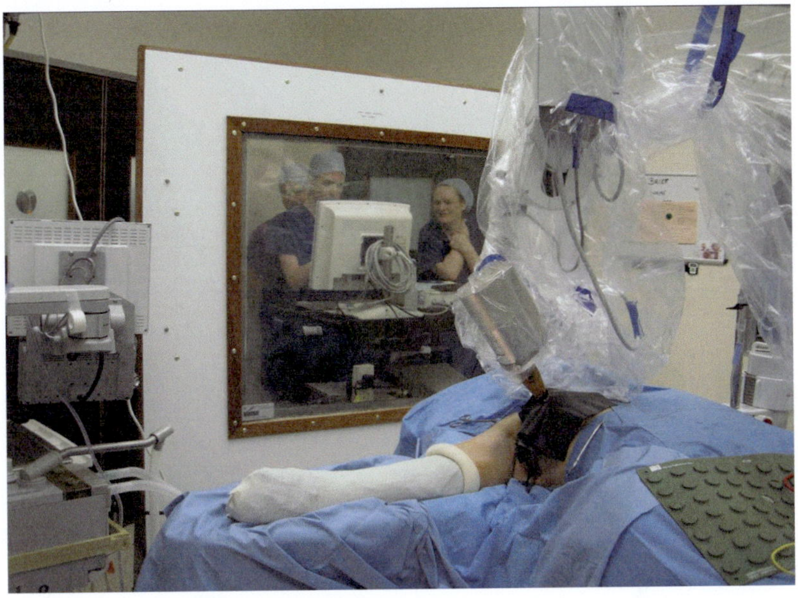

Fig. 5.3 Typical theatre setup, with staff behind a thick lead screen with window, and tungsten-rubber shielding sheets (*black*) placed over the treatment area to reduce external dose rates (Figure reproduced from Eaton et al. 2011)

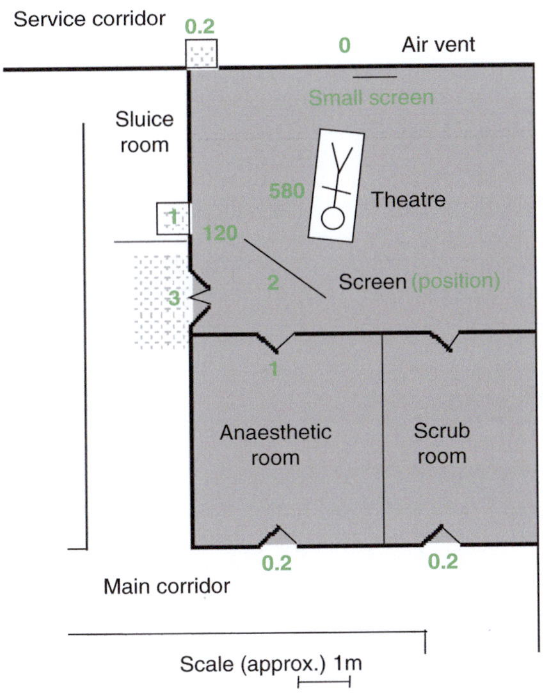

Fig. 5.4 Dose rates (in μSv/h) measured around theatre for the first 20 clinical patients, showing the effect of the small screen and optimised positioning of the large screen (Figure modified from Eaton et al. 2011)

measures implemented can be found in Eaton et al. (2011).

5.4.2 Example 2: Mannheim, Germany

Measurements were performed in a simulated treatment setup, as shown in Fig. 5.5. Readings were symmetrical either side of the patient, except at 30 cm, where the value on the nearside (point 8) was 80 mSv/h. With the addition of the shielding sheets, all values were reduced by a factor of 10.

Therefore, in theatre an individual such as the anaesthetist standing 2 m away could receive:

$$1{,}000\ \mu\text{Sv}/\text{h} \times 0.1(\text{shielding}) = 0.1\ \text{mSv}/\text{h}$$

If one 30-min procedure were performed per day for all 260 working days of the year, the total dose would be:

$$0.1\ \text{mSv}/\text{h} \times 0.5\ \text{h} \times 260 = 13\ \text{mSv}/\text{year}$$

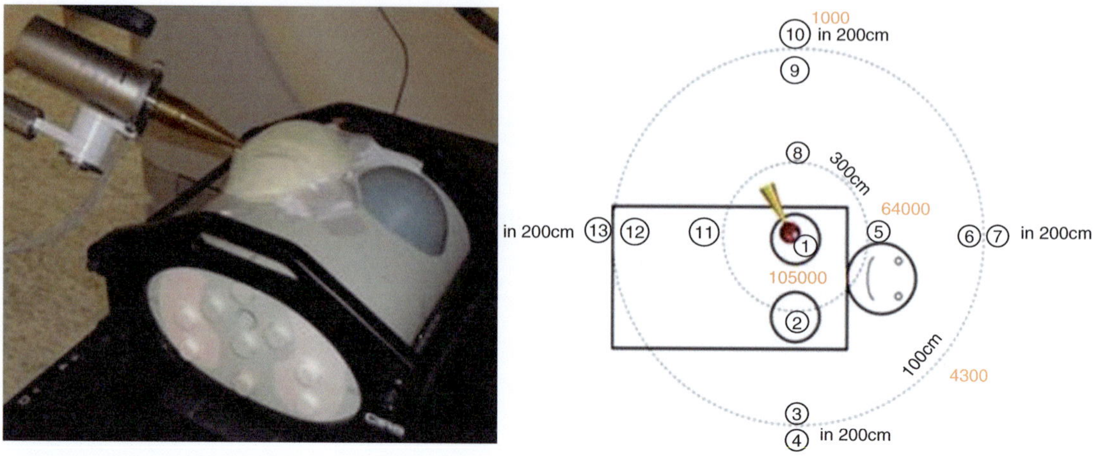

Fig. 5.5 Measurement setup (*left*) and readings (in μSv/h) at various distances from the unshielded source (*right*) (Figure modified from Schneider 2011)

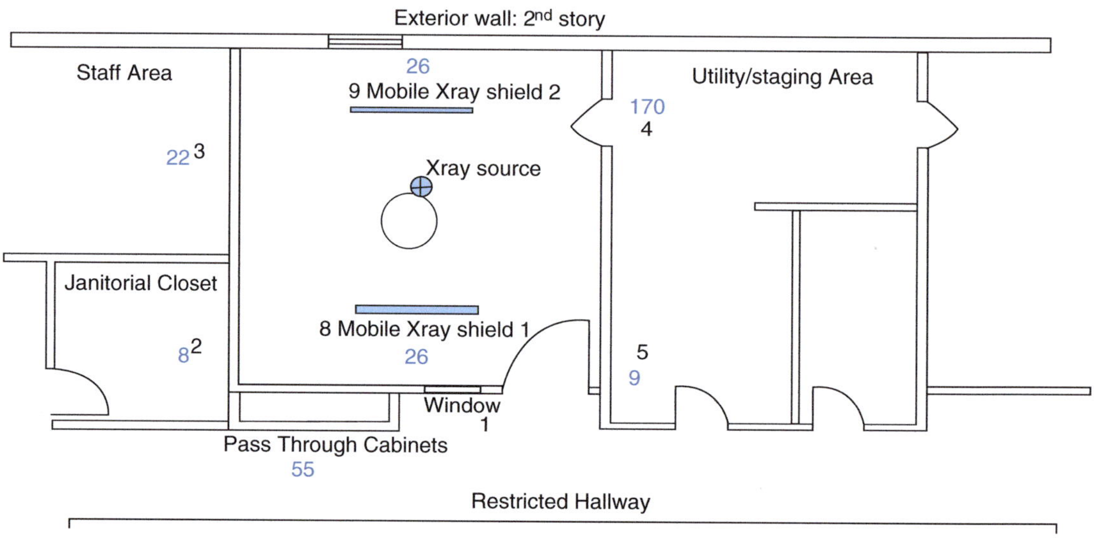

Fig. 5.6 Dose rates (in μSv/h) measured around theatre for simulated treatment (*blue*)

Table 5.6 Calculations of the worst case exposure for points around theatre shown in Fig. 5.6

Point	Dose rate (μSv/h)	Procedures (h)	Occupancy	Total (mSv/year)
1	55	130	0.25	1.8
4	170	130	0.125	2.7
8/9	26	130	1	3.4

Since the national limit for a controlled area is 6 mSv/year, the whole theatre was designated as controlled.

Measurements taken around the theatre are shown in Fig. 5.6. None of these points gave an expected annual dose greater than 6 mSv/year (Table 5.6), so it was not necessary to control any areas outside of the theatre itself.

Further details of all these measurements and the justification for measures implemented can be found in Schneider (2011).

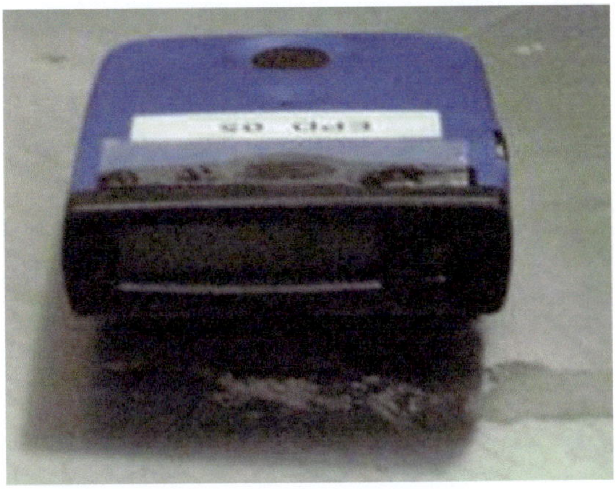

Fig. 5.7 Example of a personal dosimeter

5.5 Other Practical Measures

With appropriate shielding, the risk to staff is very low, with doses to staff involved in the procedure at potentially negligible levels compared to natural background.[3] Direct reading personal dosimeters (Fig. 5.7) can be used to monitor staff remaining to operate the equipment or the anaesthetist. These have the advantage of instantaneous feedback of any higher doses.

Application of the principles of time and distance leads to the following practical measures:

- All non-essential staff to leave the treatment area during irradiation
- Doors to be locked to restrict access
- No pregnant staff to be involved in the irradiation, unless a specific individual risk assessment has been carried out.

[3] For the first example, the dose rate behind the screen is 2 μSv/h, so ten procedures is equivalent to three days of natural background exposure.

5.6 Key Points

- INTRABEAM can be used safely in standard operating theatres.
- Medical physicists should be closely involved.
- Radiation protection is straightforward but important.

References

Daves JL, Mills MD (2001) Shielding assessment of a mobile electron accelerator for intraoperative radiotherapy. J Appl Clin Med Phys 2:165–173

Eaton DJ, Gonzalez R, Duck S, Keshtgar M (2011) Radiation protection for an intraoperative X-ray device. Br J Radiol 84:1034–1039

Institute of Physics and Engineering in Medicine (2002) Medical and dental guidance notes. IPEM, York

Khan FM (2003) The physics of radiation therapy. Lippincott, Williams and Wilkins, Philadelphia

Park CC, Yom SS, Podgorsak MB, Harris E, Price RA, Bevan A et al (2010) American Society for Therapeutic Radiology and Oncology (ASTRO) emerging technology committee report on electronic brachytherapy. Int J Radiat Oncol Biol Phys 76:963–972

Schneider F (2011) Radiation protection. In: Wenz F, Kraus-Tiefenbacher U (eds) Intraoperative radiotherapy for breast cancer. UNI-MED, Bremen

Soriani A, Felici G, Fantini M, Paolucci M, Borla O, Evangelisti G et al (2010) Radiation protection measurements around a 12 MeV mobile dedicated IORT accelerator. Med Phys 37:995–1003

Thomadsen BR, Biggs PJ, DeWerd LA, Coffey CW, Chiu-Tsao S-T, Gossman MS et al (2009) The 2007 AAPM response to the CRCPD request for recommendations for the CRCPD's model regulations for electronic brachytherapy. Report 152. AAPM, College Park

Radiobiology

6

Frederik Wenz, Katia Pasciuti, and Carsten Herskind

The principal aim of radiotherapy is to sterilise all tumour stem cells, resulting in permanent local control. When radiotherapy treatment is delivered after surgery, the aim is to eliminate any residual (microscopic) tumour cells in the tumour bed in order to prevent local recurrence. In the last few years, there has been interest in delivering a high dose of radiation in only one fraction at the time of surgery (IORT – intraoperative radiotherapy), to try to improve local tumour control and reduce damage to surrounding tissue, and to allow greater accuracy in the delivery of treatment.

The IORT technique has the advantages of:

- making the treatment more radical because it enables the elimination of possible residual tumour cells;
- increasing the antitumour effects of ionising radiation because it enables the delivery of a higher local tumour dose not feasible with external beam radiotherapy due to normal tissue tolerance;
- reducing the time interval between surgery and external beam radiotherapy treatment, thereby avoiding regrowth of neoplastic cells in the interval.

The development of more and more sophisticated linear accelerators and the use of robotic arms have promoted the widespread use of this technique.

6.1 Ionising Radiation Damage

Photon radiation can best be described as small packets of energy which are absorbed by biological tissue via the photo-effect, the Compton effect or pair production. The fast electrons realeased by these interactions produce a track of ionisations (loss of an electron from an atom) in the tissue. These ionisation events can occur either in the target molecules (i.e. DNA, direct radiation effect) or in the cellular water leading to DNA damage via the formation of hydroxyl radicals (indirect radiation effect). The number of ionisation events produced at therapeutic dose levels is very high (10^5 ionisations per cell per Gy) but the vast majority of these produce no severe damage. The main, biologically relevant damage to the DNA can be classified as base damage, single strand breaks (ssb) or double strand breaks (dsb). Cells have very sophisticated and efficient mechanisms to allow for the recognition and repair of DNA damage. Thus most lesions

F. Wenz (✉) • C. Herskind
Department of Radiation Oncology, University Medical Center Mannheim, University of Heidelberg, Theodor-Kutzer-Ufer 1-3, D-68167 Mannheim, Germany
e-mail: frederik.wenz@umm.de, http://www.umm.de; carsten.herskind@umm.de, http://www.umm.de

K. Pasciuti
Department of Radiotherapy, Royal Free London Foundation Trust, Pond Street, Hampstead, London NW3 2QG, UK
e-mail: katia.pasciuti@nhs.net

M. Keshtgar et al. (eds.), *Targeted Intraoperative Radiotherapy in Oncology*, DOI 10.1007/978-3-642-39821-6_6, © Springer-Verlag Berlin Heidelberg 2014 are repaired, and the major lethal lesion is considered to be a small fraction of unrepaired or incorrectly repaired dsb.

According to their biological effect, the different types of damage can be described as:

- No damage: if it is repaired so that the cell preserves its reproductive ability.
- Non-lethal damage: the cell preserves reproductive ability after a period of recovery but the rate of proliferation may be affected, and the cell may become more sensitive to subsequent irradiation.
- Lethal damage: the cell loses its reproductive ability. This type of damage is irreversible, irreparable and leads to cell death.
- Sub-lethal damage: appears in general at low doses and can be repaired in hours unless additional sub-lethal damage is added, eventually leading to lethal damage.

6.2 The Linear Quadratic Model

The linear quadratic model is one of the most useful ways to describe cell survival fraction as function of dose (SF, Fig. 6.1). It uses a negative exponential function depending on two components: the first is proportional to the radiation dose, D, and the second is proportional to D^2:

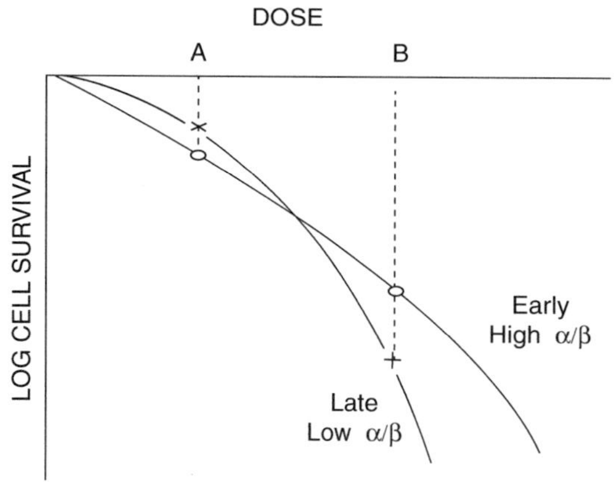

Fig. 6.1 Cell survival curves representing early-reacting/high α/β (e.g. tumour, mucosa) and late-reacting/low α/β (e.g. brain, lung, breast) tissues have a different shape. At low doses (*A*) there is relatively more tumour cell kill, i.e. lower tumour cell survival as compared to normal cell kill. At higher doses (*B*), the relation is reversed and comparatively more late radiation damage is induced

$$SF = e^{-(\alpha D + \beta D^2)} \quad (6.1)$$

where α and β are two variable parameters (Joiner and van der Kogel 2009).

The α/β ratio is a measure of the relative contributions of these two components to the overall cell killing.

The characteristic SF shape includes a low-dose shoulder region followed by a steeply sloped or more continuously bending portion at higher doses. A frequently used interpretation of the shoulder region is the accumulation of sub-lethal damage at low doses and lethality resulting from the interaction of two or more such sub-lethal lesions.

6.3 Early and Late Effects

Cell toxicity, in terms of side-effects, differs depending on the radiotherapy treatment (radical, palliative or adjuvant) and on the dose and fractionation used. Usually side-effects are classified as early and late, with the latter sometimes being chronic.

Early effects occur during the first days following the start of a radiotherapy treatment and inflammation is their dominant characteristic due to the radiation-induced damage to the healthy tissues. Late effects appear months or even years after the end of radiotherapy, resulting in hardening and loss of tissue elasticity such as fibrosis, atrophy, ulceration, stenosis and necrosis.

Since normal tissue reactions after irradiation depend on radiation effects in a relevant cell population, radiation effects in these tissues are frequently described by the linear quadratic model. Survival curves for early-reacting normal tissues and tumours are less curved than those for late-reacting normal tissues (Fig. 6.1). Early-reacting normal tissues and tumours often have a lower sensitivity to dose per fraction and a higher α/β ratio than late-responding normal tissues. The biological effects observed increase faster with increasing dose per fraction in late-responding tissues than in early-reacting tissues and tumour, whereas small doses per fraction are associated with a lower risk of complications and a better therapeutic ratio. This difference in fractionation sensitivity between early- and late-reacting tissues is interpreted as reflecting differences in DNA damage repair capacity and constitutes the basis for the differential effect of fractionation or low dose rate.

6.4 Biologically Effective Dose

The linear quadratic model provides a simple way to describe the dose response of different fractionation schemes in terms of biologically effective dose (BED). The BED is regarded as a measure of the true biological dose delivered using a particular combination of dose per fraction *d* (Gy) and total dose *D* (Gy) to a given tissue characterised by a specific α/β ratio. It can be written as:

$$BED = D\left(1 + \frac{d}{\alpha/\beta}\right) \tag{6.2}$$

BED represents the dose that is calculated to be required to reach a certain level of effect when a total dose *D* is given in very small fractions with full recovery between fractions. The BED value increases with increasing dose per fraction and its increment is greater for tissues with a low α/β ratio than for tissues characterised by a high α/β value. The classic BED equation cannot be applied to describe different fractionation schemes obtained using different radiation qualities because the value of α is not the same (Dale and Jones 1999; Herskind et al. 2005).

6.5 Linear Energy Transfer Effect and Relative Biologic Effectiveness

The radiation quality is characterized by the ionisation density in the track given as the Linear Energy Transfer (LET). The differences in tumour cell survival values reported in Fig. 6.2 for the same absorbed dose delivered by different types of radiation suggests different biological effectiveness for each type of radiation.

The reason behind the different effectiveness of differing types of radiation is to be found at the microscopic level, where the energy is deposited in different patterns for each type.

Figure 6.3 shows the major differences between low LET and high LET radiation. The interactions that occur in a biological system with low LET radiation are relatively far apart from each other; therefore they will be spread throughout the cell, delivering a more uniform distribution of ionisations. In contrast, high LET radiation

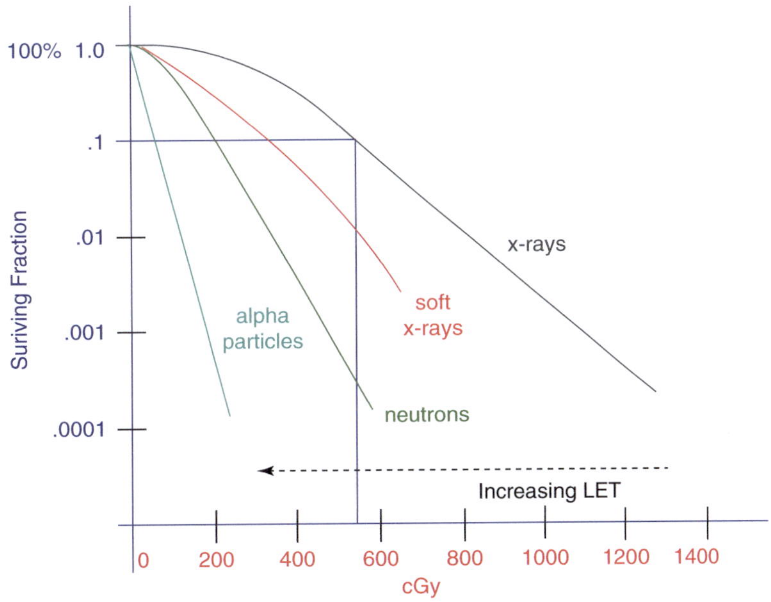

Fig. 6.2 Beams of different radiation quality may have different biological effects at the same physical dose. The same dose kills more cells when delivered as higher LET radiation

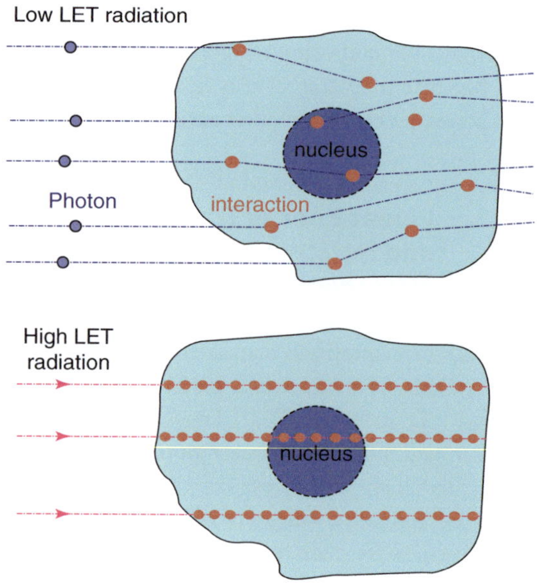

Fig. 6.3 Low and high LET radiation effect on a biological system. The dose required to kill a cell using high LET radiation is smaller than that needed when using low LET radiation

shows well-defined dense tracks of ionisation that cause more extensive damage along the track.

These differences in energy distribution form the basis of the concept of relative biologic effectiveness (RBE). The RBE is defined as the ratio of the absorbed dose of a reference radiation to the absorbed dose of a test radiation to produce the same level of biological effect, other conditions being equal (ICRP 2003; ICRU 1998).

$$RBE = \frac{Dose\ of\ Standard\ Radiation}{Dose\ of\ Test\ Radiation}\ for\ a\ given\ effect$$

RBE is strongly affected by different factors:

- RBE increases with decreasing dose per fraction.
- RBE values depend on tissue type.
- RBE depends on particle LET: increasing clustering of radiation is known to produce higher lethality.

When a new type of radiation modality is introduced in therapy, it is necessary to determine its RBE relative to the radiation beams already in use and for which the radiation-oncologist has accumulated clinical experience. The aim of the RBE calculations is to help the radiation oncologist to prescribe the right dose with the new type of radiation. Two different formalisms have been developed to calculate the RBE from the LQ model under certain assumptions (Brenner et al. 1999; Dale and Jones 1999). The former formalism including the effect of protracted irradiation has been applied to tumour-bed IORT with Intrabeam (Herskind et al. 2005) as outlined in the appendix (see Sect. 6.10). These calculations are performed using different biological systems and different experimental conditions (Herskind et al. 2005; 2008; Herskind and Wenz 2010).

6.6 Biological Effectiveness of the INTRABEAM System

IORT using low-energy X-rays differs in some specific aspects from IORT using electrons from linear accelerators or dedicated IORT machines. The 50-kV X-rays of the INTRABEAM system have an increased RBE and a steeper dose fall-off. Furthermore, the dose is delivered with a low dose rate over a prolonged time.

Soft X-rays (kV) have an increased RBE compared to standard linear accelerator X-rays (MV). Irradiation types which produce more locally concentrated ionisations, although at the same total amount of ionisations, are more effectively killing tumour cells and thus have an increased RBE. This is especially true for high LET irradiations like neutrons or heavy ions. Although soft X-rays have a somewhat higher LET than high-energy X-rays from linear accelerators, they are not considered to be high LET irradiation. The increased RBE of soft X-rays is most likely a consequence of the fact that the total energy of the beam is deposited within a relatively short distance of the track ends, which means that the ionisation events are locally more concentrated within this area. The absolute value of the RBE of 50 kV X-rays depends on the dose, endpoint, tissue and many other factors. For clinical practice with spherical tumour-bed applicators one may assume a range of 1.2–1.5 based on experimental data for different cell types although the RBE may vary with the distance from the source (Liu et al. 2013).

6.7 High Single Doses with the INTRABEAM System

Stereotactic radiosurgery (SRS) for brain tumours using the gamma knife was introduced almost 50 years ago. High single doses are currently used more frequently in clinical radiation oncology, for example in intraoperative radiotherapy (IORT) or stereotactic body radiotherapy (SBRT). The radiobiology of high single dose treatment differs in many aspects from the standard fractionated application of radiotherapy over several weeks. In addition, the INTRABEAM system uses low-energy X-rays in the range of 30–50 kV instead of, for example, 6 MV (6,000 kV) in standard linear accelerators.

When the INTRABEAM system was initially introduced into clinical practice and especially into the treatment of breast cancer 10–15 years ago, there were several challenges for modelling the radiobiological effects to guide clinical practice:

- effects of high single vs. fractionated doses;
- no proliferation of tumour cells between surgery and initiation of radiotherapy;
- no proliferation of tumour cells during radiotherapy;
- effect on the tumour bed/microenvironment of IORT using high single doses;
- new radiation quality (low-energy X-rays);
- repair of normal tissue cells during protracted delivery of radiotherapy over 30–45 min.

Some of the challenges are generic to high single dose treatment and to IORT per se, whereas the aspects of beam quality and protracted delivery are specific to the INTRABEAM system.

Radiation oncologists are typically reluctant to use high single dose treatment because classic radiobiological modelling predicts a higher rate of late damage after high single dose treatment as compared to fractionated treatment using low daily doses, especially in so-called late-reacting tissues like brain, lung, liver and breast. This concept is based on the different sensitivity of tissues to changes in the dose per fraction as described above (see Fig. 6.1). Acute-reacting tissues like tumours and mucosal cells typically show less sparing at low doses (e.g. dose A) than the late-reacting tissue. This means that the therapeutic index is favourable because at the same radiation dose, more tumour cells are killed compared with late-reacting tissue cells. At higher doses, the therapeutic index is reversed, because the cell survival curve of late-reacting tissues bends more strongly. Therefore, at higher doses (e.g. dose B), late-reacting normal tissue cells are damaged more compared to tumour cells. This is theoretically a less favourable situation, which would clinically be unacceptable. However, we know from clinical experience, especially from brain radiosurgery, that there is a strong relation of late damage to the irradiated volume and one may safely irradiate a small volume to single doses higher than 20 Gy which are capable of sterilising macroscopic tumours. More recently, it has been demonstrated that using SBRT and three to five high single doses of 12–20 Gy, even non-small cell lung cancer can be controlled in up to 90 % of cases, which cannot be achieved using fractionated radiotherapy even up to 90 Gy. Finally, all this modelling is based on the linear-quadratic model, which is only validated for doses up to 6–8 Gy. The model has limitations in predicting the effects of single doses in the range of 15 Gy and higher, which are typically used for IORT.

6.8 Temporal Effects with the INTRABEAM System

The negative effects of delaying the beginning of radiotherapy are well known, in that such delay allows proliferation of remaining tumour cells; this situation has been termed a "temporal miss" (Wenz et al. 2012). Quantification of this effect has been attempted for breast cancer in a systematic review (Huang et al. 2003), and it was estimated to be responsible for a loss in local control of about one-third (local recurrence rate of about 6 % vs. 9 %) when the delay exceeded 8 weeks. This loss of local control is considerable and comparable to the effect of an additional tumour bed boost of 16 Gy. An additional loss of local control, although not in the same magnitude, can be observed when fractionated radiotherapy is delivered over 5–6 weeks instead of one single dose. One may estimate that a single dose of

20 Gy given at surgery is equally effective to a fractionated course of 60–70 Gy given over 6 weeks with a delay of 6 weeks after surgery.

The tumour bed effect, i.e. late radiation damage to the stromal tissue in which a tumour is growing, has been known for a long time. The delayed regrowth of tumours in previously irradiated tissues is presumably based mainly on the chronic vascular effects of radiation, in that it leaves behind atrophic tissue which represents a hostile soil. This effect, based on the "seed and soil hypothesis", which has also been popularised by novel anticancer drugs like bevacizumab, is not only pronounced after high single doses but seems to have a threshold dose in the range of 8–10 Gy (Kirkpatrick et al. 2008). Novel effects such as endothelial cell apoptosis in small vessels after high single dose irradiation have recently been reported and may be an explanation for the observed effects. Also recently, there has been a report on a novel biological phenomenon resulting in a changed cytokine microenvironment in the tumour bed wound. Surgical excision of the tumour and the subsequent wound healing process lead to local production of cytokines, stimulating cell proliferation, migration and vessel formation. This cytokine cocktail is modified into a less stimulating composition by application of IORT during surgery (Belletti et al. 2008).

6.9 Normal Tissue Effects

The INTRABEAM system emits a spherical dose distribution around the tip of the drift tube. This dose fall-off is modified by the spherical applicators which are used for IORT of breast cancer. The steep dose fall-off (Fig. 6.4) and the thickness of the chest wall of about 2 cm shield the lung and the heart, which receive maximal total doses of less than 2 Gy. Therefore, no additional shielding in the form of tungsten shields, which are available from the manufacturer, is necessary for breast cancer treatment though it may be used to shield large peripheral nerves for IORT of, for instance, pelvic tumours. Radiobiological modelling predicts in addition that a distance of 5–10 mm to the skin should be respected to keep the dose below the threshold for severe fibrosis of about 13–14 Gy (of conventional high-energy photons).

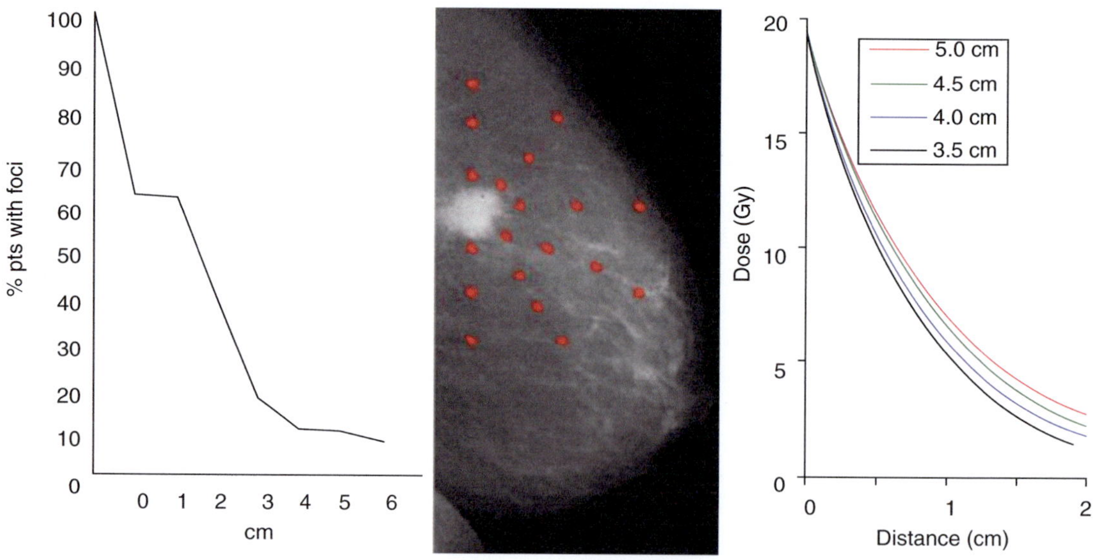

Fig. 6.4 The spherical dose distribution has a steep fall-off. When 20 Gy is prescribed to the applicator surface, there is a dose of about 5–7 Gy at 1 cm distance depending on the diameter of the applicator (*right panel*). The probability of tumour cell foci (*left panel*) and the tumour cell density (*middle panel*) are mimicked by the dose fall-off characteristics (Modified after Wenz et al. 2012)

When using the breast applicators, the INTRABEAM system delivers the radiation dose over a prolonged period in the range of 20–45 min. This is a relevant time span for normal tissue repair, which typically has a half-life time of 15–20 min. Therefore, during the protracted irradiation, there is a considerable amount of repair in the normal tissue, whereas in general tumours are less proficient in repairing DNA damage. This effect leads to an improved therapeutic index.

In conclusion, before the INTRABEAM system was used in clinical practice, starting in around the year 2000, it was necessary to perform radiobiological modelling in order to guide clinical practice. This was a difficult challenge because of the unique type of irradiation, the low dose rate, the increased RBE and the non-standard spherical dose distribution. Now, 10 years and many thousands of patients later, one can conclude that the modelling provided a reliable basis for a series of clinical trials which demonstrated the safety and effectiveness of this type of treatment.

6.10 Appendix – Detailed Mechanism

It is important to consider that, generally, the enhancement in the biological effect at greater distances from the IORT low-energy photon source, due to the increase in RBE with decreasing dose, will be reduced by cellular recovery occurring during a typical 20–50 min treatment irradiation time.

According to Brenner (Brenner et al. 1999) the equivalence in the observed effect relative to two types of radiation of high (*H*) and low (*L*) biological effectiveness delivered over the same time implies:

$$\zeta_H D_H + G D_H^2 = \zeta_L D_L + G D_L^2 \qquad (6.3)$$

where ζ_H and ζ_L are the α/β ratios for the test and reference radiation respectively and G is the generalised Lea–Catcheside time factor which accounts for dose protraction (Brenner et al. 1998):

Thus the RBE, D_L/D_H is given by:

$$RBE = \frac{\varsigma_L}{2GD_H}\left[\sqrt{1+\frac{4G}{\varsigma_L}\left(\frac{\alpha_H}{\alpha_L}D_H+\frac{G}{\varsigma_L}D_H^2\right)}-1\right] \qquad (6.4)$$

where the same duration was assumed for test (*H*) and reference (*L*) radiation.

A modification to the Brenner formula when considering a protracted (*H*) irradiation versus an acute (*L*) irradiation leads Eq. (6.3) to become:

$$\zeta_H D_H + G D_H^2 = \zeta_L D_L + D_L^2 \qquad (6.5)$$

as in Herskind et al. (2005).

Solving Eq. (6.5) for D_L and dividing by D_H, the RBE becomes:

$$RBE = \frac{\varsigma_L}{2D_H}\left[\sqrt{1+\frac{4}{\varsigma_L}\left(\frac{\alpha_H}{\alpha_L}D_H+\frac{G}{\varsigma_L}D_H^2\right)}-1\right] \qquad (6.6)$$

In the same paper, Herskind (Herskind et al. 2005) estimated the RBE variation with dose for four different applicator sizes (2, 3.5, 4.5 and 5 cm), assuming a 15-min recovery time. The results showed that for the largest applicator the RBE varied between 0.92 at the applicator surface and 1.45 at a distance of 20 mm and that the recovery effect was greater for large applicators due to longer irradiation times.

Studies suggest, moreover, that the steep decrease in the delivered dose with the increasing tissue depth using an INTRABEAM source ("photon radiosurgery system") implies that the system capability in killing tumour cells is strongly correlated with distance from the applicator surface, i.e. with depth in the tumour bed.

References

Belletti B, Vaidya JS, D'Andrea S, Entschladen F, Roncadin M, Lovat F et al (2008) Targeted intraoperative radiotherapy impairs the stimulation of breast cancer cell proliferation and invasion caused by surgical wounding. Clin Cancer Res 14:1325–1332

Brenner DJ, Hlatky LR, Hahnfeldt PJ, Huang Y, Sachs RK (1998) The linear-quadratic and most other common radiobiological models result in similar predictions of time-dose relationships. Radiat Res 150:83–91

Brenner DJ, Cheng-Shiun L, Beatty JF, Sheferk RE (1999) Clinical relative biological effectiveness of low-energy X-rays emitted by miniature X-ray devices. Phys Med Biol 44:323–333

Dale RG, Jones B (1999) The assessment of RBE effect using the concept of biologically effective dose. Int J Radiat Oncol Biol Phys 43:639–645

Herskind C, Wenz F (2010) Radiobiological comparison of hypofractionated accelerated partial breast irradiation (APBI) and single-dose intraoperative radiotherapy (IORT) with 50 kV x rays. Strahlenther. Onkol. 186:444–51

Herskind C, Steil V, Kraus-Tiefenbacher U, Wenz F (2005) Radiobiological aspect of intraoperative radiotherapy (IORT) with isotropic low-energy X ray for early-stage breast cancer. Radiat Res 163:208–215

Herskind C, Griebel J, Kraus-Tiefenbacher U, Wenz F (2008) Sphere of equivalence - a novel target volume concept for intraoperative radiotherapy using low-energy x-rays. Int J Radiat Oncol Biol Phys 72: 1575–81

Huang J, Barbera L, Brouwers M, Browman G, Mackillop WJ (2003) Does the delay in starting treatment affect the outcome of radiotherapy? A systematic review. J Clin Oncol 21:555–563

ICRP (2003) Publication 92: Relative Biologcal Effectiveness and Radiation Weighting and Quality Factor. www.icrp.org

ICRU (1998) Report 60: Fundamental Quantities and Units for ionizing Radiation. www.icru.org

Joiner M, van der Kogel A (eds) (2009) Basic Clinical Radiobiology. 4th edn. Hodder Arnold, London

Kirkpatrick JP, Meyer JJ, Marks LB (2008) The linear-quadratic model is inappropriate to model high dose per fraction effects in radiosurgery. Semin Radiat Oncol 18:240–243

Liu Q, Schneider F, Ma L, Wenz, Herskind C (2013) Relative Biologic Effectiveness (RBE) of 50 kV X-rays measured in a phantom for intraoperative tumor-bed irradiation. Int J Radiat Oncol Biol Phys 85:1127–33

Wenz F, Blank E, Welzel G, Hofmann F, Astor D, Neumaier C et al (2012) Intraoperative radiotherapy during breast-conserving surgery using a miniature x-ray generator (Intrabeam) theoretical and experimental background and clinical experience. Womens Health 8:39–47

7 Surgical Aspects of the TARGIT Technique in Breast Cancer

Mohammed Keshtgar

Targeted intraoperative radiotherapy (IORT) is a simple and straightforward technique, but its success depends on attention to detail and the concerted efforts of a multidisciplinary team of surgeons, radiation oncologists, physicists, radiotherapy technicians, and operating theatre and nursing staff.

The rationale, justification and methodology of the technique have been previously described. In brief, the equipment used is the INTRABEAM® system (Carl Zeiss Surgical, Oberkochen, Germany). This is a mobile, miniature X-ray generator which is powered by a 12-V supply and is taken to the operating theatre at the time of surgery. Accelerated electrons strike a gold target at the tip of a 10-cm-long drift tube with a diameter of 3 mm, resulting in the emission of low-energy X-rays (50 kV) in an isotropic dose distribution around the tip. The irradiated tissue is kept at a distance from the source by spherical applicators to ensure a more uniform dose distribution. Applicator spheres of various size are available, to be used in accordance with the size of the surgical cavity (Fig. 7.1). The dose rate depends on the diameter of the applicator and the distance of the tumour bed tissue from the applicator surface. The steep attenuation of the radiation dose protects normal tissues and allows the treatment to be safely carried out in an unmodified operating theatres.

7.1 Obtaining Informed Consent

During the consent process, it is important to mention some important facts about IORT based on the evidence obtained from the randomised controlled trial. In the pre-pathology group, in around 15 % of cases, it may be necessary to recommend external beam radiotherapy (EBRT) to patients who had received IORT due to untoward histological features in the primary tumour or the lymph nodes, as outlined previously. This point needs to be mentioned to patients during preoperative counselling. Patients should also be informed about the possibility of some hardening/induration of breast tissue around the area that receives IORT. This usually settles after 18–24 months. There is also a higher incidence of postoperative development of a seroma in the IORT group as compared with the EBRT group, although it is relatively uncommon in both treatments.

7.2 Scheduling

As IORT is a multidisciplinary procedure, it requires close collaboration between members of the team. The radiotherapy and the physics team need to be informed well in advance to ensure that they are available in theatre without affecting the routine activity of the department.

M. Keshtgar, BSc, FRCSI, FRCS (Gen), PhD
Division of Surgery and Interventional Sciences, Department of Breast Surgery, University College London Medical School, Royal Free London Foundation NHS Trust, Pond Street, Hampstead, London NW3 2QG, UK
e-mail: m.keshtgar@ucl.ac.uk

M. Keshtgar et al. (eds.), *Targeted Intraoperative Radiotherapy in Oncology*,
DOI 10.1007/978-3-642-39821-6_7, © Springer-Verlag Berlin Heidelberg 2014

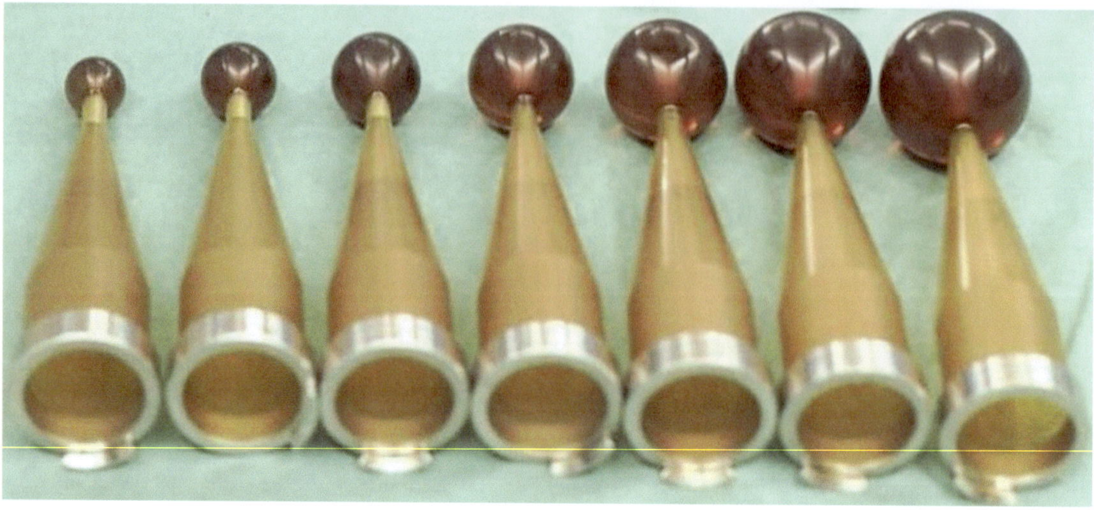

Fig. 7.1 Various sizes of applicators are available which can be used according to the size of the surgical cavity after WLE

It is preferable to schedule the IORT cases earlier on the operating list in order to avoid keeping the whole extended team in the hospital out of hours. Routinely scheduling IORT on certain days of the week (e.g. every Tuesday morning) also helps all staff to plan their time.

7.3 Choice of Operating Theatre

During the commissioning process, it is important to choose an operating room with sufficient space to manoeuvre the INTRABEAM hydraulic arm in order to avoid risk of accidental damage to the electron drift tube. After it has been connected to the INTRABEAM, the protective guard for the electron drift tube should be maintained at all times and the hydraulic arm is kept in the "parking position" while the INTRABEAM is not in use in order to avoid accidental damage (Fig. 7.2).

7.4 Applicator Availability/ Sterilisation

It is good practice to sterilise the applicators individually so that the appropriate size is chosen and used without opening other applicators. This approach will allow scheduling more than one case on the operating list, and other sterile applicators can be available for other scheduled cases. This also avoids repeated sterilisation of unused applicators.

7.5 Step-by-Step Description of the Procedure

7.5.1 Standard Wide Local/ Segmental Excision and Mobilisation

After standard wide local excision (WLE) of the primary tumour, the remaining breast tissue is mobilised by dissecting the breast tissue from the overlying skin and subcutaneous tissue, as shown in Fig. 7.3.

Gentle mobilisation of the breast tissue avoids application of tension to the tissue during pulling of the purse-string suture. It will also ensure that after application of the purse-string suture, the skin is not drawn in close to the applicator, thereby avoiding the risk of radiation-induced skin necrosis. One needs to ensure that the skin is kept at a minimum distance of 5 mm from the applicator surface, otherwise skin necrosis may result.

Use of broad-spectrum intravenous antibiotics is recommended during the perioperative period.

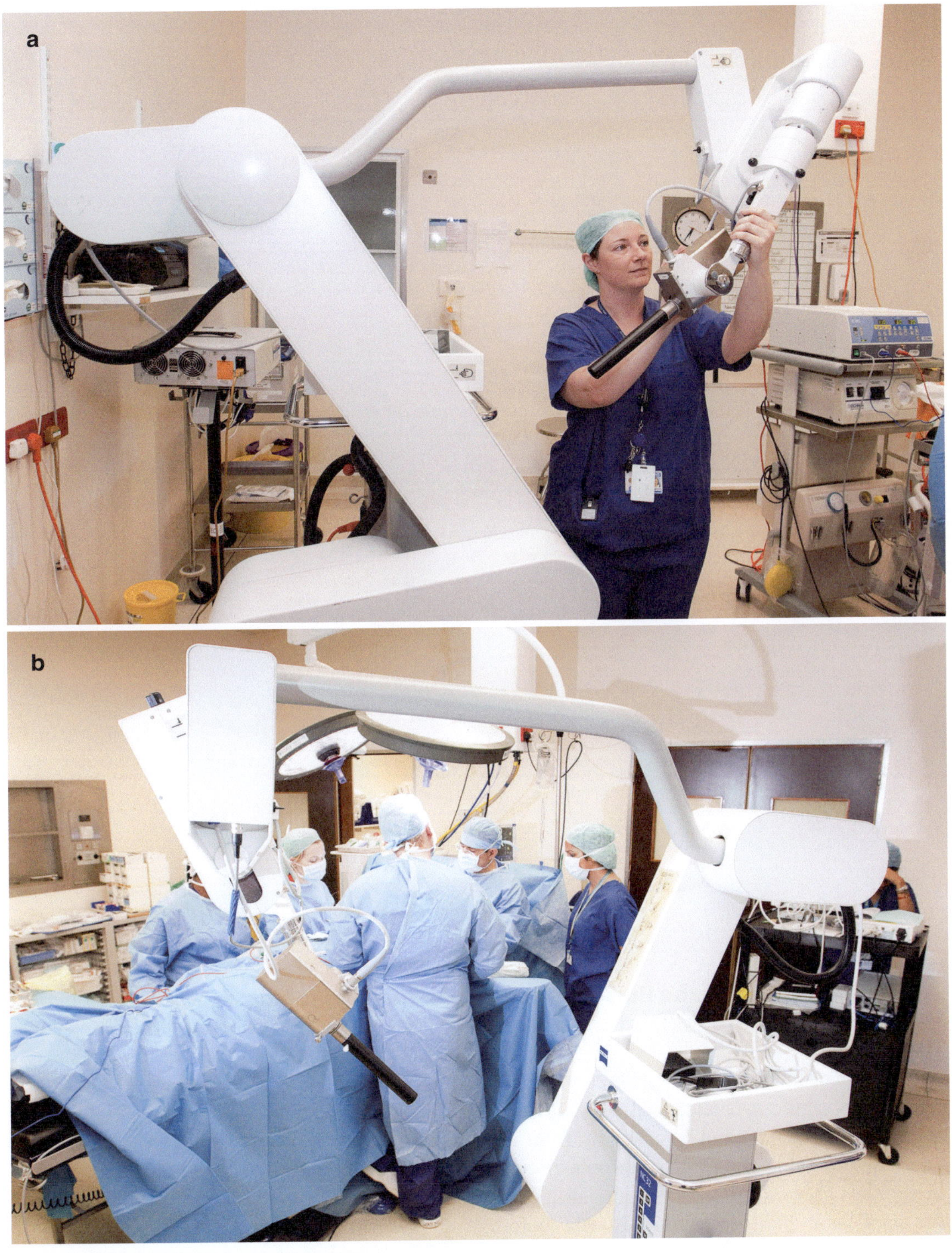

Fig. 7.2 (**a**) A protective guard should be inserted before use to minimize accidental damage to the drift tube. (**b**) The hydraulic arm is maintained in the "parking position" at all times while the INTRABEAM is not in use in order to avoid accidental damage

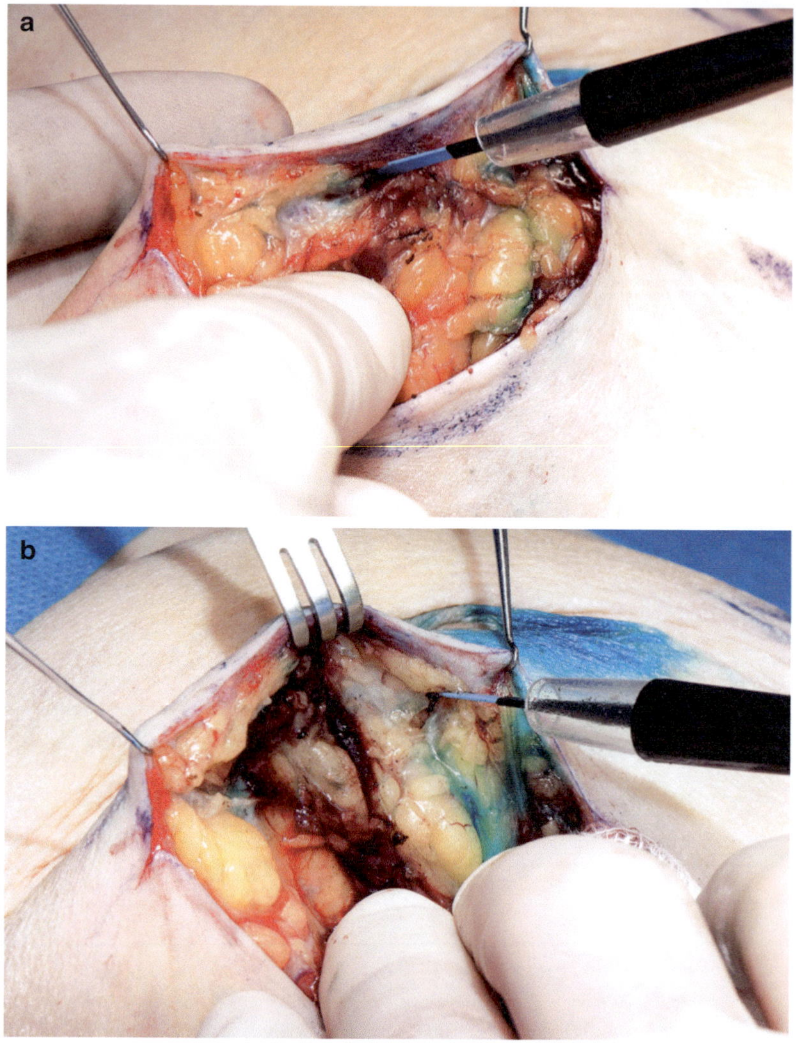

Fig. 7.3 (**a**, **b**) Gentle mobilisation of breast tissue from the overlying skin

7.5.2 Application of the Purse-String Suture

After adequate mobilisation of the breast tissue, a purse-string suture is applied to the breast tissue at the tumour bed, around 5 mm away from the edge, at 10-mm intervals until the whole circumference has been covered. It is important to place the applicator and perform a test run before inserting it onto the INTRABEAM in order to ensure that it fits properly and that the purse-string suture draws all the tissue within the tumour bed and conforms the target tissue adequately to the surface of the applicator. When applying the purse-string suture to a fatty breast, special care must be exercised to take good full thickness bites in order to avoid cutting through ("cheese wiring") the tissue when the purse-string suture is pulled. We recommend using a monofilament material (1/0 prolene) suture with an adequately sized needle. It is preferable to use a blunt needle (Ethiguard blunt point needles) to minimise risk of needle stick injury (Fig. 7.4).

7.5.3 Choice of an Appropriately Sized Applicator

After removal of the primary tumour, the WLE specimen and the resultant cavity are measured in three dimensions to guide the choice of applicator

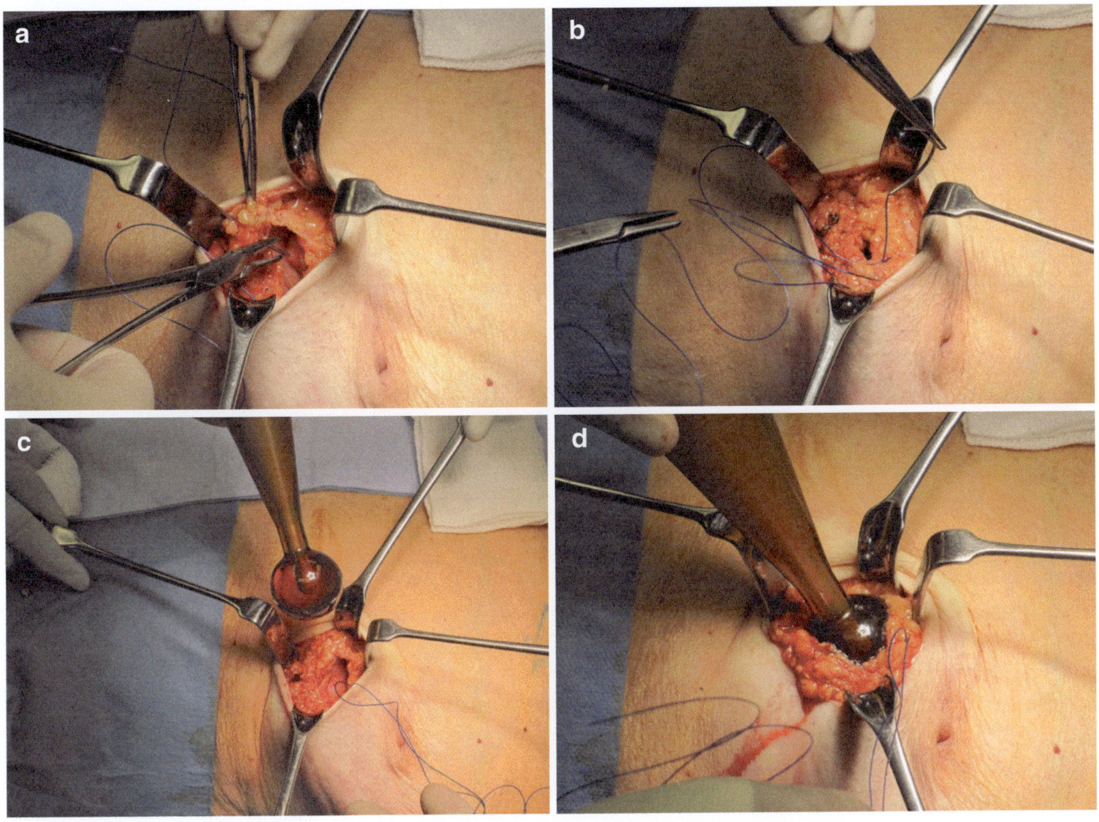

Fig. 7.4 (a–d) Application of the purse string using 1/0 prolene suture. The purse string is tested before the applicator is inserted

size (Fig. 7.5). The applicator should not be too tight, since for radiotherapy to be effective, adequate tissue oxygenation is required. On the other hand, the applicator should not be too loose as the breast tissue needs to be in direct contact with the applicator without any dead space to ensure that an adequate radiation dose is delivered to the tumour bed. If intraoperative ultrasound is available, proximity of the breast tissue to the applicator can be checked during surgery.

Careful attention to haemostasis is extremely important, since poor haemostasis causes the geometry of the cavity to change due to collection of blood, which can lead to delivery of a suboptimal radiation dose to the target tissue. It can also create a tense and hypoxic environment, which can compromise the treatment.

It is the responsibility of the surgeon to check that the applicator is intact without any damage before insertion.

7.5.4 Draping of the INTRABEAM

Although the applicators are sterile, the INTRABEAM and the hydraulic arm need to be covered by a sterile plastic drape, which is specifically designed for this purpose. Care needs to be taken that the sheet is properly orientated to ensure that the blue straps are on the outside part when the applicator is inserted through the opening at the centre of the drape. After this, the blue straps are tied around the hydraulic arm. It is important to leave some slack over the INTRABEAM to allow manoeuvring of the device during insertion into the tumour bed (Fig. 7.6).

7.5.5 Positioning of the INTRABEAM

The applicator is inserted onto the INTRABEAM after aligning the projection on the applicator

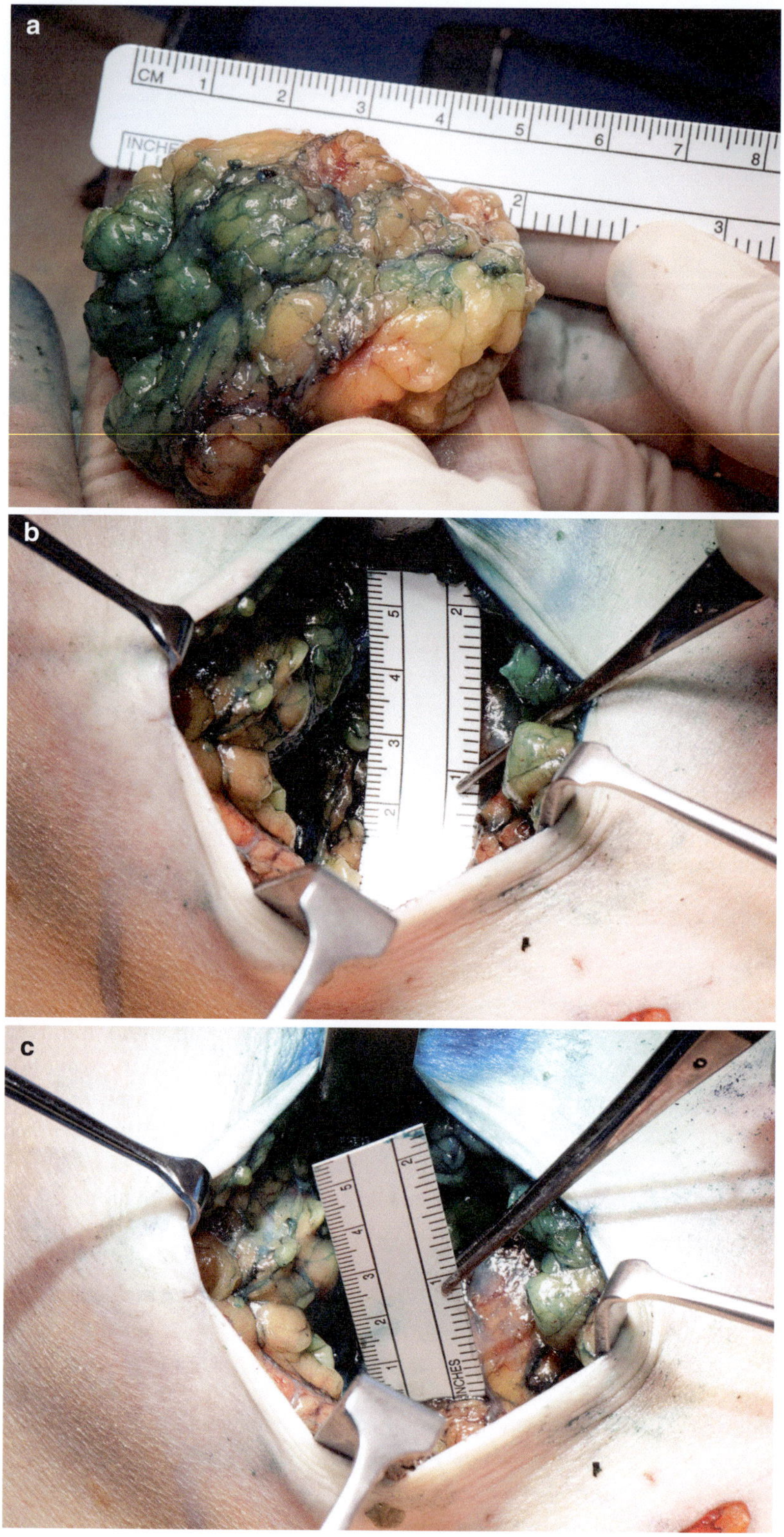

Fig. 7.5 (**a–c**) Measurement of the specimen and the cavity after WLE to assist in choice of the applicator size

with the notch at the base (Fig. 7.7). Care needs to be taken that the fragile electron drift tube is not touched during this process. Upon application of firm pressure, one can feel a click, which indicates that the applicator is securely applied to the INTRABEAM device. It is imperative that the applicator is snugly fitted to the INTRABEAM, which ensures that the optical interlock system within the device registers that the applicator has been applied correctly and allows the device to deliver the radiation.

The hydraulic arm can be positioned on the same side as the surgery or on the opposite side, depending on the design of the operating room and the surgeon's preference (Fig. 7.8).

The applicator, which is connected to the INTRABEAM, is then inserted into the tumour bed and the purse-string suture is pulled and tied snugly at the neck of the applicator. In this way the breast tissue (the target) is conformed around the applicator (the source) and therefore this type of radiotherapy can be referred to as conformal radiotherapy. If required, additional sutures can be applied at this stage to ensure that all the tumour bed tissue is approximated to the applicator (Fig. 7.9).

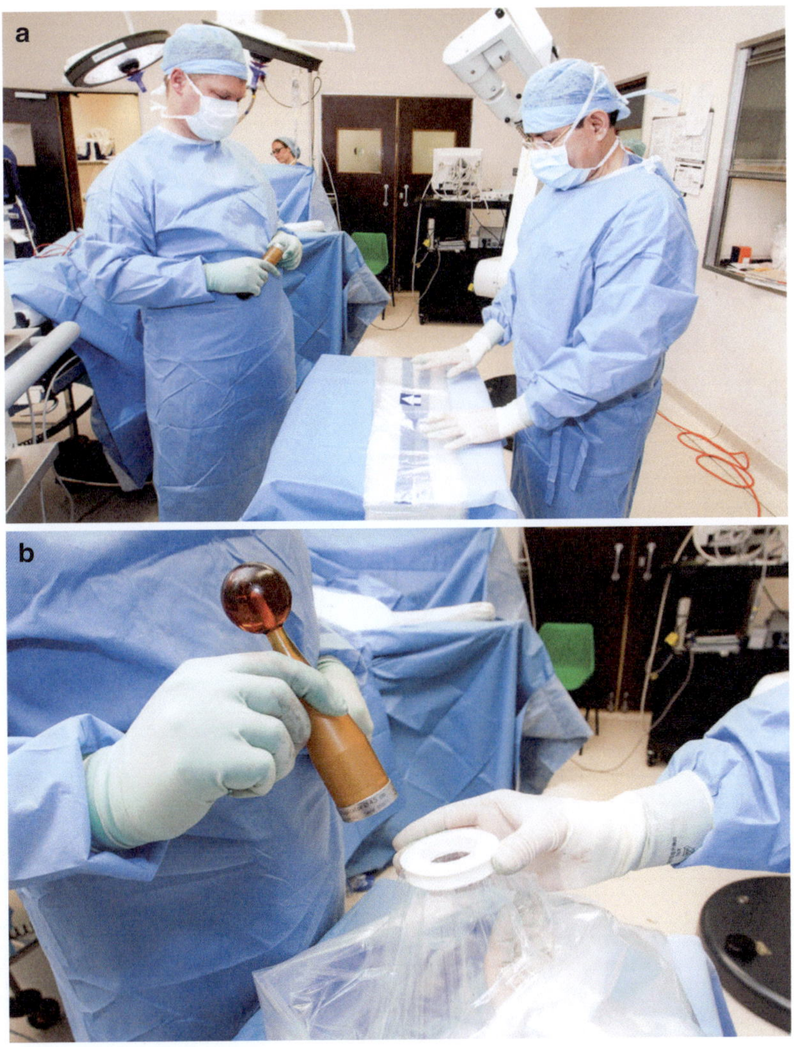

Fig. 7.6 (**a–d**) Steps in draping of the INTRABEAM, ensuring that the blue straps are on the outside of the drape

Fig. 7.6 (continued)

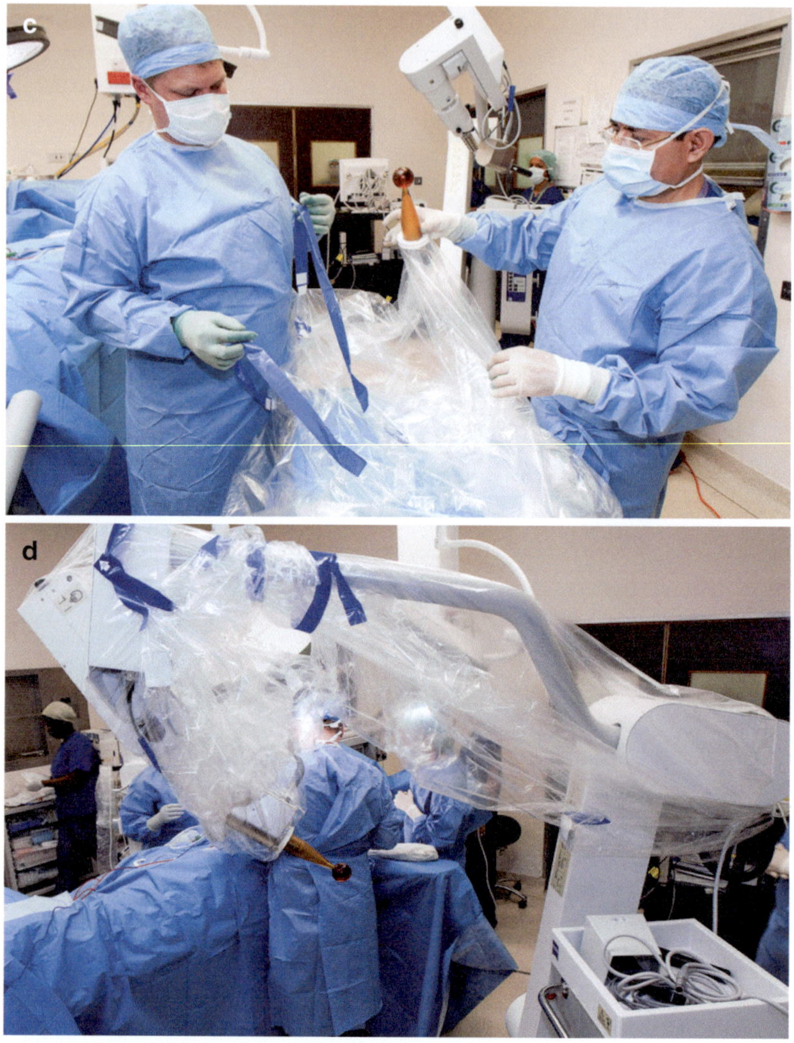

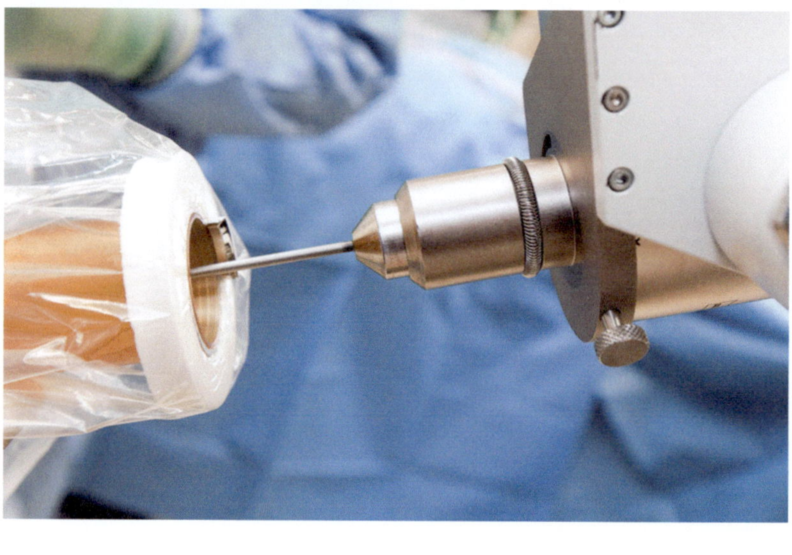

Fig. 7.7 Insertion of the applicator onto the INTRABEAM, ensuring that the projection on the applicator is aligned with the notch on the INTRABEAM

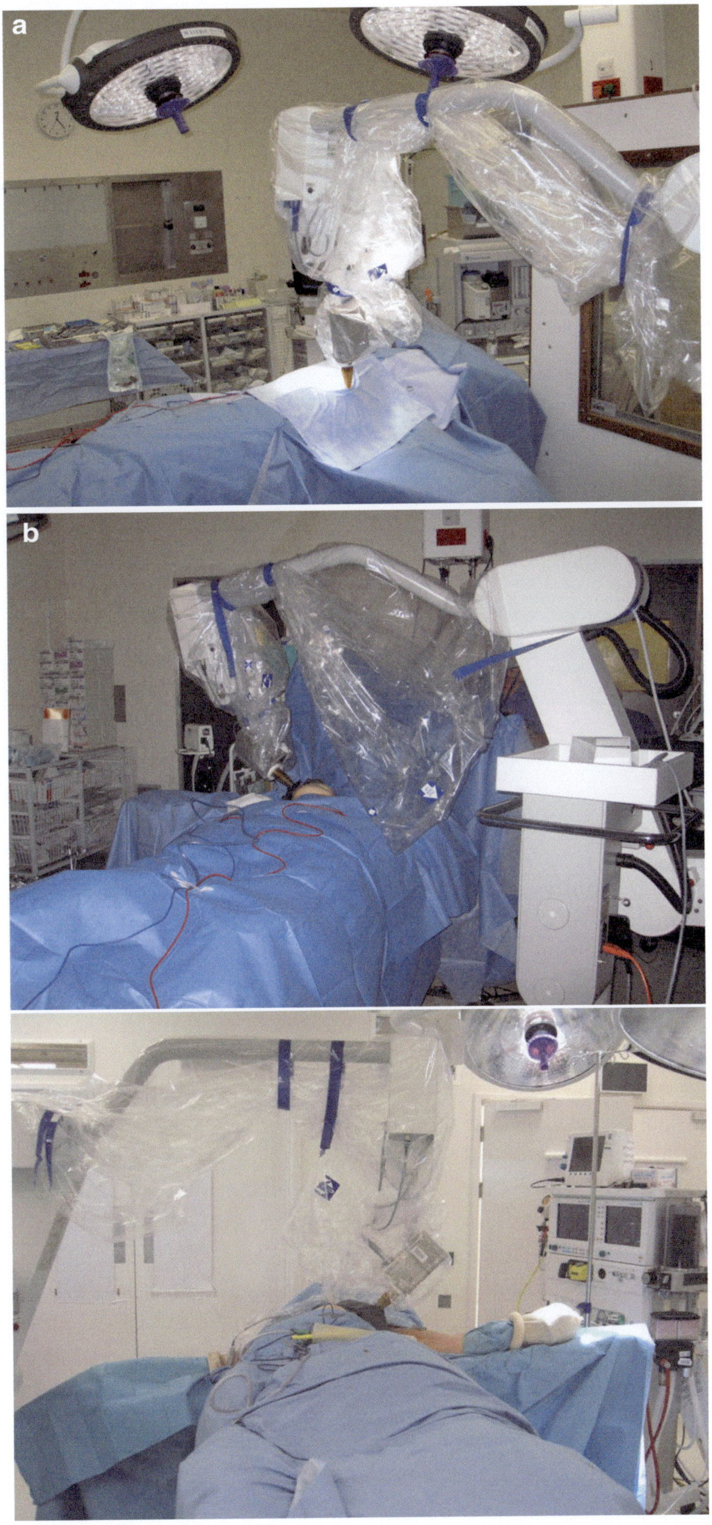

Fig. 7.8 The hydraulic arm is very versatile and can be used from the same side (**a**) or from the opposite side (**b**) as the surgery

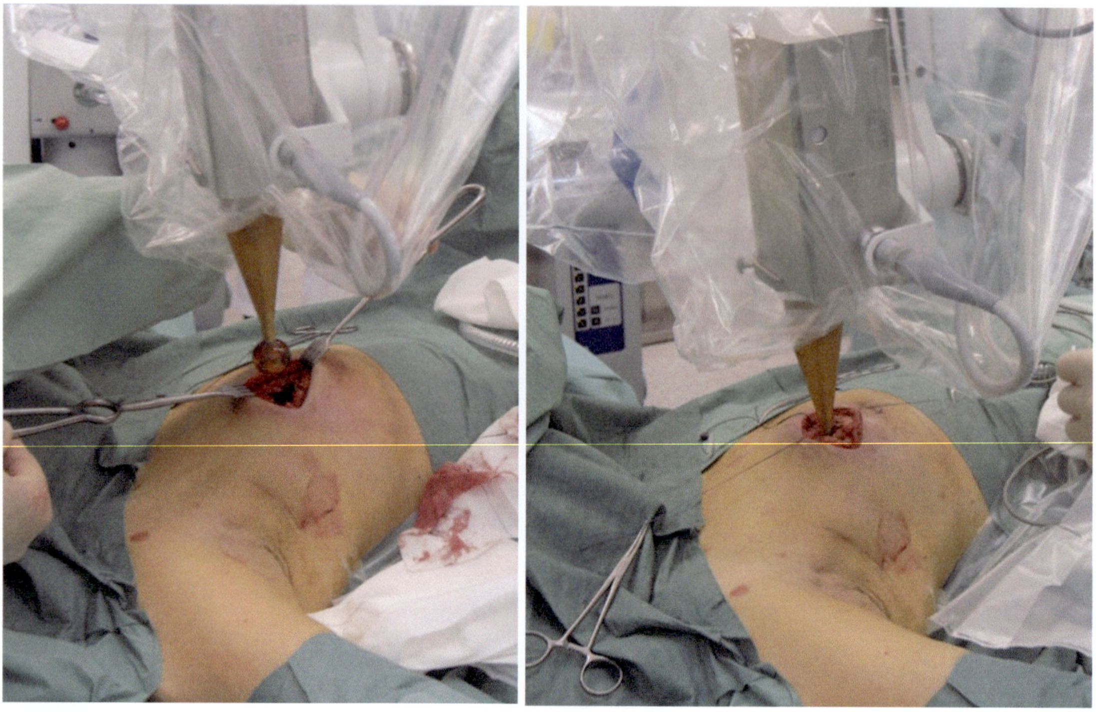

Fig. 7.9 Conformal radiotherapy: the breast tissue is conformed around the applicator by pulling the purse-string suture

At this time, some fine-tuning of the position of the INTRABEAM is done. It should be established that it is at right angles to the treatment area, and the hydraulic arm should be pulled gently upwards to ensure that the applicator does not press on the chest wall during the respiratory movements. After satisfactory placement, the hydraulic arm is locked into position to avoid inadvertent movements.

At this stage, stay sutures (3/0 silk) or a self-retaining retractor are used to retract the skin edges from the dome of the applicator. As outlined earlier, it is important that there is at least 5 mm distance between the applicator and the skin to avoid radiation damage to the skin. We recommend use of a thin wet gauze over the wound to keep the tissue moist and also maintain a minimum distance between the skin and the applicator (Fig. 7.10).

Finally, two sheets of external shielding are placed over the wound as demonstrated in Fig. 7.11. For radiation safety reasons, it is important that they are applied snugly to the neck of the applicator, avoiding any gaps.

7.5.6 Delivery of Radiotherapy

At this stage, the surgeon needs to sign a document confirming the applicator size used, which determines the time required for IORT. The members of the surgery and nursing team leave the operating room after this, while the anaesthetist and radiotherapy team can remain in the operating theatre and continue with the delivery of the radiotherapy.

After completion of the IORT, the surgical team returns to the operating room, and after removal of the external shielding and the purse-string suture, the applicator and the INTRABEAM are removed from the tumour bed. The sterile draping is removed from the hydraulic arm which is cleaned with disinfectant wipe by the theatre staff.

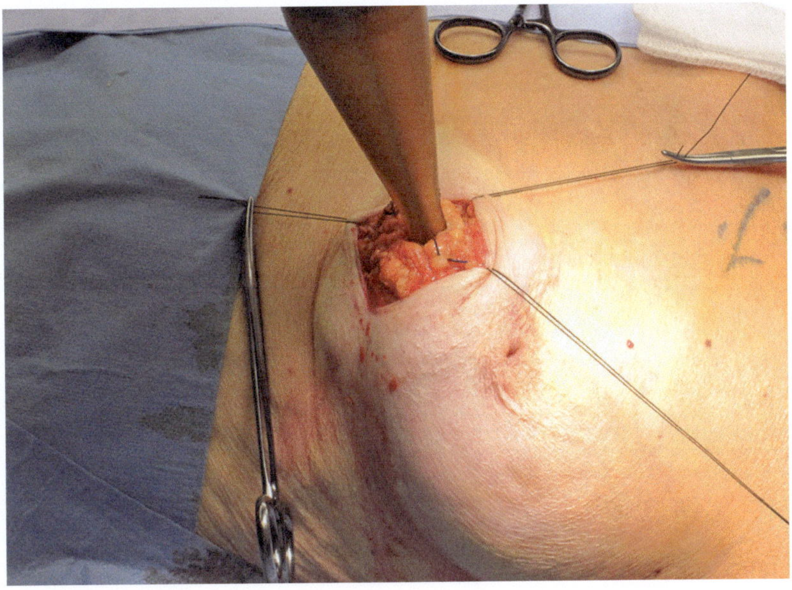

Fig. 7.10 Stay sutures are applied to ensure that the skin edges are retrac ted from the applicator

The breast tissue, which has been mobilised, is approximated and the resultant cavity is closed in a form of glanduloplasty, which enhances the cosmetic outcome.

7.6 What Happens If the Patient Needs Attention from the Anaesthetist During IORT?

If the patient needs attention during the delivery of radiotherapy, there is an emergency stop button on the control console of the unit which can be pressed. The clinical needs of the patient can then be attended to by the anaesthetist and the remaining duration of radiotherapy is then delivered.

7.7 Intraoperative Diagnosis of the Sentinel Lymph Node

As most patients who undergo IORT are candidates for sentinel node biopsy, we take advantage of the time required to deliver the radiotherapy and perform intraoperative testing of the (histological) status of the sentinel lymph nodes. Various intraoperative testing techniques are available, and at our centre we are using the one-step nucleic acid (OSNA) test. Before the completion of IORT, the result of the OSNA test is received and acted upon. It is therefore possible for a woman to have complete removal of the tumour, staging of the axilla (clearance if required) and radiotherapy all in a single session.

7.8 Use of Internal Shielding

As the INTRABEAM generates low-energy X-rays, the radiation dose attenuates steeply and the risk of radiation-induced damage to the underlying structures within the chest wall is minimal; therefore, use of internal shielding is not usually recommended. This is in contrast to devices that use electron beam and megavoltage radiotherapy, where use of internal shielding is mandatory. However, in very thin patients with a left-sided breast lesion, specially designed internal shielding is available and can be used if there are any concerns regarding the proximity of the heart to the applicator. It is important that only this specially designed internal shield is used in this situation and that it is removed at the end of the procedure.

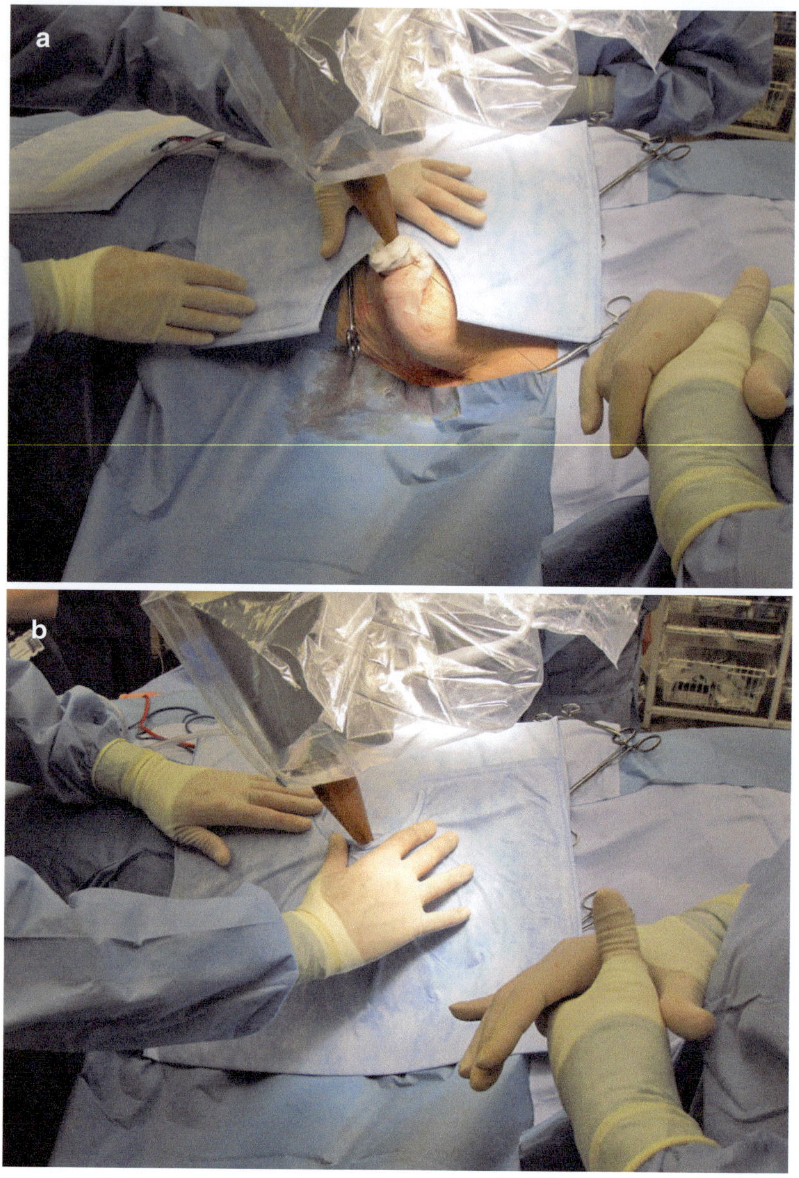

Fig. 7.11 (**a**, **b**) Insertion of external radiation shields

7.9 Upper Inner Quadrant Breast Cancer

Sometimes, lesions within the periphery of the upper inner quadrant of the breast pose a specific problem in that there is no breast tissue on the medial aspect to be mobilised and wrapped around the applicator. In these circumstances, the practice at UCL is to apply the purse-string suture as described above and to use a folded wet gauze as a spacer on the medial aspect of the applicator in order to ensure that a minimum distance of 5 mm is maintained between the skin and the dome of the applicator (Fig. 7.12).

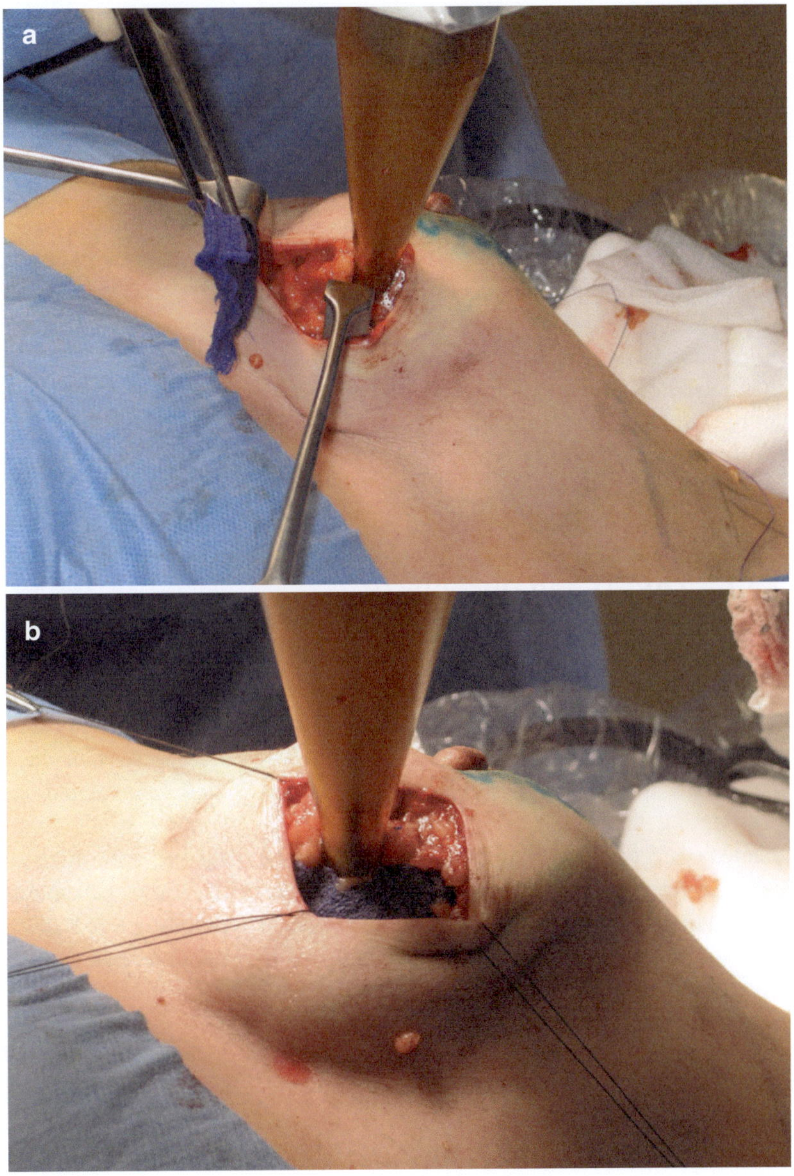

Fig. 7.12 (**a**, **b**) In the case of upper inner quadrant tumours, if there is no breast tissue on the medial aspect to be mobilised and wrapped around the applicator, a folded wet gauze can be used as a spacer to ensure maintenance of a minimum distance of 5 mm between the skin and the dome of the applicator

7.10 Breast Tumours that Are Too Close to the Skin

Some centres consider IORT to be contraindicated in situations where the breast tumour is close to the skin. At UCL, we do not regard this as a contraindication, provided an ellipse of the overlying skin can be excised without concerns regarding adequacy of the excision margins. If there are any concerns regarding close proximity of the skin to the applicator, wet gauze can be used as a spacer, as described above.

7.11 Intraoperative Determination of the Tumour Margins

Intraoperative determination of margins (frozen section histology) can be used if the required facilities are available; however, most centres rely on the definitive histology. If, on final histology, the margins are involved or deemed too close based on the local protocol of each unit, further re-excision of the margins can be performed. In these circumstances, the patient is offered EBRT to the whole breast, omitting the boost radiation (as in this situation IORT is regarded as a replacement for the boost radiation).

7.12 TARGIT and Oncoplastic Surgery

Targeted IORT can be used in conjunction with oncoplastic procedures. The only limiting factor in these circumstances is the size of the resultant cavity after removal of the primary tumour. Considering that the largest available applicator diameter is 5 cm, if the tumour bed tissue can be easily conformed around the applicator, IORT can be used in this setting. However, if the cavity is too large for this, EBRT needs to be considered. When using IORT in these circumstances, it is good practice to use marker clips at the tumour bed to mark the area in case the patient needs EBRT in future.

7.13 Post-pathology IORT

In some centres, because of the referral pattern and the local practice, targeted radiotherapy is delivered as a second procedure after the primary tumour has been excised. Within our randomised trial more than 1,000 patients were in the post-pathology stratum. The advantage of this approach is that the final histology, nodal status, margin clearance and receptor status of the tumour are known and the patient's eligibility for IORT can be verified. However, in our randomised trial, the pre-pathology group performed better than the post-pathology stratum for the primary outcome of ipsilateral breast recurrence. For the whole cohort the absolute difference at 5 years was 2.0 %, which was higher with TARGIT and reached the conventional levels of statistical significance ($p=0.042$), but was within the pre-specified non-inferiority margin. In the pre-pathology arm the absolute difference at 5 years for ipsilateral breast recurrence was 1 % and in the post-pathology arm it was higher, at 3.7 %. We therefore advocate the use of IORT at the same time as tumour excision if at all possible.

Sometimes, accurate determination of the tumour bed can be challenging in this cohort, especially if there has been a long interval between surgery and IORT. Use of preoperative ultrasound for accurate determination of the tumour cavity is recommended. We also recommend use of markers within the tumour cavity (sutures or titanium clips) to ensure accurate identification of the tumour cavity.

The tumour cavity in these circumstances is well capsulated and contracted and usually smaller applicators are required as compared to the pre-pathology stratum.

Use of perioperative intravenous antibiotics is recommended in these circumstances to minimise the risk of postoperative wound infection.

7.14 Key Points

- Surgical aspects of the IORT are simple and straightforward
- Attention to detail is important
- Meticulous haemostasis
- Team working
- Appropriate scheduling
- Choice of appropriately sized applicator
- Ensuring good approximation of the tumour bed tissue to the applicator
- Maintaining a minimum distance of 5 mm between the skin and the dome of the applicator
- Use of folded wet gauze as a spacer if required
- Use of IORT at the same time as WLE is preferable to use of IORT as a second procedure

8 Follow-Up Findings in the Tumour Bed After IORT – What the Radiologist Needs to Know

Klaus Wasser and Elena Sperk

Since the establishment of breast-conserving therapy 20 years ago it has become well known that structural changes like parenchymal scarring, local oedema, seroma, fat necroses and dystrophic calcification occur at the original tumour site. Physicians have learned to handle these alterations and to differentiate them from local recurrence (Krishnamurthy et al. 1999). Currently, for radiologists it is important to know whether IORT, as a result of the local radiation effect, causes increased or other forms of structural changes in the tumour bed that need to be accounted for in follow-up examinations.

To date, a few studies have reported on the findings in the tumour bed after IORT with low-energy x-rays. The first study dealing with this topic, by Wasser et al. (2007), was focussed on the first 2 years of follow-up after IORT as a boost. Applying mammography and ultrasound, haematomas or seromas as well as fat necroses were seen significantly more frequently compared to a conventionally treated control group (breast-conserving surgery and external radiation therapy). Generally, these findings were confirmed by another study of the same working group (Ruch et al. 2009) that included patients receiving IORT as single radiation or as boost and a follow-up period of at least 3 years. In this study, changes occurring in the tumour bed over time were observed very carefully on both mammography and ultrasound. After IORT, patients had a higher incidence of fat necroses/oil cysts (Fig. 8.1a) on the late follow-up mammograms compared to the conventionally treated control group (57 % vs. 17 %). The oil cysts were significantly larger in the IORT group (median 4.5 cm^2 vs. 1.4 cm^2). In nearly all IORT patients the oil cysts arose from partially organised haematomas/seromas, which in this group were generally more frequent (76 % vs. 37 %) and larger (median 3.6 cm^2 vs. 1.8 cm^2). After IORT a decreasing incidence of haematomas/seromas (defined on ultrasound) was reciprocal to an increasing incidence of oil cysts (defined on mammography), and the size of both entities correlated with each other. Liquid lesions with polypoid inner wall thickening on ultrasound (Fig. 8.1b) appeared more frequently in the tumour bed after IORT (28 % vs. 2 %). According to their previous experiences after additional diagnostic procedures in a few patients (e.g. core cut biopsy or magnetic resonance mammography), the authors assumed that the latter finding correlates with different kinds of inert scar tissue at the lesion margin (e.g. fat necrosis, fibrosclerosis). Thus, they concluded that the radiologist is confronted with large and organised wound cavities in most cases after IORT in early postoperative

K. Wasser (✉)
Institute of Clinical Radiology and Nuclear Medicine, University Medical Center Mannheim, University of Heidelberg, Theodor-Kutzer-Ufer 1-3, D-68167, D-68167 Mannheim, Germany
e-mail: klaus.wasser@umm.de, http://www.umm.de

E. Sperk
Department of Radiation Oncology, University Medical Centre Mannheim, University of Heidelberg, Theodor-Kutzer-Ufer 1-3, D-68167, D-68167 Mannheim, Germany
e-mail: elena.sperk@umm.de, http://www.umm.de

M. Keshtgar et al. (eds.), *Targeted Intraoperative Radiotherapy in Oncology*,
DOI 10.1007/978-3-642-39821-6_8, © Springer-Verlag Berlin Heidelberg 2014

follow-up studies (<3 years). In further follow-ups, fat necroses arise from these cavities, and about 60 % of patients likewise show large oil cysts on late follow-up mammograms. A further aim of the study by Ruch et al. (2009) was to identify influencing factors associated with the above-mentioned findings in the tumour bed. Neither the applicator size nor the tumour size nor the texture of the breast parenchyma correlated with the incidence and extent of post-treatment changes in the tumour bed.

Rivera et al. (2012) observed the mammographic changes in the tumour bed in patients treated with IORT as single radiation in a randomised trial (TARGIT-A). They found a higher incidence of fat necroses in comparison to

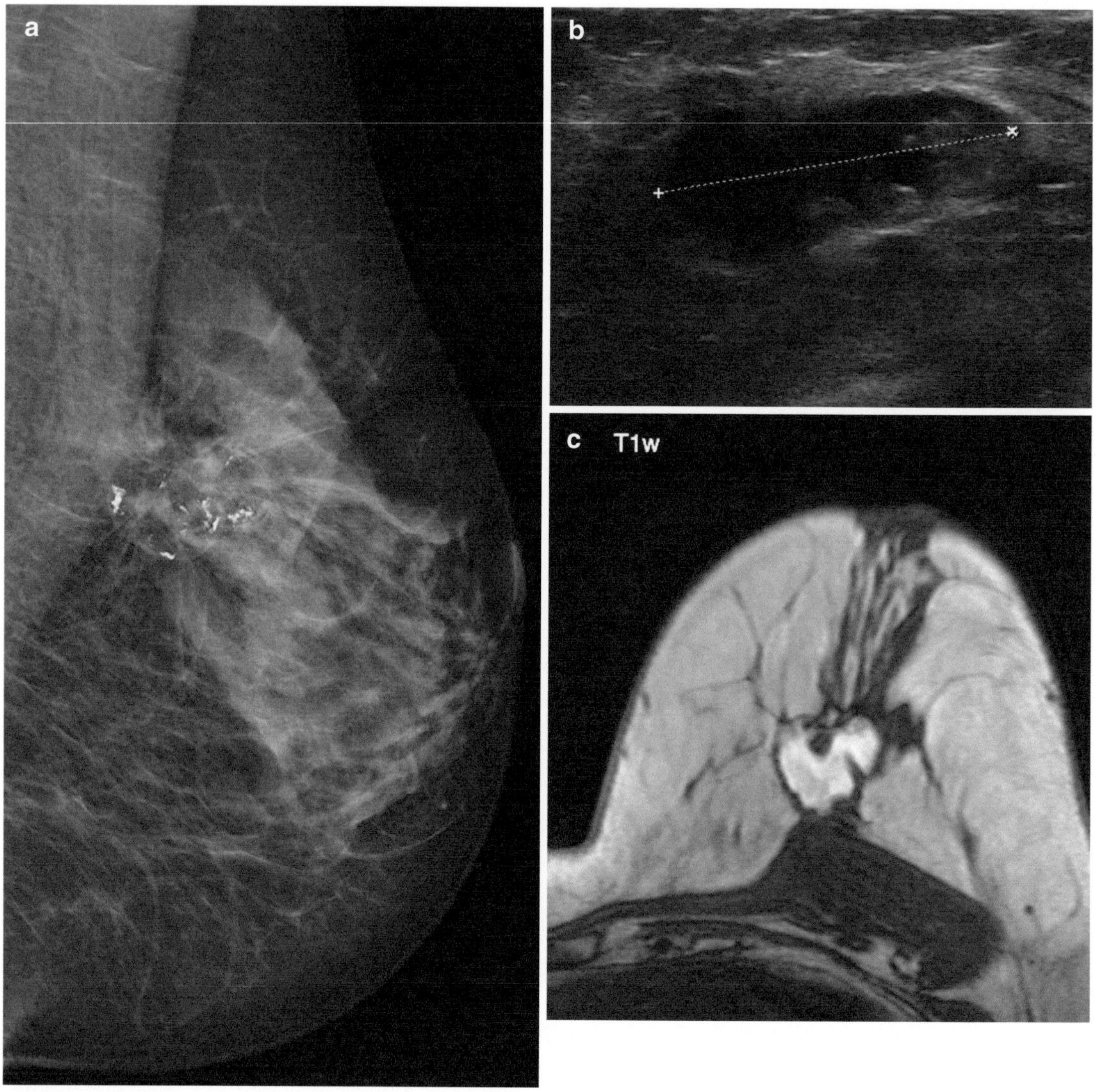

Fig. 8.1 Mammogram (**a**) of a patient with breast cancer who had received breast-conserving therapy and IORT as a boost 5 years previously. A well-circumscribed and partially calcified mass of 3.5 cm was seen at the original tumour site, defined as an oil cyst-like lesion. On ultrasound (**b**) the lesion appeared as a well-circumscribed liquid formation with polypoid inner wall thickening. On magnetic resonance mammography (**c**–**e**) the formation consisted of fat-equivalent material in most parts (**c**, **d**) and was surrounded by a smooth and subtle rim enhancement (**e**), rather consistent with an oil cyst-like lesion

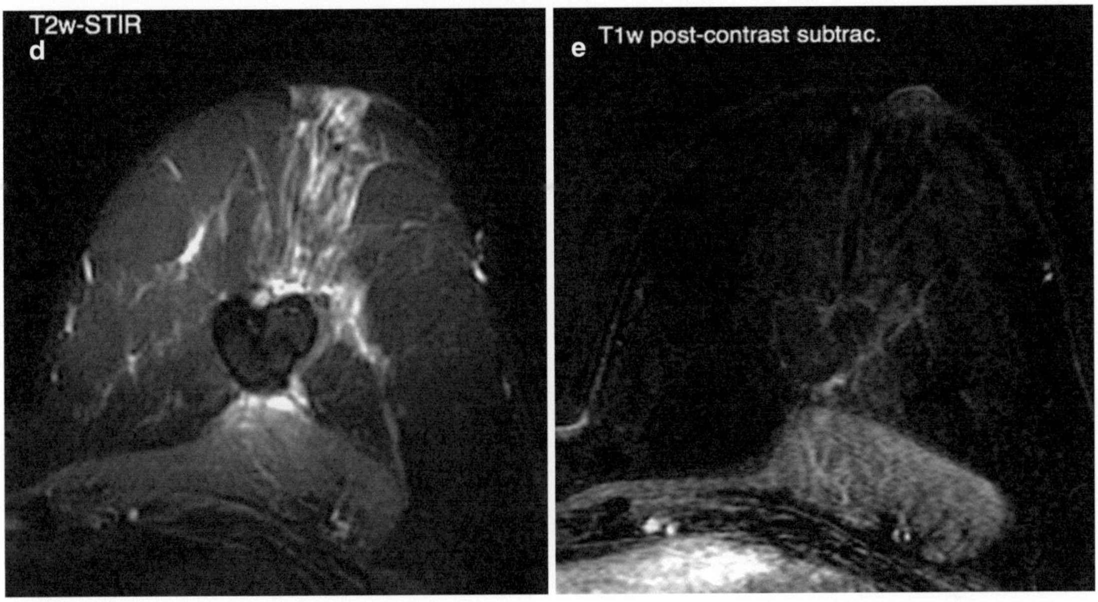

Fig. 8.1 (continued)

Table 8.1 Patients with fat necroses seen on postoperative follow-up mammograms after IORT (low-energy x-rays) compared to conventionally treated control groups: results of different studies

	Year	No. of patients (IORT)	No. of patients (control)	Fat necroses: IORT (%)	Fat necroses: control (%)
Wasser et al. (2007)[a]	2007	27	27	52	15
Ruch et al. (2009)[b]	2009	54	48	57	17
Rivera et al. (2012)[c]	2012	15	16	36	12

[a]IORT as boost
[b]IORT as boost or as single radiation
[c]IORT as single radiation

the control group. The extent of the fat necroses was not investigated in this study. Other changes such as architectural distortion, skin thickening, skin retraction, calcifications and mass density were not found to have a higher incidence. Taking all above-mentioned studies together (Wasser et al. 2007; Ruch et al. 2009; Rivera et al. 2012), a common finding is the higher incidence of fat necroses in the tumour bed after IORT (Table 8.1 demonstrates the incidence of fat necroses in the different studies). From the clinical point of view it is of interest whether the structural changes after IORT complicate the radiological follow-up and trigger further diagnostic procedures.

The above-mentioned studies by Wasser et al. (2007) and Rivera et al. (2012) additionally gave attention to this question. In the study by Wasser et al. (2007), findings in the tumour bed were not judged to have a significantly higher impact on interpretation. Additional diagnostic procedures (e.g. magnification mammography, magnetic resonance mammography, core cut biopsy) due to unclear findings were performed with similar frequency in both groups, IORT and control. Also, Rivera et al. (2012) pointed out that the changes in the tumour bed did not interfere with mammographic interpretation. Another study by Wasser et al. (2012a) focussed especially on this question. After IORT, compared to conventional treatment, sole mammographic follow-up evaluation was significantly more often judged to be distinctly complicated owing to postoperative changes in the tumour bed. Overall, however, such difficulty occurred in a rather small percentage of patients (16–21 % in the IORT group vs. 0–8 % in the control group). Retrospectively, analysing the ultrasound-supported mammographic follow-ups, it was found that further non-routine diagnostic procedures due to unclear findings in the tumour bed became necessary in 7 % (IORT) vs. 8 % (control group) of the patients.

The first study on magnetic resonance mammography after IORT analysed the changes in the tumour bed in comparison to a conventionally treated historical control group (Wasser et al. 2012b). The results were in line with the reports of mammography and ultrasound findings and showed a high incidence of wound cavities with fat necrosis (81 %). The contrast enhancement of these changes normally presented as rim enhancement and did not cause any diagnostic uncertainty if viewed together with other tissue characteristics (Fig. 8.1c, d). The authors concluded that the value of magnetic resonance mammography for follow-up diagnosis after IORT remains similar to that after conventional breast-conserving therapy.

In conclusion, all previous studies have pointed out that structural changes in the tumour bed, especially fat necroses, are increased after IORT with low-energy x-rays. To date, there is no evidence that those changes might significantly interfere with the radiological follow-up examinations.

Finally, it remains unclear whether the abovementioned changes in the tumour bed have to be defined as other than classical oil cysts or seromas, i.e. whether a new kind of wound cavity formation might need to be considered. To elucidate this issue, further studies with correlation of radiological and histopathological findings will be necessary.

References

Krishnamurthy R, Whitman GJ, Stelling CB, Kushwaha AC (1999) Mammographic findings after breast conservation therapy. Radiographics 19 Spec No:S53-62, quiz S262-3

Rivera R, Smith-Bronstein V, Villegas-Mendez S, Rayhanabad J, Sheth P, Rashtian A, Holmes DR (2012) Mammographic findings after intraoperative radiotherapy of the breast. Radiol Res Pract 2012:758371

Ruch M, Brade J, Schoeber C, Kraus-Tiefenbacher U, Schnitzer A, Engel D et al (2009) Long-term follow-up-findings in mammography and ultrasound after intraoperative radiotherapy (IORT) for breast cancer. Breast 18:327–334

Wasser K, Schoeber C, Kraus-Tiefenbacher U, Bauer L, Brade J, Teubner J et al (2007) Early mammographic and sonographic findings after intraoperative radiotherapy (IORT) as a boost in patients with breast cancer. Eur Radiol 17:1865–1874

Wasser K, Ruch M, Brade J, Schoeber C, Kraus-Tiefenbacher U, Schnitzer A et al (2012a) Do structural changes in the tumour bed after intraoperative radiotherapy (IORT) of breast cancer complicate the evaluation of mammograms in a long-term follow-up? Eur J Radiol 81:e255–e259

Wasser K, Schnitzer A, Engel D, Krammer J, Wenz F, Kraus-Tiefenbacher U et al (2012b) First description of MR mammographic findings in the tumor bed after intraoperative radiotherapy (IORT) of breast cancer. Clin Imaging 36:176–184

9 Quality of Life and Late Radiation Toxicity

Elena Sperk and Grit Welzel

9.1 Quality of Life (G. Welzel)

Health-related quality of life (QoL) is a subjective (self-perceived) multidimensional health assessment on the part of the patient. QoL as a scientific concept was accepted by Index Medicus in 1977 and later by the World Health Organisation and the *New England Journal of Medicine* (Beth 1992). Today, QoL is an accepted part of medical research, and an important end-point of cancer treatment. Commonly used QoL instruments are the Functional Assessment of Cancer Therapy - General Questionnaire (FACT-G) (Cella et al. 1993) and the European Organisation for Research and Treatment of Cancer QoL Questionnaire Core 30 (EORTC QLQ-C30) (Aaronson et al. 1993). Both questionnaires contain questions, or items, that are organised into scales. Each scale measures a different domain of QoL. The QLQ-C30 concentrates largely on physical functioning and clinical symptoms, whereas the FACT-G has a stronger focus on social and emotional aspects (Kemmler et al. 1999).

E. Sperk (✉) • G. Welzel
Department of Radiation Oncology,
University Medical Centre Mannheim,
University of Heidelberg, Theodor-Kutzer-Ufer 1-3,
D-68167 Mannheim, Germany
e-mail: elena.sperk@umm.de, http://www.umm.de;
grit.welzel@umm.de, http://www.umm.de

9.1.1 QoL After IORT in General

Up to now very few studies have assessed the potential impact of intraoperative radiation therapy (IORT) on patient QoL. In 1996, Magrini et al. (1996) reported on a non-randomised study of nine patients with locally advanced or recurrent rectal or anal cancer who had had surgical exploration, sacrectomy and intraoperative electron irradiation. A non-standardised questionnaire was used to collect information on current health status, including QoL. Eight of the nine patients reported a reduction in pain and improved QoL 2–37 (median, 18) months postoperatively. Other studies (Shibata et al. 2000; Mannaerts et al. 2002) suggest unfavourable functional and QoL outcomes after IORT-containing multimodality treatment for locally advanced primary and recurrent rectal cancer. However, the combination of surgery with external beam radiotherapy (EBRT), IORT and chemotherapy has improved local control and survival for these patients.

Ohtsuka and colleagues (2001) conducted a small non-randomised prospective study in 20 Japanese patients who underwent pylorus-preserving pancreatoduodenectomy (PPPD), three of them were treated with IORT. The aims of this study were to assess the subjective QoL before PPPD and in the short and long term after PPPD and to analyse factors predicting delayed recovery of QoL. The QoL questionnaire assessed two domains: physical and psychosocial aspects. IORT was a significant factor in

M. Keshtgar et al. (eds.), *Targeted Intraoperative Radiotherapy in Oncology*,
DOI 10.1007/978-3-642-39821-6_9, © Springer-Verlag Berlin Heidelberg 2014

predicting delayed recovery of QoL after PPPD by univariate analysis, but not by multivariate analysis.

9.1.2 QoL After IORT in Breast Cancer Patients

Most of the studies assessing QoL after IORT have focussed on breast cancer survivors. QoL has been assessed using the EORTC QLQ-C30 and breast module QLQ-BR23. In 2006, Lemanski et al. (2006) reported a series of 26 women with early breast cancer treated with 9–20 Gy (median 10 Gy) IORT with 9-MeV electron beams followed by postoperative EBRT (50 Gy in 2-Gy fractions). They found an excellent general cancer-specific QoL and few symptoms at a median follow-up of 9 years. Four years later, Lemanski et al. (2010) reported the QoL results of 42 patients in a single-centre phase II trial of IORT evaluating a dose of 21 Gy delivered to the tumour bed as a one-shot procedure. Again, at a median follow-up of 30 months, the QoL questionnaire scores indicated an excellent QoL and few symptoms.

Our group assessed QoL in breast cancer patients treated with IORT alone, IORT followed by EBRT or EBRT alone (Welzel et al. 2010, 2013; Blank et al. 2010a). In all studies, QoL was collected using the EORTC QLQ-C30 and the breast module QLQ-BR23. In addition, fatigue, anxiety, depression, self-esteem and body image parameters were controlled. In a cross-sectional sample of 103 women treated with an IORT boost dose of 20 Gy followed by EBRT (46–50 Gy in 2-Gy fractions), we assessed QoL and LENT-SOMA toxicities at a median follow-up of 32 (range, 6–65) months (Blank et al. 2010a). Compared with an age-adjusted general population sample, the patients showed a significant impairment in the following domains of the QLQ-C30: QoL, cognitive, emotional, fatigue, pain, dyspnoea, insomnia and financial difficulties. Patients with higher grade LENT-SOMA toxicities rated significantly more breast and arm symptoms such as breast fibrosis, lymphoedema, telangiectases and breast pain and worse general health.

In a matched-pair study (Welzel et al. 2010), we assessed the QoL of 69 other patients with early breast cancer treated with IORT as a single treatment, IORT given as a boost plus EBRT (IORT-EBRT) or conventional EBRT. The patients were randomly matched for age and time since breast-conserving surgery in a 1:1:1 ratio. IORT was given with 50-kV X-rays (INTRABEAM® system, Carl Zeiss Surgical, Oberkochen, Germany) delivering 20 Gy at the applicator surface. EBRT (46–50 Gy in 2-Gy fractions in the IORT-EBRT group and 56 Gy in 2-Gy fractions in the EBRT group) was initiated after completion of wound healing and/or chemotherapy. The median follow-up was 47 (range, 18–70) months, and all patients were disease free at the time of survey. We found only a few QoL differences between the three groups: There was a non-significant trend towards more general pain and reduced global health after IORT-EBRT as compared to EBRT alone. IORT tended to induce fewer breast symptoms compared with EBRT, and IORT alone induced significantly fewer breast and general pain symptoms compared with IORT-EBRT.

In 2010 and 2011, we mailed questionnaires to the first 123 TARGIT-A patients from the University Medical Center Mannheim sample, and compared IORT-EBRT patients with two non-randomised control groups of patients treated with (a) IORT as a tumour bed boost followed by EBRT outside of TARGIT-A (IORT-boost) or (b) EBRT followed by an external beam boost to the tumour bed (EBRT-boost) (Welzel et al. 2013). The primary end points were global health status, restrictions in daily activities (role functioning) and general pain subscales from the QLQ-C30 and the breast symptoms and arm symptoms subscales from the QLQ-BR23. Two hundred and thirty women with stage I-III breast cancer were entered into the study: 87 women from the two arms of the TARGIT-A trial, 90 women receiving IORT as a tumour bed boost followed by EBRT outside of TARGIT-A (IORT-boost group) and 53 women treated with EBRT followed by an external beam boost (EBRT-boost group). The mean follow-up period in the TARGIT-A groups was 32 (range,

9–94) months versus 39 (range, 8–64) months in the non-randomised control groups. All patients were disease-free at the time of QoL assessment. TARGIT-A patients receiving IORT alone reported less general pain, fewer breast and arm symptoms, and better role functioning compared with patients receiving EBRT. TARGIT-A patients receiving IORT also had fewer breast symptoms than TARGIT-A patients receiving IORT followed by EBRT for high-risk features on final pathology. There were no significant differences between TARGIT-A patients receiving IORT-EBRT and non-randomised IORT-boost or EBRT-boost patients. A summary of the QoL scores from the Mannheim matched pair analysis and the Mannheim TARGIT-A QoL trial (Welzel et al. 2010, 2013) is provided in Table 9.1. Similar QoL scores were noted in both studies for patients after IORT, IORT-EBRT and IORT boost, respectively. The variations in the EBRT group are probably due to differences in medical co-morbidities. However, in the TARGIT-A QoL trial, multiple regression analyses revealed that both having two or more medical co-morbidities and being treated without IORT predicted general pain symptoms and limitations in daily activities, i.e. worse role functioning.

9.1.3 Conclusion

To summarise, in contrast to toxicity reports, very few studies have investigated QoL after IORT. The available research is limited by its focus on

Table 9.1 Summary of the QoL scores from the Mannheim matched pair analysis and the Mannheim TARGIT-A QoL trial

	Matched pair analysis (I)				
	Mannheim TARGIT-A QoL trial (II)			EBRT + boost (III)	
	IORT	EBRT	IORT-EBRT	IORT-boost	EBRT-boost
	Mean (SD)	Mean (SD)	Mean (SD)	Mean (SD)	Mean (SD)
General pain					
I	23.9 (24.5)	27.5 (34.7)	42.8 (32.9)	36.5 (35.0)	26.7 (29.8)
II	21.3 (33.2)	40.9 (32.3)	43.8 (32.1)		
Breast symptoms					
I	8.6 (12.3)	19.2 (23.8)	26.1 (27.6)	27.0 (24.4)	21.9 (24.1)
II	7.0 (14.0)	19.0 (20.0)	29.7 (22.8)		
Arm symptoms					
I	22.2 (25.9)	21.7 (27.7)	37.2 (36.5)	32.5 (28.7)	27.6 (29.1)
II	15.1 (22.2)	32.8 (28.6)	32.6 (25.8)		
Role functioning					
I	71.7 (30.7)	73.2 (25.7)	65.9 (26.8)	63.7 (31.8)	70.8 (30.8)
II	78.7 (35.2)	60.5 (29.5)	65.6 (29.5)		
Global health status					
I	70.3 (23.0)	70.3 (23.9)	57.6 (20.7)	59.6 (21.7)	72.0 (20.2)
II	63.3 (24.2)	52.4 (22.1)	60.9 (19.9)		
Medical co-morbidities ≥2					
I	56 %	39 %	56 %	54 %	17 %
II	56 %	80 %	69 %		
ALND					
I	74 %	65 %	100 %	61 %	79 %
II	16 %	30 %	25 %		

TARGIT-A TARGeted Intra-operative radioTherapy versus whole breast radiotherapy for breast cancer, *IORT* intraoperative radiotherapy, *EBRT* external beam whole breast radiotherapy, *ALND* axillary lymph node dissection, I results of the patients from the matched pair analysis, II results of the patients from the Mannheim TARGIT-A QoL trial, III results of the patients receiving an IORT or EBRT boost outside of TARGIT-A breast cancer patients. Patients with early breast cancer treated with breast-conserving surgery and IORT +/– EBRT present with excellent QoL scores and few symptoms compared with patients receiving EBRT without a boost. In the randomised setting, several general health-related and disease-specific QoL domains (restrictions in daily activities, i.e. role functioning, general pain, breast and arm symptoms) are superior after IORT than after EBRT. Non-randomised comparisons show equivalent parameters in the IORT-EBRT group and the IORT-boost or EBRT-boost control group.

9.2 Late Radiation Toxicity (E. Sperk)

Understanding of the indications for and use of IORT has grown as increasing numbers of patients have been treated. In 2004 the level of evidence was scored IV in regard to the postoperative complications seen in 25 patients treated with IORT using INTRABEAM (Cuncins-Hearn et al. 2004). During the past 10 years, the TARGIT-A trial has recruited a total of 3,451 patients, randomised consistently into the experimental arm with IORT (n = 1,721) or the standard arm with EBRT (n = 1,730). The first results, presented in 2010, showed non-inferiority of IORT as a sole treatment in early stage breast cancer within the scope of a randomised, international, multi-centre phase 3 trial (Vaidya et al. 2010).

Generally, late toxicity is classified as toxicity occurring 90 days or more after treatment. Different scores exist to assess late toxicity, and all of them have specific advantages and drawbacks. Some are detailed while others are less precise in definition of the differences from 0 to I, II, III or IV. The most common toxicity scores are the CTCAE (Common Terminology Criteria of Adverse Events) defined by the EORTC (European Organisation for Research and Treatment of Cancer), the RTOG (Radiation Therapy Oncology Group) or other leading organisations. For late toxicities the LENT SOMA (Late Effects of Normal Tissue; Subjective, Objective, Management, and Analytic) scales are usually used. The LENT SOMA tables were well described in 1995 and are used for almost all entities (No authors listed 1995). With these tables it is possible to achieve a high level of objectivity, though a certain subjectivity will always remain. Hoeller et al. compared the RTOG and LENT SOMA scores in a group of breast cancer patients (n = 259). The impact of the classification system on grading late effects was evaluated. The study group concluded that LENT SOMA criteria seem to be a better tool than the RTOG scale for grading and recording late radiation toxicity because use of the LENT/SOMA criteria resulted in some upgrading of skin toxicity in comparison with the RTOG score. In contrast, fibrosis scores correlated very well (Hoeller et al. 2003).

IORT for breast cancer is used in a number of situations: (a) breast cancer recurrence during second breast-conserving surgery to avoid mastectomy, (b) as an advanced boost followed by external whole breast radiotherapy or (c) as a single treatment in early stage breast cancer. Table 9.2 gives an overview of all applications for IORT in breast cancer and the available toxicity data until December 2012.

9.2.1 IORT for Breast Cancer Recurrence

In general, mastectomy is recommended for patients suffering from recurrent breast cancer within the pre-irradiated breast. Normal tissue tolerance does not permit a further full-dose course of radiotherapy to the entire breast after second breast-conserving surgery. With IORT it is possible to offer these patients second breast-conserving surgery followed by IORT to the site of the tumour without causing significant normal tissue damage. The first results regarding toxicity in pre-irradiated patients were reported in 2007 by Kraus-Tiefenbacher et al. (2007). The group reported no local recurrences in 17 patients after a median follow-up of 26 months. Acute toxicities were reported as mild, with no grade III or IV toxicities and an excellent or good cosmetic

Table 9.2 Late toxicity after IORT: an overview for all applications

Study	Year	N	F-U (months)	LR (%)	Chronic skin toxicity	Toxicity
Pre-irradiated						
Kraus-Tiefenbacher et al.	2007	15	26	0 (0)		RTOG °III–IV: 0 %
Keshtgar et al.	2011	21	42	0 (0)		No unexpected
Kraus-Tiefenbacher et al.	2011	20	37	2 (10)	T: 5 % H: 5%	Fibrosis° II–III: 45 %
IORT as a boost						
Kraus-Tiefenbacher et al.	2006	73	25		T: 0 %	RTOG °III–IV: 0 %
Wenz et al.	2008	48	36		T: 6 % H: 8 %	°0–I: 63 % Fibrosis °II–III: 23 %
Wenz et al.	2010	155	34	2 (1.3) @5 years K-M: 98.5 %	T: 6 % H: 6 %	Fibrosis °III: 5 % Fibrosis °II: 30 %
Blank et al.	2010a, b	197 (@5 years: 58)	37 (60)	5 (2.5) @5 years K-M: 97.0 %	T: 13.5 % H: 0.5 %	Fibrosis °0–I: 62 % Fibrosis °II: 34.6 % Fibrosis °III: 3.4 %
IORT alone						
Vaidya et al.	2010	1,113	48	6 (0.5)		RTOG °III–IV: 0.5 %
Sperk et al.	2012	54 (IORT n=34, IORT+EBRT n=20)	40	0 (0)	T: 5.8 % (IORT alone 0 %) H: 5.6 %	Fibrosis °II: 17 % (5.9 % IORT alone) Fibrosis °III: 0 %

Abbreviations: *N* number of patients, *F-U* Follow-up, *LR* Local recurrence, *T* Telangiectases, *H* Hyperpigmentation, *K-M* Kaplan-Meier estimates

outcome in 82 %. Fibrosis as a late toxicity occurred in 35 % in a limited volume of tissue and 17.6 % had grade II or III fibrosis.

A follow-up report of these patients along with additional three cases was reported in 2011 (Kraus-Tiefenbacher et al. 2011). Median follow-up was 37 months and two recurrences were seen (10 %). Grade II and III toxicities were observed in nine patients, at a peak after 18 months. Telangiectasia, grade II fibrosis and retraction were observed in one patient after longer follow-up. Seven patients developed retraction, two had breast pain and one showed hyperpigmentation and breast oedema.

Keshtgar et al. (2011) reported the results of IORT as sole treatment in 80 patient with breast cancer who could not be treated with EBRT. They demonstrated a reduction in fibrosis in the IORT group compared to patients treated with standard EBRT (15 % vs. 25 %).

9.2.2 IORT as a Boost

Most experience and results are available for IORT as a boost followed by a shortened course of EBRT for 4.5 weeks (Wenz et al. 2012). The first results of a single-centre experience were reported in 2006 by Kraus-Tiefenbacher et al. (2006). No grade III or IV toxicities (CTC score and LENT SOMA score for telangiectases) were seen in 73 patients with a median follow-up of 25 months. Fibrosis of the entire breast was seen in 5 %. Circumscribed fibrosis around the tumour bed was palpable in up to 27 %, with a peak around 18 months after therapy and a decline thereafter. The observed toxicity rates were not influenced by age, tumour stage or systemic therapy. The cosmetic outcome was good to excellent in ≥90 % of cases.

Another detailed analysis of late toxicities after IORT as a boost (n=48) showed chronic skin toxicities in 6-8 % regarding telangiectases and hyperpigmentation after a median follow-up of 36 months (Wenz et al. 2008). Grade II-III fibrosis was found in 23 %. A subanalysis showed that starting EBRT about 5–6 weeks after IORT appeared to be associated with a decreased risk of chronic late toxicity compared with a shorter interval. In detail, the median interval between IORT and EBRT was significantly shorter in patients with higher grade toxicities (n = 18) than in the 30 patients without higher grade toxicities (29.5 days vs. 39.5 days, p = 0.023). Of the 18 patients with higher grade toxicities at 3 years, 12 developed higher grade fibrosis (II-III), three telangiectasia, one breast oedema of grade II, six retraction, four hyperpigmentation and five pain of grade II or III.

Five years' experience of the same centre with the IORT boost was available for 155 cases, with a median follow-up of 34 months in 2010 (Wenz et al. 2010), at which time low recurrence rates were seen (Kaplan-Meier estimate at 5 years: 98.5 % recurrence free). A systematic analysis of 79 patients with a minimum follow-up of 3 years was done to evaluate late toxicity according to the LENT SOMA scales. Consistent low chronic skin toxicities were detected, with telangiectases and hyperpigmentation each seen in 6 %. Grade III fibrosis was observed in 5 % and grade II fibrosis in 30 %, which was in line with other reports of fibrosis after (accelerated partial) breast irradiation. Breast oedema was seen in 8 %.

A further analysis was undertaken of 77 patients to correlate late toxicity with the presence (n = 56) or absence (n = 21) of a seroma at the time of CT planning (Kraus-Tiebenbacher et al. 2010). Large breast volume and greater applicator sizes were significantly associated with a visible seroma during planning CT. Seroma size, breast volume and applicator size correlated significantly with fibrosis of the breast.

Recent results from a single centre were reported for 197 patients treated with an IORT boost with a median follow-up of 37 months. There was a local recurrence-free rate of 97 % (Kaplan-Meier estimates at 5 years) (Blank et al. 2010b). The disease-free survival reached 81.0 % and overall survival 91.3 % at 5 years. Among 58 patients with a median follow-up of 60 months, chronic skin toxicities were seen in 13.5 %. No or barely palpable fibrosis was seen in 62 %. Marked increase in density (grade III) was detected in 3.4 % and grade II fibrosis in 34.6 %. Other toxicities included severe pain (6.9 %), retraction (29.3 %), oedema of the breast (1.7 %) and lymphoedema in general (3.4 %). Figure 9.1 shows a patient with 3 years follow-up after IORT boost.

9.2.3 IORT as Sole Treatment

Within the TARGIT-A trial (n = 2,232), peri- and postoperative complications did not differ significantly between the two groups (IORT 3.3 % vs. EBRT 3.9 %) (Vaidya et al. 2010). Toxicities were documented according to the RTOG scales. There were significantly fewer patients with RTOG grade III-IV in the experimental arm than in the standard arm (0.5 % vs. 2.1 %). One may doubt, however, whether this difference represents a clinically relevant impact.

The first detailed toxicity results for patients randomised within the TARGIT-A trial were published in 2012 as a single-centre experience (Sperk et al. 2012). In this trial, 54 patients were treated with IORT in arm A (34 IORT alone, 20 IORT + EBRT) and 55 patients were treated with EBRT in arm B. Patients treated with IORT as a planned boost (n = 196) served as a control group. Median follow-up was 40 months in arm A and 42 months in arm B. Late toxicities were assessed with the LENT SOMA scale. In general there were no significant differences regarding fibrosis, breast oedema, retraction, ulceration, lymphoedema of the arm, hyperpigmentation or pain. There were significantly fewer telangiectases in arm A (5.8 %) than in arm B (17.7 %), and in the subanalysis the fibrosis rate for IORT alone (in arm A) was 5.9 % compared with 37.5 % after IORT + EBRT (arm A) and 18.4 % after EBRT alone (arm B). No telangiectases were seen after IORT alone. Patients receiving IORT alone had about half the risk of developing higher grade toxicities (hazard ratio 0.46; p = 0.010). No recurrences or deaths were seen in either in arm A or arm B after a maximum follow-up of 10 years.

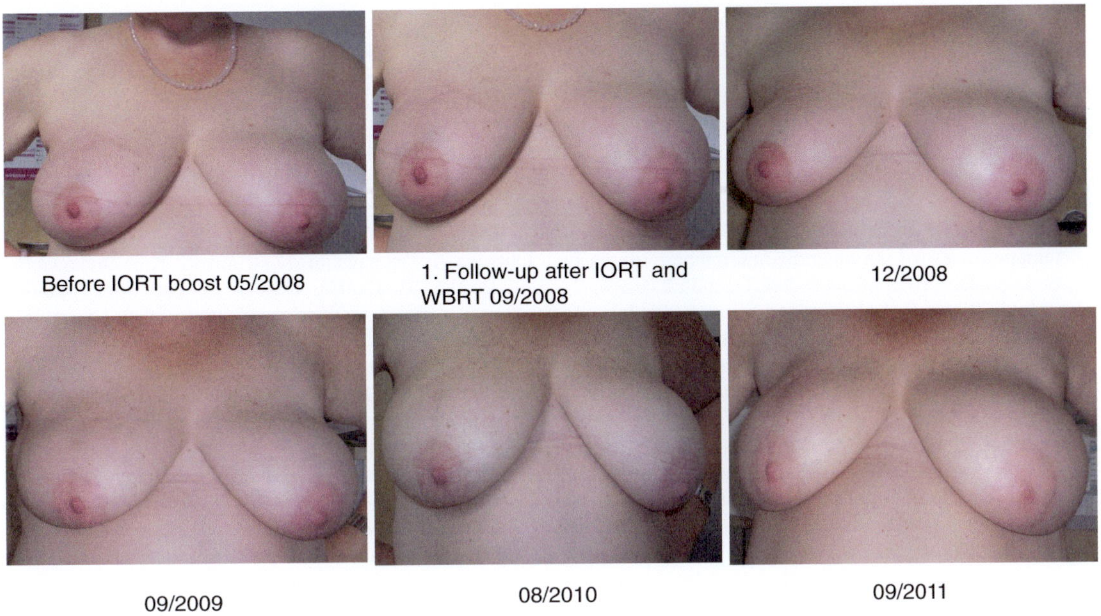

Fig. 9.1 Patient after IORT as a boost (*right breast*) 05/2008 followed by WBRT 06-07/2008. No chronic skin toxicities appeared during 3 years of follow-up

9.2.4 Summary

In summary, very low rates of chronic skin toxicities (telangiectases and hyperpigmentation) were seen after IORT for all applications (re-irradiation for breast recurrence, IORT as a boost and IORT as a sole treatment in early breast cancer), ranging between 0 and 13.5 %. Other late toxicities were also low or similar to results seen after standard breast irradiation. Grade II-III fibrosis was seen in up to 38 % after IORT as a boost. The rate of higher grade fibrosis in patients treated with IORT alone is very low, at less than 6 %. Patients with IORT alone have about half the risk of developing higher grade toxicities in general. A prospective assessment of IORT-boost patients was started in 2011 (TARGIT BQR). Furthermore, the TARGIT-E trial started recruiting patients in April 2011. In this trial, elderly patients aged >70 years with early breast cancer are treated with IORT alone without randomisation. When indicated (risk factors in final histopathology), EBRT is added as done in the TARGIT-A trial (Wenz et al. 2012). A phase III trial is in preparation to evaluate the superiority of the IORT boost in comparison to the standard percutaneous boost with electrons or photons (TARGIT-B).

Conclusion

Breast cancer patients treated with IORT in general have an excellent quality of life, with few late radiation toxicities. In the randomised setting both quality of life and late radiation toxicity seem to be superior in patients with IORT alone compared to a standard treatment with EBRT.

References

Aaronson NK, Ahmedzai S, Bergmann B, Bullinger M, Cull A, Duez NJ et al (1993) The European Organisation for Research and Treatment of Cancer QLQ-C30: a quality-of-life instrument for use in international clinical trials in oncology. J Natl Cancer Inst 85:365–376

Beth P (1992) Measuring quality of life: the medical perspective. Nord J Psychiatry 46:85–89

Blank E, Welzel G, Sütterlin M, Wenz F (2010a) Quality of life after intraoperative radiotherapy (IORT) as a boost in patients with early breast cancer. Geburtsh Frauenheilk 70:803–811

Blank E, Kraus-Tiefenbacher U, Welzel G, Keller A, Bohrer M, Sütterlin M, Wenz F (2010b) Single-center long-term follow-up after intraoperative radiotherapy as a boost during breast-conserving surgery using low-kilovoltage x-rays. Ann Surg Oncol 17(Suppl 3): 352–358

Cella DF, Tulsky DS, Gray G, Sarafian B, Linn E, Bonomi A et al (1993) The functional assessment of cancer therapy scale: development and validation of the general measure. J Clin Oncol 11:570–579

Cuncins-Hearn A, Saunders C, Walsh D, Borg M, Buckingham J, Frizelle F, Maddern G (2004) A systematic review of intraoperative radiotherapy in early breast cancer. Breast Cancer Res Treat 85:271–280

Hoeller U, Tribius S, Kuhlmey A, Grader K, Fehlauer F, Alberti W (2003) Increasing the rate of late toxicity by changing the score? A comparison of RTOG/EORTC and LENT/SOMA scores. Int J Radiat Oncol Biol Phys 55:1013–1018

Kemmler G, Holzner B, Kopp M, Dünser M, Margreiter R, Greil R, Sperner-Unterweger B (1999) Comparison of two quality-of-life instruments for cancer patients: the functional assessment of cancer therapy-general and the European Organization for Research and Treatment of Cancer Quality of Life Questionnaire-C30. J Clin Oncol 17:2932

Keshtgar MR, Vaidya JS, Tobias JS, Wenz F, Joseph D, Stacey C et al (2011) Targeted intraoperative radiotherapy for breast cancer in patients in whom external beam radiation is not possible. Int J Radiat Oncol Biol Phys 80:31–38

Kraus-Tiefenbacher U, Bauer L, Scheda A, Fleckenstein K, Keller A, Herskind C et al (2006) Long-term toxicity of an intraoperative radiotherapy boost using low energy X-rays during breast-conserving surgery. Int J Radiat Oncol Biol Phys 66:377–381

Kraus-Tiefenbacher U, Bauer L, Scheda A, Schoeber C, Schaefer J, Steil V, Wenz F (2007) Intraoperative radiotherapy (IORT) is an option for patients with localized breast recurrences after previous external-beam radiotherapy. BMC Cancer 7:178

Kraus-Tiebenbacher U, Welzel G, Brade J, Hermann B, Siebenlist K, Wasser KS et al (2010) Postoperative seroma formation after intraoperative radiotherapy using low-kilovoltage X-rays given during breast-conserving surgery. Int J Radiat Oncol Biol Phys 77:1140–1145

Kraus-Tiefenbacher U, Blank E, Wenz F (2011) Intraoperative radiotherapy during a second breast-conserving procedure for relapsed breast cancer after previous external beam radiotherapy. Int J Radiat Oncol Biol Phys 80:1279–1280

Lemanski C, Azria D, Thezenas S, Gutowski M, Saint-Aubert B, Rouanet P et al (2006) Intraoperative radiotherapy given as a boost for early breast cancer: long-term clinical and cosmetic results. Int J Radiat Oncol Biol Phys 64:1410–1415

Lemanski C, Azria D, Gourgon-Bourgade S, Gutowski M, Rouanet P, Saint-Aubert B et al (2010) Intraoperative radiotherapy in early-stage breast cancer: results of the Montpellier phase II trial. Int J Radiat Oncol Biol Phys 76:698–703

Magrini S, Nelson H, Gunderson LL, Sim FH (1996) Sacropelvic resection and intraoperative electron irradiation in the management of recurrent anorectal cancer. Dis Colon Rectum 39:1–9

Mannaerts GH, Rutten HJ, Martijn H, Hanssens PE, Wiggers T (2002) Effects on functional outcome after IORT-containing multimodality treatment for locally advanced primary and locally recurrent rectal cancer. Int J Radiat Oncol Biol Phys 54:1082–1088

No authors listed (1995) LENT SOMA tables. Radiother Oncol 35:17–60

Ohtsuka T, Yamaguchi K, Chijiiwa K, Kinukawa N, Tanaka M (2001) Quality of life after pylorus-preserving pancreatoduodenectomy. Am J Surg 182: 230–236

Shibata D, Guillem JG, Lanouette N, Paty P, Minsky B, Harrison L et al (2000) Functional and quality-of-life outcomes in patients with rectal cancer after combined modality therapy, intraoperative radiation therapy, and sphincter preservation. Dis Colon Rectum 43:752–758

Sperk E, Welzel G, Keller A, Kraus-Tiefenbacher U, Gerhardt A, Sütterlin M, Wenz F (2012) Late radiation toxicity after intraoperative radiotherapy (IORT) for breast cancer: results from the randomized phase III trial TARGIT. A. Breast Cancer Res Treat 135:253–260

Vaidya JS, Joseph DJ, Tobias JS, Bulsara M, Wenz F, Saunders C et al (2010) Targeted intraoperative radiotherapy versus whole breast radiotherapy for breast cancer (TARGIT-A trial): an international, prospective, randomised, non-inferiority phase 3 trial. Lancet 376:91–102, Erratum in: Lancet. 2010;376:90

Welzel G, Hofmann F, Blank E, Kraus-Tiefenbacher U, Hermann B, Suetterlin M, Wenz F (2010) Health-related quality of life after breast-conserving surgery and intraoperative radiotherapy for breast cancer using low-kilovoltage X-rays. Ann Surg Oncol 17:S359–S367

Welzel G, Boch A, Blank E, Kraus-Tiefenbacher U, Keller A, Hermann B et al (2013) Radiation-related quality of life parameters after targeted intraoperative radiotherapy vs. Whole breast radiotherapy in patients with breast cancer: results from the randomized phase III trial TARGIT-a. Radiat Oncol 8(1):9

Wenz F, Welzel G, Keller A, Blank E, Vorodi F, Herskind C et al (2008) Early initiation of external beam radiotherapy (EBRT) may increase the risk of long-term toxicity in patients undergoing intraoperative radiotherapy (IORT) as a boost for breast cancer. Breast 17:617–622

Wenz F, Welzel G, Blank E, Hermann B, Steil V, Sütterlin M, Kraus-Tiefenbacher U (2010) Intraoperative radiotherapy as a boost during breast-conserving surgery using low-kilovoltage X-rays: the first 5 years of experience with a novel approach. Int J Radiat Oncol Biol Phys 77:1309–1314

Wenz F, Blank E, Welzel G, Hofmann F, Astor D, Neumaier C et al (2012) Intraoperative radiotherapy during breast-conserving surgery using a miniature x-ray generator (INTRABEAM (®)): theoretical and experimental background and clinical experience. Womens Health (Lond Engl) 8:39–47

Cosmetic Outcome Following TARGIT

10

Norman R. Williams and Mohammed Keshtgar

10.1 Body Image

The evaluation of cosmetic outcome following treatments for early breast cancer has its roots in the concept of body image (Chan 2010). In the 1980s, research (Goin 1982) showed how physical aspects of the body can have an effect on emotional well-being, and the positive effects when body image is restored after it has been altered by disease (Goin and Goin 1988).

Cosmetic outcome therefore has an important psychological aspect in addition to the physiological wound healing process. An understanding of factors that influence cosmetic outcome is essential if progress is to continue in offering women the best possible therapeutic options.

N.R. Williams, BSc, PhD, MICR, CSci (✉)
Clinical Trials Group, Division of Surgery and Interventional Science, Faculty of Medical Sciences, University College London, Charles Bell House, 67-73 Riding House Street, London W1W 7EJ, UK
http://www.ucl.ac.uk/ctg

M. Keshtgar, BSc, FRCSI, FRCS (Gen), PhD
Division of Surgery and Interventional Sciences, Department of Breast Surgery, University College London Medical School, Royal Free London Foundation NHS Trust, Pond Street, Hampstead, London NW3 2QG, UK
e-mail: m.keshtgar@ucl.ac.uk

Royal Free London Foundation Trust, The Breast Unit, University College London, Pond Street, Hampstead NW3 2QG, UK
e-mail: christine.williams13@nhs.net, m.keshtgar@ucl.ac.uk

10.2 Factors Affecting Cosmetic Outcome

The cosmetic effects of breast conservation therapy (lumpectomy plus radiotherapy, as an alternative to mastectomy) have been studied for decades (Harris et al. 1979). The evidence indicates that cosmetic outcome is the result of many factors, including those related to surgery (volume of tissue resected, type of surgery), radiotherapy (dose) and other factors (skin colour, age of patient) (Taylor et al. 1995). Pre-surgical psychological factors are also important, as demonstrated by a study of more than 200 women who had reconstructive breast surgery and were followed up for 2 years (Roth et al. 2007). Women who had a negative body image before surgery were more likely to be dissatisfied with the cosmetic outcome of surgery.

10.3 Evaluation of Cosmetic Outcome

The usual methods for evaluating cosmetic outcome are assessments made by the clinical care team, including the surgeon who performed the operation. Although this is an important source of feedback, such information is obviously biased and cannot be used reliably to compare techniques carried out by different clinicians, perhaps at different centres, using different techniques. Some researchers utilise a blinded assessment of outcome, usually by an independent panel examining

M. Keshtgar et al. (eds.), *Targeted Intraoperative Radiotherapy in Oncology*,
DOI 10.1007/978-3-642-39821-6_10, © Springer-Verlag Berlin Heidelberg 2014

photographs, but this is time consuming and too cumbersome to be used in routine practice.

From the patient's perspective, subjective assessment is, of course, unavoidable, and ideally should form a part of any cosmetic assessment.

10.4 Turning Subjective into Objective

Advances in surgery, oncoplasty and radiotherapy are happening regularly. Part of the assessment of the balance of risks and benefits must include an assessment of cosmetic outcome. Standard, reproducible evaluations are required, which should ideally be inexpensive and easy to use, and give meaningful results. This will ensure the data are both scientifically robust and important to the patient.

BCCT.core 2.0 (INESC Porto, Portugal; http://medicalresearch.inescporto.pt/breastresearch/index.php/BCCT.core) is a software application for the automated prediction of the aesthetic result of treatments for early breast cancer, and overcomes the drawbacks of subjective evaluation. The software algorithm is based on pattern recognition, validated on a dataset of digital photographs classified into four groups (excellent, good, fair, poor) by a panel of international experts, using established criteria. Objective features relevant to the aesthetic evaluation are as follows:

- Asymmetry

  Dimensionless. Breast retraction assessment (BRA), Lower breast contour (LBC), Upward nipple retraction (UNR), Breast compliance evaluation (BCE), Breast contour difference (BCD), Breast area difference (BAD)
- Colour

  Eight different indices portraying global colour dissimilarity.
- Scar

  Eight different indices based on localised colour differences.

See Fig. 10.1 for examples.

Although patient-reported outcome measures are increasingly used and quality of life is a key measure of clinical effectiveness, the measures used fall short of those required for evidence-based medicine. A review of 227 outcome studies for aesthetic and reconstructive breast surgery found only one study that was validated, specific and reproducible (Pusic et al. 2007). The use of objective measurement of the patient's perception and expectations is needed to assist in the development of accurate predictive tools to better enable clinicians and patients to choose the optimal treatment.

10.5 Experience from the TARGIT-A Trial

Data from 114 women over 50 years old participating in the TARGIT-A Trial (ISRCTN34086741) from one centre (Perth, Australia) were analysed. Frontal view digital photographs were assessed, blind to treatment, using BCCT.core. Data on patient and tumour characteristics were obtained from hospital notes. Statistical analysis was by generalised estimating equations on all data, and logistic regression analysis at year 1 only.

Photographs were taken at baseline (before surgery) and 1, 2, 3 and 4 years after initial breast-conserving surgery; none of the 114 patients had subsequent breast surgery. Median age at randomisation was 62 years (IQR 56–68). The composite scores were dichotomised into excellent and good (EG), and fair and poor (FP). There was a non-significant 45 % increase in the odds of having an outcome of EG for patients in the TARGIT group relative to the external beam radiotherapy (EBRT) group (OR = 1.45, 95%CI 0.78–2.69, $p = 0.245$) after adjusting for tumour size. The results were similar when adjusted for tumour grade and age of the patient. For year 1 there was a statistically significant 2.35-fold increase in the odds of having an outcome of EG for patients in the TARGIT group relative to the EBRT group (OR = 2.35, 95%CI 1.02–5.45, $p = 0.047$) after adjusting for age of the patient, tumour size and grade.

These results showed a significantly better cosmetic outcome with TARGIT compared to EBRT in the first year after surgery (Fig. 10.2) (Keshtgar et al. 2011).

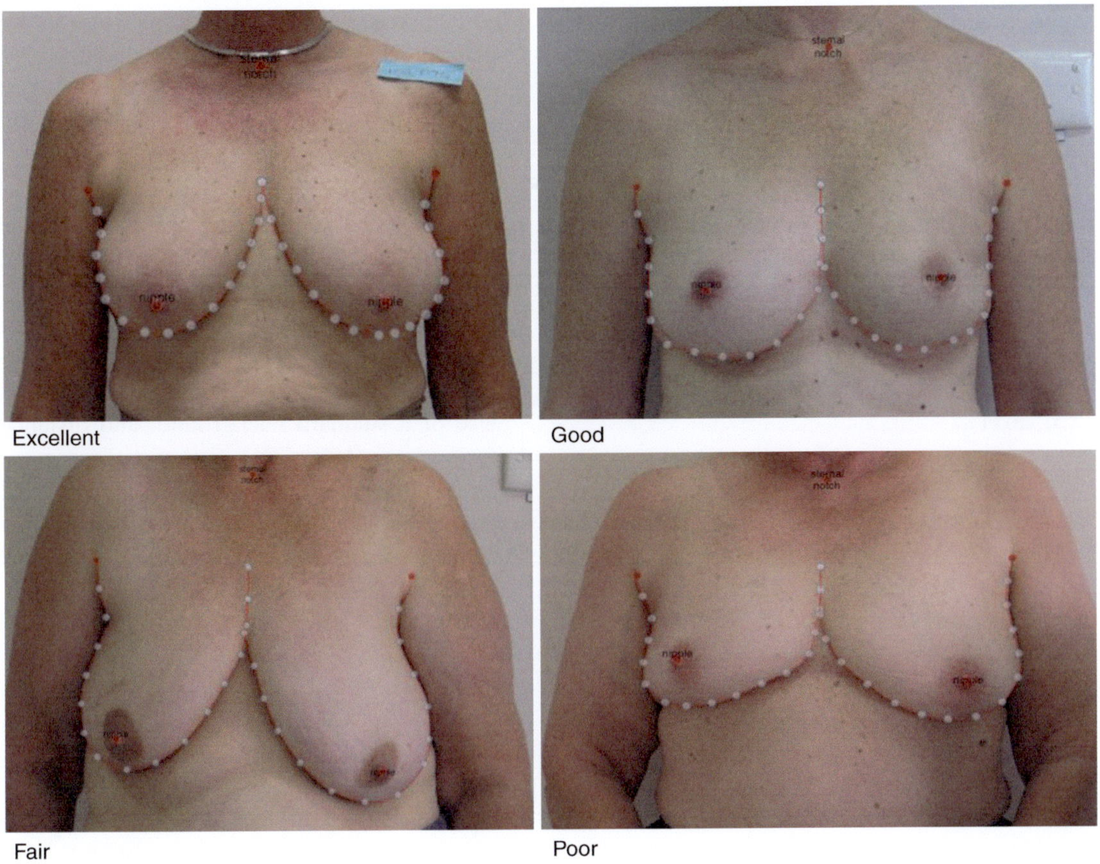

Fig. 10.1 Examples of assessment using BCCT.core

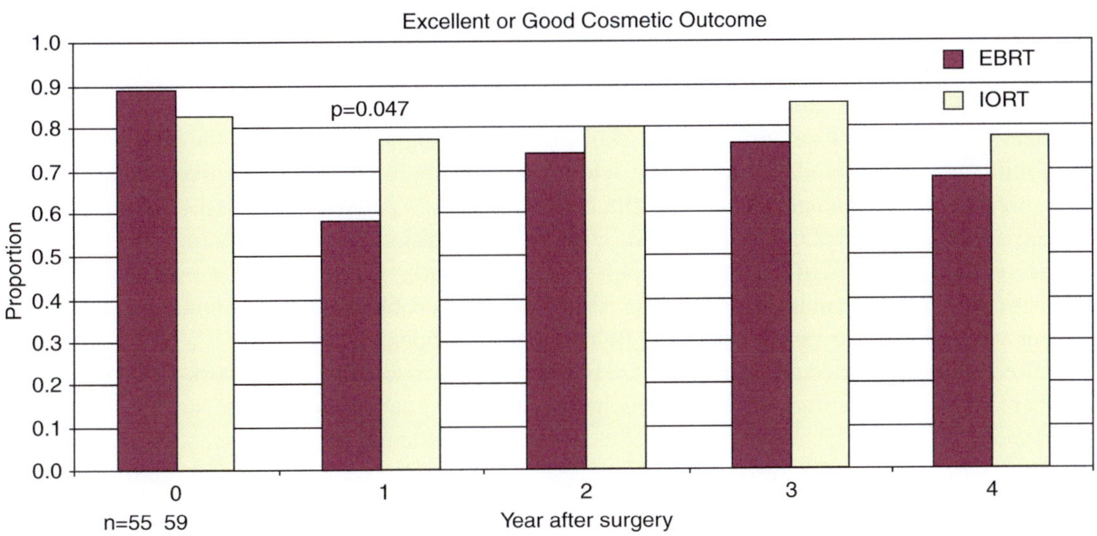

Fig. 10.2 Results from patients in the TARGIT trial

There are few published studies on the measurement of cosmesis after IORT. In the MSKCC Series (Sacchini et al. 2008), where quadrant IORT of 18–20 Gy was given, the cosmetic outcome was acceptable. In the Montpellier phase II trial (Lemanski et al. 2010) IORT was given as electrons (21 Gy). At a median follow-up of 30 months of 94 patients, all showed excellent or good cosmesis. In a study of IORT using Axxent, a balloon-based electronic brachytherapy (20 Gy), a median follow-up of 12 months of 11 patients showed excellent cosmesis in 10 (Ivanov et al. 2011).

10.6 Why Is TARGIT Better?

A more detailed analysis of the data provided by BCCT.core was used to measure the corresponding change in skin appearance in the treatment area. The colour histograms of the treated and untreated breasts were recorded in the CIE L*a*b* colour space. Like the more common RGB (red, green, blue) colour space, CIE L*a*b* is also a three-channel colour space, but more perceptually uniform. L* is the lightness, a* is the redness or greenness, and b* is yellowness or blueness. The histogram was computed for each channel individually (one-dimensional histograms) and over the complete colour space (3D histogram). The dissimilarity between corresponding histogram signatures of the two breasts were compared with the chi square statistic and Earth Mover's Distance (EMD) (Cardoso and Cardoso 2007). A significant change in skin appearance when measured in the a* channel, both with the chi square statistic and EMD, was observed, with higher values in the EBRT group. The effectiveness of the a* channel in capturing skin colour changes due to radiotherapy in BCCT has already been reported (Oliveira et al. 2010). Higher dissimilarity values in the a* channel correspond to higher changes in the redness/greenness of the skin. Therefore it seems that most of the difference between the TARGIT and EBRT groups was due to a reddening of the skin after EBRT.

10.7 Future Work

Further research is needed regarding the objective aesthetic evaluation of treatments for early breast cancer. Some of the challenges include:

- Incorporation of 3D techniques, not only to improve visualisation but also to make better use of volumetric estimations, for example breast size and volume of the tumour bed cavity
- Optimal use of lighting for the avoidance of shadows, enhancement of contrast and standardisation of colour balance
- Use of a standard background, and distance from camera to patient
- Determination of the best views (frontal and lateral, with possible inclusion of acute angles); stance of patient (standing or sitting, hands on hips or relaxed by side)
- Markings for reference, e.g. sternal notch, or inclusion of scales
- Data security and anonymisation of photographs by not including the face or identifying jewellery in the photograph, and non-identifiable labelling of digital files
- Optimal timing for image capture, e.g. the largest differences between EBRT and TARGIT appear to be within the first year
- Inclusion of an assessment of texture
- More information on the effect of baseline skin colour and texture; breast volume, size and shape
- Inclusion of assessments with patient wearing a bra and/or usual clothing
- Inclusion of assessments of treatment impacts on the sensation of the nipple and areola and the weight or position of the breast
- Development of objective measures of patient's perception and expectations

In addition, the clinical team must communicate clearly to the patient the expected result; tools to enable effective communication need to be developed.

There is clearly much work to be done. The ultimate goal is for clinical staff to be able to enable patients to make choices with better information so that they have a more realistic expectation of outcome, in an effort to minimise the impact of breast cancer treatments on their psychological well-being.

References

Cardoso JS, Cardoso MJ (2007) Towards an intelligent medical system for the aesthetic evaluation of breast cancer conservative treatment. Artif Intell Med 40:115–126

Chan LK (2010) Body image and the breast: the psychological wound. J Wound Care 19:133–134, 136, 138

Goin MK (1982) Psychological reactions to surgery of the breast. Clin Plast Surg 9:347–354

Goin MK, Goin JM (1988) Growing pains: the psychological experience of breast reconstruction with tissue expansion. Ann Plast Surg 21:217–222

Harris JR, Levene MB, Svensson G, Hellman S (1979) Analysis of cosmetic results following primary radiation therapy for stages I and II carcinoma of the breast. Int J Radiat Oncol Biol Phys 5:257–261

Ivanov O, Dickler A, Lum BY, Pellicane JV, Francescatti DS (2011) Twelve-month follow-up results of a trial utilizing Axxent electronic brachytherapy to deliver intraoperative radiation therapy for early-stage breast cancer. Ann Surg Oncol 18:453–458

Keshtgar M, Williams NR, Corica T, Saunders C, Joseph DJ, Bulsara MK et al (2011) Cosmetic outcome one, two, three and four years after intra-operative radiotherapy compared with external beam radiotherapy for early breast cancer: an objective assessment of patients from a randomised controlled trial. Breast 20:S63

Lemanski C, Azria D, Gourgon-Bourgade S, Gutowski M, Rouanet P, Saint-Aubert B et al (2010) Intraoperative radiotherapy in early-stage breast cancer: results of the Montpellier phase II trial. Int J Radiat Oncol Biol Phys 76:698–703

Oliveira HP, Magalhaes A, Cardoso MJ, Cardoso JS (2010) An accurate and interpretable model for BCCT.core. Conf Proc IEEE Eng Med Biol Soc 2010:6158–6161

Pusic AL, Chen CM, Cano S, Klassen A, McCarthy C, Collins ED et al (2007) Measuring quality of life in cosmetic and reconstructive breast surgery: a systematic review of patient-reported outcomes instruments. Plast Reconstr Surg 120:823–837

Roth RS, Lowery JC, Davis J, Wilkins EG (2007) Psychological factors predict patient satisfaction with postmastectomy breast reconstruction. Plast Reconstr Surg 119:2008–2015

Sacchini V, Beal K, Goldberg J, Montgomery L, Port E, McCormick B (2008) Study of quadrant high-dose intraoperative radiation therapy for early-stage breast cancer. Br J Surg 95:1105–1110

Taylor ME, Perez CA, Halverson KJ, Kuske RR, Philpott GW, Garcia DM et al (1995) Factors influencing cosmetic results after conservation therapy for breast cancer. Int J Radiat Oncol Biol Phys 31:753–764

Targeted Intraoperative Radiotherapy and Persistent Pain After Treatment

11

Kenneth Geving Andersen and Henrik Flyger

11.1 Introduction

Persistent pain has been established to be a significant problem following various surgical procedures (Kehlet et al. 2006; Aasvang et al. 2010; Wildgaard et al. 2009), including those used for breast cancer (Andersen and Kehlet 2011). Factors that may modify the risk of developing persistent pain are age, preoperative pain, nerve injury, acute postoperative pain, psychosocial factors, type of surgery, adjuvant treatment, type of analgesia and genetics; these are often divided into pre-, intra- and postoperative risk factors (Kehlet et al. 2006; Andersen and Kehlet 2011). A review of persistent pain following breast cancer treatment (PPBCT) has recently been published (Andersen and Kehlet 2011). This chapter discusses radiotherapy as a risk factor for the development of PPBCT, describes the results of a cross-sectional questionnaire study on PPBCT and examines avenues for further research.

K.G. Andersen, MD (✉)
Section for Surgical Pathophysiology, 7621, Rigshospitalet, Copenhagen University, Blegdamsvej 9, DK-2100 Copenhagen, Denmark

Department of Breast Surgery, Rigshospitalet, Copenhagen University, Copenhagen, Denmark
e-mail: kenneth.geving.andersen@rh.regionh.dk

H. Flyger, MD, PhD
Department of Breast Surgery, Herlev Hospital, Copenhagen University, Herlev Ringvej 75, DK-2730 Herlev, Denmark
e-mail: henrik.flyger@regionh.dk

11.2 Definition

The condition of pain following breast cancer treatment was formerly termed post-mastectomy pain syndrome (Andersen and Kehlet 2011), defined as a typical neuropathic pain with unpleasant sensations in the form of numbness, pins and needles, burning or stabbing. The pain is located in the axilla, arm, shoulder or chest wall on the side of surgery and may last more than 3 months after surgery (Smith et al. 1999). Jung et al. criticised this definition and proposed four distinct neuropathic pain syndromes (Jung et al. 2003). While neuropathic pain may be a prominent part of PPBCT, clear evidence for the pathogenic mechanisms is still missing from the literature (Andersen and Kehlet 2011). This, taken together with recent discussions on the definition of neuropathic pain (Haanpaa et al. 2011), argues for a more pragmatic definition of PPBCT. Radiation therapy and chemotherapy may induce various side-effects, such as chemotherapy-induced neuropathy (Jung et al. 2005), and pain occurring up to 3 months after surgery may be one of the accepted side-effects of adjuvant therapy. A more operational definition would take this into account and define PPBCT as pain 3 months or more after adjuvant therapy has ended, but such a definition has not been employed in any previous study. Thus, PPBCT in this chapter refers to patients with persistent pain at least 3 months after surgery.

M. Keshtgar et al. (eds.), *Targeted Intraoperative Radiotherapy in Oncology*,
DOI 10.1007/978-3-642-39821-6_11,

11.3 Prevalence

The nature of surgical and adjuvant treatment, as well as definition, measurement method and anatomical localisation, has influenced reporting of the prevalence of PPBCT. Studies using the post-mastectomy pain syndrome definition have reported the prevalence to be around 25 %, whereas studies using the conventional International Association for the Study of Pain definition, i.e. pain lasting for >3 months after surgery, report a prevalence of ca. 50 % across all treatments (Andersen and Kehlet 2011). A large Danish nationwide study, including 3,253 patients, divided patients into 12 well-defined treatment groups and found the prevalence to range from 25 % (in patients treated with mastectomy and sentinel lymph node biopsy without chemotherapy or radiation therapy) to 60 % (in patients treated with breast-conserving surgery, axillary lymph node dissection and a radiation field extending to the periclavicular lymph nodes) (Gärtner et al. 2009).

11.4 Radiotherapy as a Risk Factor for Persistent Pain

It has been shown that radiotherapy may cause neuropathy and neuropathic pain (Jung et al. 2005; Cross and Glantz 2003). It is also important to consider the extension of the radiation field as radiation to the axilla may cause brachial plexopathy. Current evidence tends to indicate that radiotherapy is a risk factor for PPBCT but findings are discrepant, with several studies reporting an association (Gärtner et al. 2009; Ishiyama et al. 2006; Kairaluoma et al. 2006; Peuckmann et al. 2009; Poleshuck et al. 2006; Tasmuth et al. 1995, 1997, 1999; Vilholm et al. 2008) but others finding no correlation (Fecho et al. 2009; Hack et al. 1999; Jud et al. 2010; Johansen et al. 2000). In explaining these discrepant findings, methodological issues must be considered (Andersen and Kehlet 2011).

Three studies, although not examining pain in detail, have investigated pain as an adverse effect in randomised trials. From the SWEBCG91-RT trial, it was shown that in patients treated with radiotherapy to residual breast tissue the relative risk of reporting pain in the breast occasionally was 1.80 (95%CI 1.26–2.57), while the relative risk of reporting pain in the breast on at least a weekly basis was 15.1 (95%CI 2.03–112) (Lundstedt et al. 2010). Hughes et al. reported that, compared with non-irradiated patients, significantly more patients treated with breast radiation therapy reported breast pain 2, 3 and 4 years after treatment (Hughes et al. 2004). A study from the Ontario Oncology Group found that significantly more irradiated patients reported troublesome pain in the breast 6 months later, but failed to observe any difference between irradiated and non-irradiated patients after 2 years (Whelan et al. 2000). The aforementioned three studies were, however, conducted in patients treated some years ago and may not reflect modern treatment regimens. In many other studies, timing and dosage regimens have not been well described, and thus it is difficult to draw conclusions (Andersen and Kehlet 2011).

11.5 How IORT May Be Beneficial in Relation to Persistent Pain, and Supporting Evidence

As stated above, a number of studies have suggested that radiotherapy is a risk factor for PPBCT, but the pathophysiological mechanisms responsible for persistent pain are unclear and have not been well documented in animal models (Bennett 2010). Pathophysiologically, persistent postsurgical pain is currently understood to be complex and to involve pre-, intra- and postoperative risk factors. Nerve injury is necessary but is not sufficient to cause persistent pain (Kehlet et al. 2006). Intraoperative radiotherapy (IORT) represents an interesting model to test the influence of radiotherapy on the development of PPBCT, as IORT limits the radiation field and thus the radiation exposure of nerves. To date, however, only one study has examined in detail the influence of IORT on persistent pain (Andersen et al. 2012). This was a cross-sectional questionnaire study in patients enrolled in the TARGIT-A (Vaidya et al. 2010) trial from the Copenhagen University Hospitals. The results of the study are summarised below.

11.5.1 Patients

Patients identified in the local TARGIT database from March 2007 to January 2010 were examined for eligibility. Inclusion criteria were: female sex, postmenopausal status with age 50 years or older, primary unifocal and unilateral breast cancer, T1, N0 [N0(i+) and N1(mi)], M0, oestrogen receptor-positive status confirmed by cytological or histological examination, suitability for breast-conserving surgery and availability for regular follow-up for at least 10 years. Exclusion criteria were: presence of bilateral breast cancer at the time of diagnosis, previous cancer in and/or irradiation to the ipsilateral breast, known presence of the BRCA2 gene mutation, lobular cancer or an extensive intraductal component (≥25 % of the tumour) and administration of primary medical treatments (hormones or chemotherapy). In addition, patients with previous contralateral breast surgery, local recurrence, metastatic disease, other cancer or axillary lymph node dissection were excluded to rule out any influence on pain measurement.

Randomisation was made by the TARGIT trial centre in London, UK. Patients were not blinded to treatment. In the present study, data provided from the local TARGIT database were blinded for the investigators. Data collection and analysis was undertaken at Rigshospitalet, Copenhagen, Denmark.

In the group that received IORT, the treatment was given as a secondary procedure.

11.5.2 Outcomes

The primary outcome was pain in the area of the operated breast, the side of the chest, the axilla or the arm. Secondary outcomes were: intensity and frequency of pain, pain in more than one area, use of analgesics, sensory disturbances and pain elsewhere. A detailed study questionnaire developed for a previous nationwide study of persistent pain and sensory disturbances was used (Gärtner et al. 2009). Questions addressing the prevalence of pain were dichotomous, requiring "yes" or "no" answers. Patients were then asked systematically to specify pain according to location (breast, side of the chest wall, axilla or arm) and to indicate its intensity on a 0–10 numerical rating scale (0=no pain, 10=worst imaginable pain). Frequency of pain was assessed on a three-point verbal categorical scale: (1) every day or almost every day, (2) 1–3 days a week or (3) more rarely. Treatment data were provided from the Danish Breast Cancer Cooperative Group (DBCG) and the TARGIT database.

11.5.3 Results

Eligible patients were screened from the local TARGIT database and ineligible patients discarded according to the above-mentioned exclusion criteria on the basis of registrations in the DBCG database. Questionnaires were sent out in April 2010 to a total of 244 eligible patients. Patients who had not responded after 1 month were sent a reminder. The response rate was 98 % (n=240). Two questionnaires were discarded due to incompleteness. There were no statistically significant differences between the IORT and the external beam radiotherapy (EBRT) group with respect to age, follow-up, disease characteristics or endocrine therapy (Table 11.1). All patients were treated with breast-conserving surgery and sentinel lymph node biopsy. No patients received axillary lymph node dissection or chemotherapy.

The prevalence of pain was 33.9 % in the EBRT group and 24.6 % in the IORT group ($p=0.11$) (Table 11.2). Pain localisation was similar in the two groups. Pain intensity was low for most patients and was not significantly different between the two groups: of the patients who experienced pain, 71 % in the EBRT group and 77 % in the IORT group scored 3 or lower on the numerical rating scale. As regards frequency of pain, 86.8 % of the patients reporting pain in the EBRT group said that they experienced pain on a

Table 11.1 Treatment characteristics in the EBRT and IORT groups (Andersen et al. 2012)

	EBRT	IORT	p (95 % CI)	Total
No. (%)	112 (47.1)	126 (52.9)		238
Non-responders	4	0		4
Age, years (mean)	65.74 (SD 6.17)	64.76 (SD 6.45)	0.23 (−0.64–2.60)	65.22 (SD 6.33)
Follow-up, months (mean)	17.06 (SD 10.39)	17.36 (10.64)	0.87	17.22 (SD 10.50)
Endocrine therapy, n (%)			0.28	
No ET	95 (84.8)	99 (79.4)		194 (81.9)
AI	17 (15.2)	26 (20.6)		43 (18.1)
TAM	0	0		0
Unknown	0	0		0
Tumour size, mm (mean)	10.75 (SD 3.59)	10.65 (SD 4.14)	0.85 (−0.91–1.12)	10.70 (SD 3.89)
Lymph nodes (mean)	2.32 (SD 1.44)	2.24 (SD 1.33)	0.67	2.28 (SD 1.38)
WHO, n (%)				
Invasive ductal	94 (83.9)	106 (84.1)		200 (84.0)
Invasive lobular	1 (0.9)	0		1 (0.4)
Mucinous	5 (4.5)	6 (4.8)		11 (4.6)
Medullary	0	0		0
Papillary	1 (0.9)	3 (2.4)		4 (1.7)
Tubular	5 (4.5)	8 (6.3)		13 (5.4)
Others	3 (2.7)	2 (1.6)		5 (2.1)
Unknown	3 (2.7)	1 (0.8)		4 (1.7)

EBRT external beam radiotherapy to the breast, *IORT* intraoperative radiotherapy, *ET* endocrine therapy, *AI* aromatase inhibitor, *TAM* tamoxifen

weekly basis or more often, versus 64.5 % of the IORT patients (p=0.044). The prevalence of pain elsewhere (outside the treatment area) was higher in the IORT group than in the EBRT group (40.7 % vs. 26.4 %) (p=0.027). The prevalence of sensory disturbances was similar in the two groups.

11.5.4 Discussion

The results of this randomised study suggest that treatment with IORT does not modify the risk of development of PPBCT compared with EBRT. In the EBRT group, 33.9 % of patients reported persistent pain in the breast area, side of the chest, axilla or arm, whereas in the IORT group 24.6 % reported pain in these areas (p=0.11). The OR for experiencing persistent pain was 1.57 (95 % CI 0.90–2.77) in the EBRT group compared with the IORT group, indicating that, with reasonable certainty, the treatment with IORT can be regarded to be as safe as EBRT in terms of PPBCT. A larger population will be required in order to investigate further the trend towards a positive effect of IORT on the prevalence of PPBCT and the frequency of pain. The prevalence of pain elsewhere was significantly higher in patients treated with TARGIT, but there is no pathophysiological explanation as to why IORT should produce more pain in general, given that pain elsewhere was described as headache, neck-shoulder pain and low-back pain. Such non-specific pain complaints in the joints and muscles are a common side-effect of aromatase inhibitors (Coleman et al. 2008), but the use of aromatase inhibitors in the two groups was similar. It is to be noted, however, that general pain complaints have previously been shown to be associated with a higher risk of PPBCT (Andersen and Kehlet 2011; Gärtner et al. 2009). Therefore it should be expected that TARGIT group had a

Table 11.2 Persistent pain after breast cancer treatment in the EBRT and IORT groups (Andersen et al. 2012)

	EBRT	IORT	p	Total
Reporting pain, n (%)	38 (33.9)	31 (24.6)	0.11	69 (29.0)
cont. OR (95 % CI)	1.57 (0.90–2.77)	1		
Localisation, n (%)				
Breast	31 (81.6)	26 (83.9)	0.80	57 (82.6)
Side of the chest	12 (31.6)	6 (19.4)	0.25	18 (26.1)
Axilla	19 (50.0)	12 (38.7)	0.35	31 (44.9)
Arm	5 (13.2)	7 (22.6)	0.30	12 (17.4)
Pain in more than 1 area, n (%)	21 (55.3)	15 (48.4)	0.57	36 (52.2)
NRS (median, IQR)				
Worst (overall)[a]	3 (2)	3 (1)	0.87	
Breast	2 (1)	3 (1)	0.98	
Side of the chest	2,5 (3)	2 (2)	1.00	
Axilla	2 (2)	2 (2)	0.69	
Arm	5 (6)	4 (4)	0.68	
Worst pain, n (%)[b]			0.59	
Light pain	27 (71.0)	24 (77.4)		51 (73.9)
Moderate pain	10 (26.3)	7 (22.6)		17 (24.6)
Severe pain	1 (2.6)	0		1 (1.4)
Frequency of worst pain, n (%)			0.090	
Daily	19 (50.0)	11 (35.5)		30 (43.5)
1–3 day/week	14 (36.8)	9 (29.0)		23 (33.3)
Less	5 (13.2)	11 (35.5)		16 (23.2)
Use of analgesics, n (%)	6 (15.8)	5 (16.1)	0.97	11 (15.9)
Consulting doctor, n (%)	5 (13.2)	3 (9.7)	0.65	8 (11.6)
Sensory disturbances, n (%)[c]	27 (23.2)	26 (20.6)	0.75	53 (21.8)
Pain in other locations, n (%)[d]	28 (26.4)	48 (40.7)	0.02	76 33.9)

NRS Numerical rating scale
[a]Worst pain rating across all measured localisations
[b]Worst pain across all measured localisations; light pain: NRS 1–3; moderate pain: NRS 4–7; severe pain: NRS 8–10
[c]Missing data on three patients: 1 in the EBRT group and 2 in the IORT group
[d]Missing data on 14 patients: 6 in the EBRT group and 8 in the IORT group

higher prevalence of PPCBT, while the opposite was found. Only 20 % of the patients received adjuvant endocrine therapy due to the inclusion of only patients with low-risk breast cancer. The nature of the TARGIT treatment precluded a blinding of patients, and may have introduced bias in the IORT population. However, the higher prevalence of pain elsewhere argues against this. The intensity of treatment-related pain in the two treatment groups was similar, with most patients experiencing light pain. The frequency of pain was high, with most patients experiencing pain on a weekly basis. The fact that patients treated with EBRT experienced pain more frequently (p=0.044) suggests a favourable effect of TARGIT.

As stated above, the pathophysiological background for the increased risk of PPBCT with radiation therapy is yet to be described. While with TARGIT the smaller radiation field may be expected to reduce harm to nerves (as the radiation is focussed on breast tissue), we observed the frequency of sensory disturbances to be similar, at about 22 %, in the two groups; this is somewhat lower than the prevalence of 31 % detected in a comparable population in the study by Gärtner et al. (2009). This discrepancy may be attributable to the fact that the present cohort comprised an older population and had a shorter follow-up time, 17 months versus 26 months. The late effects of radiotherapy are reported to accumulate with time (Bajrovic et al. 2004).

11.6 Directions for Future Research

Research in this field is challenging owing to incomplete understanding of the relative role of the different pathogenic mechanisms underlying PPBCT (Andersen and Kehlet 2011). Further research into persistent pain after treatment with IORT should focus on pain measurement. This should be done according to the recommendations by the "Initiative in Methods, Measurement, and Pain Assessment in Clinical Trials" (IMMPACT) (Dworkin et al. 2005), with emphasis on pain on movement as well as the consequences of pain for physical function (Srikandarajah and Gilron 2011). Questionnaires should be specific to the breast cancer population to improve comparability within the population, and to define the specific functional and psychosocial consequences of PPBCT. Suggestions on how to design a study of PPBCT have been further described in a review (Andersen and Kehlet 2011).

11.7 Summary

Persistent pain after breast cancer treatment is a significant clinical problem and affects between 25 and 60 % of patients, depending on treatment. The complex pathophysiology involves several pre-, intra- and postoperative risk factors, including young age, extensive surgery in the axilla and radiation therapy. IORT does not increase the prevalence of PPBCT compared with EBRT. The trend towards a positive effect of IORT with regard to frequency of pain warrants a larger trial to clarify the potential benefit of IORT.

Acknowledgements This work was funded by the Danish Cancer Society and the research leading to these results is part of the European Collaboration, which has received support from the Innovative Medicines Initiative Joint Undertaking under grant agreement no 115007, the resources of which are composed of a financial contribution from the European Union's Seventh Framework Programme (FP7/2007–2013) and an in kind contribution from EFPIA companies.

The authors declare no conflict of interests.

References

Aasvang EK, Gmaehle E, Hansen JB, Gmaehle B, Forman JL, Schwarz J et al (2010) Predictive risk factors for persistent postherniotomy pain. Anesthesiology 112:957–969

Andersen KG, Kehlet H (2011) Persistent pain after breast cancer treatment: a critical review of risk factors and strategies for prevention. J Pain 12:725–746

Andersen KG, Gartner R, Kroman N, Flyger H, Kehlet H (2012) Persistent pain after targeted intraoperative radiotherapy (TARGIT) or external breast radiotherapy for breast cancer: a randomized trial. Breast 21:46–49

Bajrovic A, Rades D, Fehlauer F, Tribius S, Hoeller U, Rudat V et al (2004) Is there a life-long risk of brachial plexopathy after radiotherapy of supraclavicular lymph nodes in breast cancer patients? Radiother Oncol 71:297–301

Bennett GJ (2010) Pathophysiology and animal models of cancer-related painful peripheral neuropathy. Oncologist 15(Suppl 2):9–12

Coleman RE, Bolten WW, Lansdown M, Dale S, Jackisch C, Merkel D et al (2008) Aromatase inhibitor-induced arthralgia: clinical experience and treatment recommendations. Cancer Treat Rev 34:275–282

Cross NE, Glantz MJ (2003) Neurologic complications of radiation therapy. Neurol Clin 21:249–277

Dworkin RH, Turk DC, Farrar JT, Haythornthwaite JA, Jensen MP, Katz NP et al (2005) Core outcome measures for chronic pain clinical trials: IMMPACT recommendations. Pain 113:9–19

Fecho K, Miller NR, Merritt SA, Klauber-Demore N, Hultman CS, Blau WS (2009) Acute and persistent postoperative pain after breast surgery. Pain Med 10:708–715

Gärtner R, Jensen MB, Nielsen J, Ewertz M, Kroman N, Kehlet H (2009) Prevalence of and factors associated with persistent pain following breast cancer surgery. JAMA 302:1985–1992

Haanpaa M, Attal N, Backonja M, Baron R, Bennett M, Bouhassira D et al (2011) NeuPSIG guidelines on neuropathic pain assessment. Pain 152:14–27

Hack TF, Cohen L, Katz J, Robson LS, Goss P (1999) Physical and psychological morbidity after axillary lymph node dissection for breast cancer. J Clin Oncol 17:143–149

Hughes KS, Schnaper LA, Berry D, Cirrincione C, McCormick B, Shank B et al (2004) Lumpectomy plus tamoxifen with or without irradiation in women 70 years of age or older with early breast cancer. N Engl J Med 351:971–977

Ishiyama H, Niino K, Hosoya T, Hayakawa K (2006) Results of a questionnaire survey for symptom of late complications caused by radiotherapy in breast conserving therapy. Breast Cancer 13:197–201

Johansen J, Overgaard J, Blichert-Toft M, Overgaard M (2000) Treatment of morbidity associated with the management of the axilla in breast-conserving therapy. Acta Oncol 39:349–354

Jud SM, Fasching PA, Maihofner C, Heusinger K, Loehberg CR, Hatko R et al (2010) Pain perception and detailed visual pain mapping in breast cancer survivors. Breast Cancer Res Treat 119:105–110

Jung BF, Ahrendt GM, Oaklander AL, Dworkin RH (2003) Neuropathic pain following breast cancer surgery: proposed classification and research update. Pain 104:1–13

Jung BF, Herrmann D, Griggs J, Oaklander AL, Dworkin RH (2005) Neuropathic pain associated with nonsurgical treatment of breast cancer. Pain 118:10–14

Kairaluoma PM, Bachmann MS, Rosenberg PH, Pere PJ (2006) Preincisional paravertebral block reduces the prevalence of chronic pain after breast surgery. Anesth Analg 103:703–708

Kehlet H, Jensen TS, Woolf CJ (2006) Persistent postsurgical pain: risk factors and prevention. Lancet 367:1618–1625

Lundstedt D, Gustafsson M, Malmstrom P, Johansson KA, Alsadius D, Sundberg A et al (2010) Symptoms 10–17 years after breast cancer radiotherapy data from the randomised SWEBCG91-RT trial. Radiother Oncol 97:281–287

Peuckmann V, Ekholm O, Rasmussen NK, Groenvold M, Christiansen P, Møller S et al (2009) Chronic pain and other sequelae in long-term breast cancer survivors: nationwide survey in Denmark. Eur J Pain 13:478–485

Poleshuck EL, Katz J, Andrus CH, Hogan LA, Jung BF, Kulick DI, Dworkin RH (2006) Risk factors for chronic pain following breast cancer surgery: a prospective study. J Pain 7:626–634

Smith WC, Bourne D, Squair J, Phillips DO, Chambers WA (1999) A retrospective cohort study of post mastectomy pain syndrome. Pain 83:91–95

Srikandarajah S, Gilron I (2011) Systematic review of movement-evoked pain versus pain at rest in postsurgical clinical trials and meta-analyses: a fundamental distinction requiring standardized measurement. Pain 152(8):1734–1739

Tasmuth T, von Smitten K, Hietanen P, Kataja M, Kalso E (1995) Pain and other symptoms after different treatment modalities of breast cancer. Ann Oncol 6:453–459

Tasmuth T, Kataja M, Blomqvist C, von Smitten K, Kalso E (1997) Treatment-related factors predisposing to chronic pain in patients with breast cancer – a multivariate approach. Acta Oncol 36:625–630

Tasmuth T, Blomqvist C, Kalso E (1999) Chronic post-treatment symptoms in patients with breast cancer operated in different surgical units. Eur J Surg Oncol 25:38–43

Vaidya JS, Joseph DJ, Tobias JS, Bulsara M, Wenz F, Saunders C et al (2010) Targeted intraoperative radiotherapy versus whole breast radiotherapy for breast cancer (TARGIT-A trial): an international, prospective, randomised, non-inferiority phase 3 trial. Lancet 376:91–102

Vilholm OJ, Cold S, Rasmussen L, Sindrup SH (2008) The postmastectomy pain syndrome: an epidemiological study on the prevalence of chronic pain after surgery for breast cancer. Br J Cancer 99:604–610

Whelan TJ, Levine M, Julian J, Kirkbride P, Skingley P (2000) The effects of radiation therapy on quality of life of women with breast carcinoma: results of a randomized trial. Ontario Clinical Oncology Group. Cancer 88:2260–2266

Wildgaard K, Ravn J, Kehlet H (2009) Chronic post-thoracotomy pain: a critical review of pathogenic mechanisms and strategies for prevention. Eur J Cardiothorac Surg 36:170–180

12 Other Applications of INTRABEAM®

Tina Reis, Elena Sperk, Yasser Abo-Madyan, Michael Ehmann, Frederic Bludau, and Frederik Wenz

12.1 Introduction

Intraoperative radiotherapy (IORT) permits the delivery of a high radiation dose directly to the residual tumour or tumour bed while sparing nearby normal tissues. In most cases, IORT with the INTRABEAM® system is employed as a part of multimodal treatment, with the aim of providing an additional benefit in terms of prevention of local recurrence. IORT is used to treat many tumours, the most common being:

- locally advanced or recurrent colorectal cancer
- soft tissue sarcomas
- stomach and pancreatic cancers
- primary or recurrent gynaecological cancers
- head and neck tumours

New fields of application are the treatment of symptomatic vertebral metastases, for which purpose IORT is employed in combination with balloon kyphoplasty ("kypho-IORT"), and intravaginal X-ray brachytherapy. A variety of applicators have been designed for the different treatments (Fig. 12.1).

12.2 Surgical Applications

Between January 2008 and July 2011, a total of 223 IORT procedures were performed in Mannheim, including 150 in patients with breast cancer and 73 in those undergoing surgery for other cancers (Fig. 12.2). After IORT for breast cancer, the most frequent procedures were kypho-IORT (30 cases) and IORT for sarcomas and recurrent rectal cancer (25 and 11 cases, respectively).

Sarcomas are rare cancers, accounting for only 1–3 % of all cancers. They are a very heterogeneous group of tumours, roughly divided into bone and soft tissue sarcomas. Soft tissue sarcomas are the largest subgroup and most often arise in the extremities and trunk. The mainstay of treatment is surgery. Nevertheless, the management of soft tissue sarcoma has evolved from solely surgical treatment to an interdisciplinary multimodal approach including surgery, chemotherapy and

T. Reis (✉) • M. Ehmann • E. Sperk • F. Wenz
Department of Radiation Oncology,
University Medical Center Mannheim,
University of Heidelberg, Theodor-Kutzer-Ufer 1-3,
D-68167 Mannheim, Germany
e-mail: tina.reis@umm.de;
michael.ehmann@umm.de, http://www.umm.de;
elena.sperk@umm.de, http://www.umm.de;
frederik.wenz@medma.uni-heidelberg.de,
frederik.wenz@umm.de, http://www.umm.de

Y. Abo-Madyan
Department of Radiation Oncology,
University Medical Centre Mannheim,
University of Heidelberg, Theodor-Kutzer-Ufer 1-3,
D-68167 Mannheim, Germany

Department of Clinical Oncology and Nuclear
Medicine (NEMROCK), Faculty of Medicine,
Cairo University, Cairo, Egypt
e-mail: yasser.abomadyan@umm.de, http://www.umm.de

F. Bludau
Department of Orthopaedic and Trauma Surgery,
University Medical Centre Mannheim,
University of Heidelberg, Theodor-Kutzer-Ufer 1-3,
D-68167 Mannheim, Germany

M. Keshtgar et al. (eds.), *Targeted Intraoperative Radiotherapy in Oncology*,
DOI 10.1007/978-3-642-39821-6_12, © Springer-Verlag Berlin Heidelberg 2014

Fig. 12.1 Various (spherical, needle, cylindrical) applicators for the INTRABEAM system

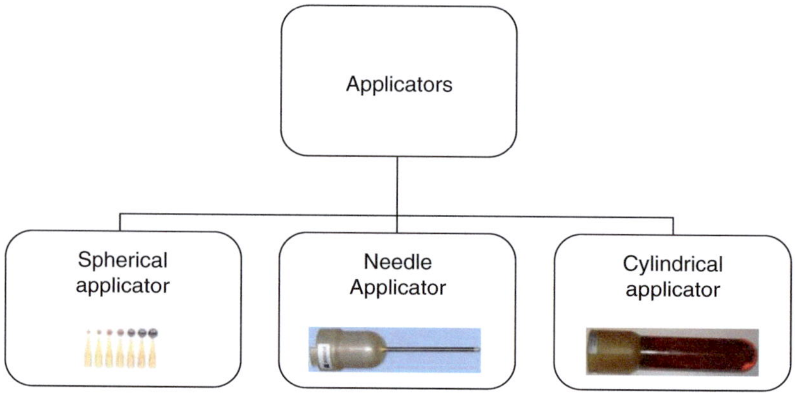

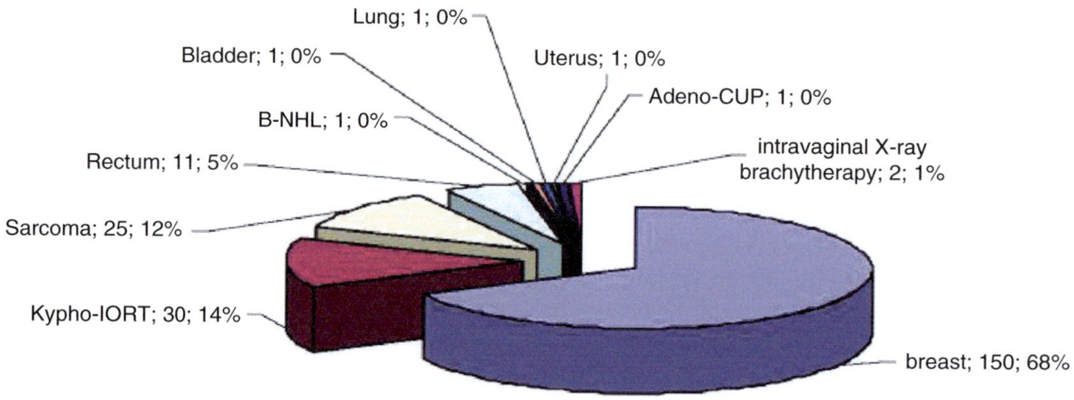

Fig. 12.2 IORT in Mannheim between January 2008 and July 2011

radiotherapy. External beam radiotherapy (EBRT) applied pre- or postoperatively improves the probability of local control and results in cure rates that are comparable to those achieved with more extensive resections or amputations (Rosenberg et al. 1982). IORT alone or followed by postoperative EBRT is also a reasonable radiotherapy treatment option. Lehnert et al. (2000) observed a 40 % reduction in local recurrence after IORT in patients with soft tissue sarcomas of the extremities, the trunk or the retroperitoneum in comparison with patients treated with surgery alone. One randomised study, by Sindelar et al. (1993), compared combined IORT and postoperative EBRT versus EBRT alone and observed a local recurrence rate of 40 % versus 80 % without any difference in overall survival after 5 years.

Among the 25 patients with sarcoma who we treated with IORT, one was an 80-year-old with a recurrent liposarcoma of the retroperitoneum. The initial diagnosis of retroperitoneal liposarcoma had been made 6 years previously. The patient initially underwent tumour resection without adjuvant therapy. After diagnosis of relapse, preoperative EBRT was first administered. Due to a lack of response, EBRT was stopped after 27 Gy and a wide excision with IORT in the field of the residual tumour (applicator size 5 cm; dose 12 Gy at the applicator surface) was performed (Fig. 12.3).

Another example was a 56-year-old patient with a high-grade sarcoma of the right thigh. In this case, multimodal treatment was delivered. The patient first underwent a wide excision with IORT (applicator size 5 cm; dose 5 Gy), followed by EBRT with 60 Gy (Fig. 12.4).

The incidence of rectal cancer is 15–25 cases per 100,000 inhabitants. Preoperative radiochemotherapy followed by surgery by means of improved techniques has become the standard of

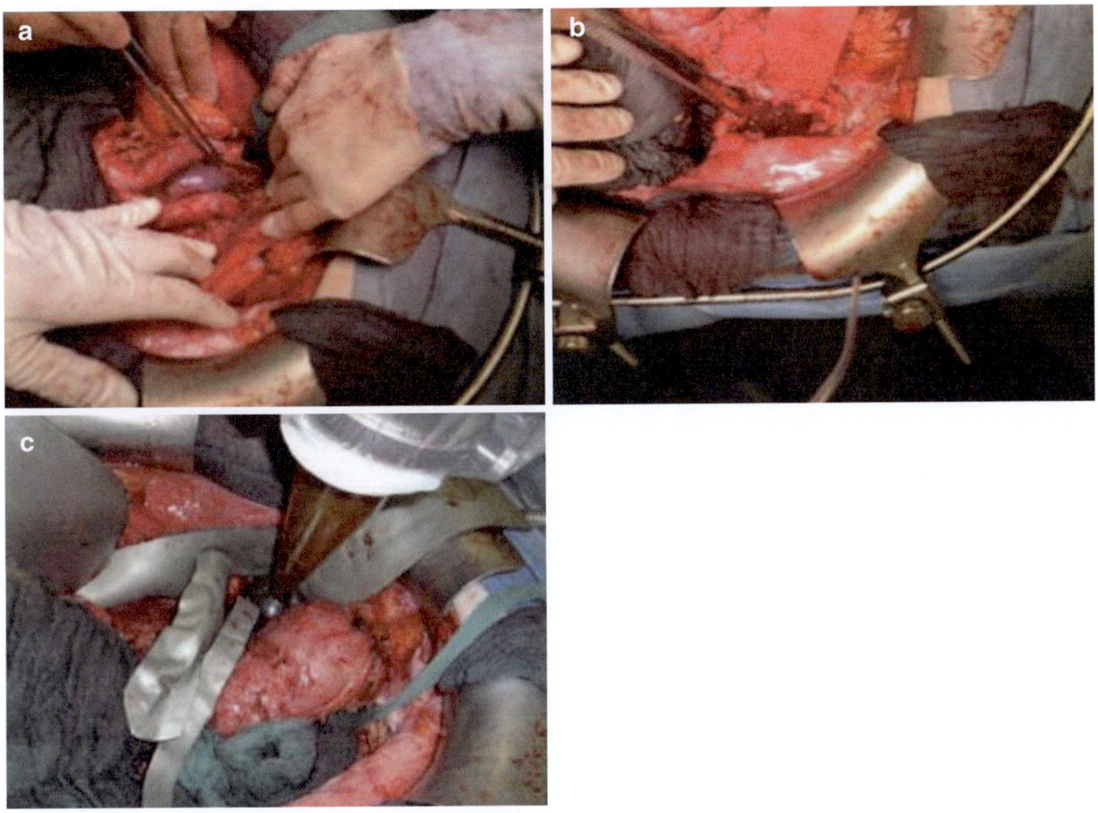

Fig. 12.3 (**a**, **b**) Retroperitoneal operating field after wide excision of a relapsed liposarcoma. (**c**) Positioning of the spherical applicator within the range of the microscopic residual tumour (R1)

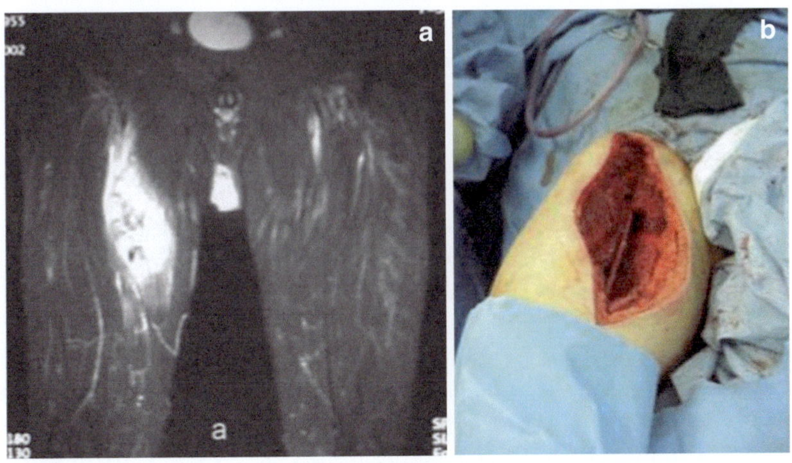

Fig. 12.4 (**a**) Preoperative coronal MRI showing a high-grade sarcoma of the right thigh. (**b**) Wound after resection of the tumour, before insertion of the applicator

care for locally advanced tumours because of improved local control and the effect of downsizing/-staging (Ferenschild et al. 2006). Recurrent rectal cancer, however, remains a very serious problem. Between 3 and 15 % of patients develop a local relapse, and without treatment the median overall survival for patients with recurrent rectal cancer is only 6 months (McDermott et al. 1985; Welch and Donaldson 1978). A particular challenge is posed by previously irradiated patients, because the required high dose cannot be administered again. Moreover, resection margin involvement has been demonstrated to be the most important prognostic factor in patients undergoing surgery for recurrent rectal cancer, but the likelihood of negative margins after resection is low.

Valentini et al. (2006) reported results of treatment with EBRT and concurrent chemotherapy with or without salvage surgery in 59 patients with previously irradiated recurrent rectal cancer. Median dosage was 30 Gy followed by a boost of 10.8 Gy (1.2 Gy twice daily with a minimum 6-h interval). During the radiation treatment, concurrent chemotherapy was delivered (5-fluorouracil, protracted intravenous infusion, 225 mg/m^2/day, 7 days per week). The overall 5-year survival was 39 %. Another treatment option for previously irradiated patients with local relapse is surgery combined with IORT. Suzuki et al. (1995) described the outcome of 106 patients who underwent palliative resection of locally relapsed disease. Forty-two patients received IORT as a component of treatment (mostly 15–20 Gy) and 41 received EBRT (mostly 45 Gy). Patients receiving IORT had a 5-year survival rate of 19 %, compared with 7 % among those without IORT. An updated Mayo Clinic analysis (Haddock et al. 2001) described 175 patients with locally recurrent colorectal cancer (123 without and 52 with prior EBRT) who underwent IORT. Five-year survival in previously irradiated patients was 12 %. The 3-year local control rate for the same group was 51 %.

Between January 2008 and July 2011, 11 patients at our centre received IORT for the treatment of recurrent rectal cancer. Figure 12.5 shows the intraoperative setting in a 73-year-old patient with metastasised rectal cancer with infiltration of the bladder and the anal skin after initial abdominoperineal rectum extirpation in 2002. A transanal excision was performed in combination with IORT (dose 4 Gy to a tissue depth of 5 mm, applicator size 4 cm) as well as a radical cystectomy. In the future a flat applicator will be available for treatment of rectal cancer recurrences while sparing the surrounding tissue. The flat design of the new applicator will allow irradiation to a depth of 0.1–1.0 cm without scattering dose to the surrounding organs at risk.

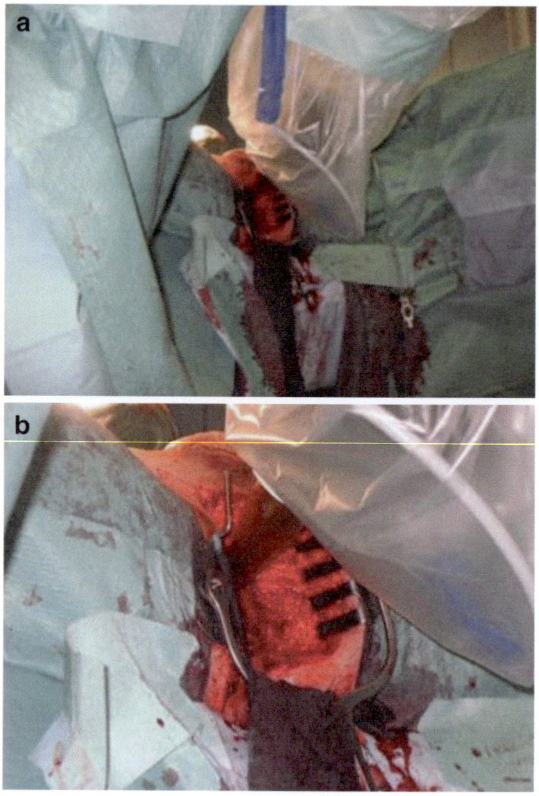

Fig. 12.5 (**a**, **b**) IORT after transanal excision and radical cystectomy with the positioned applicator inside the operative field (dose 4 Gy in a tissue depth of 5 mm, applicator size 4 cm)

All our experience in use of IORT with the INTRABEAM system for the treatment of recurrent rectal cancer or sarcomas concerns individual cases. As yet, no clinical trials have been performed on IORT in such patients.

12.3 Kypho-IORT – IORT During Kyphoplasty

12.3.1 Indications

The skeletal system is the most common site of metastases, being affected in up to 30 % of all cancer patients (Hage et al. 2000). The leading focus is the vertebral column with an incidence of 30–70 % (Wong et al. 1990; Boland et al. 1982;

Harrington 1986). Most patients (70–90 %) suffer from severe axial pain. Besides this, vertebral metastases can cause pathological fracture and neurological dysfunction by spinal cord compression (Janjan 1997; Gilbert et al. 1978; Smith et al. 2000). Although the median overall survival of patients with advanced cancer is limited, the survival time of patients with bone metastases varies depending on the primary tumour. Therefore it is necessary to optimise the palliative treatment to achieve a high quality of life.

For patients with spinal metastases but without spinal cord compression and pain or impeding or existing instability, surgery and external beam radiotherapy (EBRT) are frequently used treatment options. Furthermore, it is well established that decompressive surgery with adjuvant radiotherapy exerts analgesic effects with good local tumour control in patients with painful spinal metastases (Moulding et al. 2010; Gerszten et al. 2009; van der Linden et al. 2006). Nevertheless, pain relief takes weeks and structural stability, months. For patients with pathological fracture or vertebrae prone to fracture without epidural compression, minimally invasive surgical techniques like kyphoplasty or vertebroplasty have been shown to yield pain reduction and sufficient stabilisation (Halpin et al. 2004; Garfin et al. 2001). However these surgical therapies have no anticancer effect and postoperative radiotherapy is necessary to prevent early regrowth. Disadvantages of this combined therapy include the long treatment period, typically 1–4 weeks, which is often associated with mental and physical strain; in addition, chemotherapy and fractionated radiotherapy are typically not applied simultaneously owing to increased side-effects.

The combination of kyphoplasty and a single dose of IORT (kypho-IORT) attains sufficient stability under sterilisation of the metastasis and reduction of treatment time. Kypho-IORT could therefore be an interesting therapeutic option in the palliative setting. Patients with oligometastases who meet the following eligibility criteria can be considered suitable for kypho-IORT: (a) pathologically or cytologically proven primary tumour; (b) painful or unstable lesions between T4/5 and L5 and (c) Karnofsky index ≥60 %. Our recently published findings (Schneider et al. 2011) indicate that up to one-third of patients with spinal metastases meet these criteria. Simultaneous visceral metastases do not represent an exclusion criterion, but patients with primary bone tumours, soft tissue extension and epidural or intraspinal invasion are excluded. Prior to kypho-IORT, all patients should undergo a physical examination and a CT or MRI scan to evaluate the extension of the metastases.

12.3.2 Physical and Technical Aspects

Prior to the first clinical application, kypho-IORT was performed in a donated body in order to estimate the delivered doses in the surrounding tissue. Two ionisation chambers, one beside the vertebra and one in the spinal cord, were used (Schneider et al. 2011). Measurements revealed a maximum dose of 3.8 Gy in the spinal cord and a dose of 0.2 Gy adjacent to the vertebra. Examples of dose distributions depending on the position of the radiation source are shown in Fig. 12.6.

The procedure of balloon kyphoplasty (Medtronic, Kypho, Minnesota, USA) is done according to standard kyphoplasty with minor

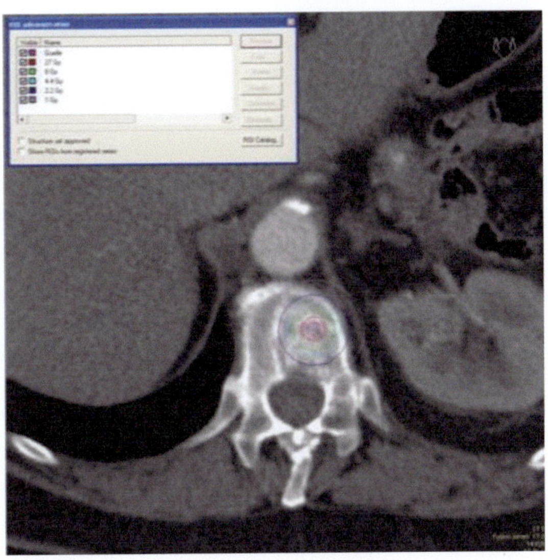

Fig. 12.6 Approximate dose distribution

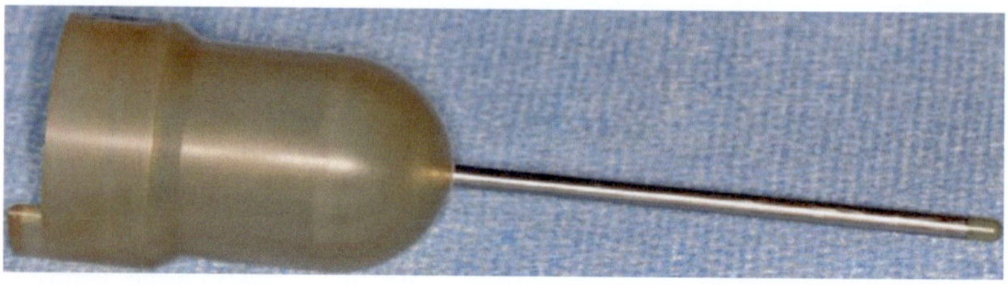

Fig. 12.7 Specially designed needle applicator for kypho-IORT

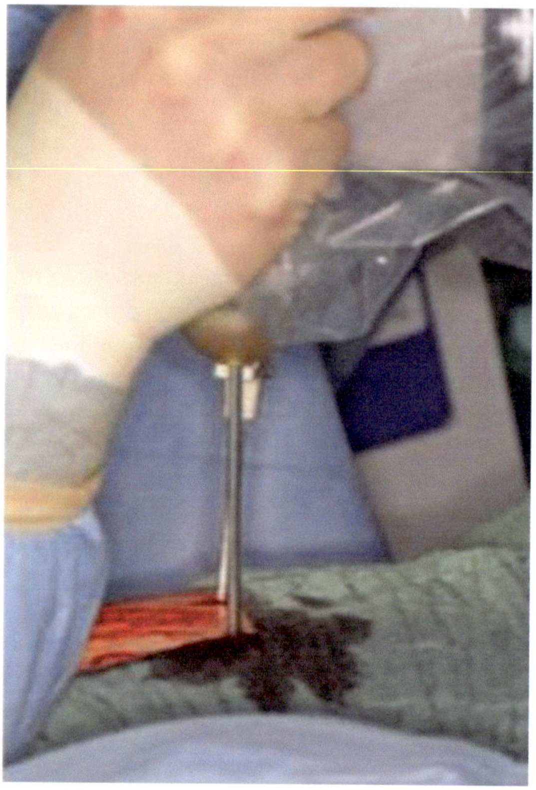

Fig. 12.8 Insertion of the applicator, including the drift tube, into the metallic sleeves

modifications. All patients are placed in the prone position on a radiolucent table under general anaesthesia. After sterile preparation, the Kirschner wire is inserted; this is followed by application of the working cannula, with a metallic sleeve designed especially for kypho-IORT, which is positioned in the pedicle. After removal of the working cannula, a drill is inserted to create a tract into the vertebra.

To permit use of the INTRABEAM system for kyphoplasty, a specially designed applicator was developed. This applicator (4.1 mm diameter) consists of a stainless steel tube with a tip made of plastic and a plastic head, which is necessary to adapt it to the X-ray source of the INTRABEAM system (Fig. 12.7). The steel tube of the applicator protects the sensitive probe from bending and the plastic tip minimises the absorption.

After removing the burr, the applicator, including the drift tube of the INTRABEAM, is guided through the specially designed metallic sleeve (5 mm diameter, 6 cm length) into the vertebral body (Fig. 12.8). For verification of the correct position of the guiding sleeve and the applicator, biplanar X-rays are used. A single radiation dose of 8 Gy in 10 mm is delivered during 2 min to the centre of the metastasis (Fig. 12.9). After application of radiation, the INTRABEAM system is removed and the working cannula is again inserted while the metallic sleeve remains in place to avoid reflow of the cement. Further steps of kyphoplasty conform to standard kyphoplasty, with inflation and deflation of the balloon followed by cement injection (Fig. 12.10).

12.3.3 First Clinical Results

In July 2009 we started a pilot phase as preparation for a phase II dose escalation study. Eighteen eligible patients with spinal metastases were enrolled, with a total of 21 vertebral lesions. The median surgical time was 70 min (range, 53–173), including 2 min for IORT. No technical problems appeared during the treatment of the seven lumbar lesions. During treatment of thoracic lesions, bending of the drift tube occurred in two of the first nine cases (22 %) and IORT could not be completed. After additional modification of the sleeves, bending of the drift tube was seen in only one of 12 further treated vertebrae (8 %). As postoperative EBRT can be administered in

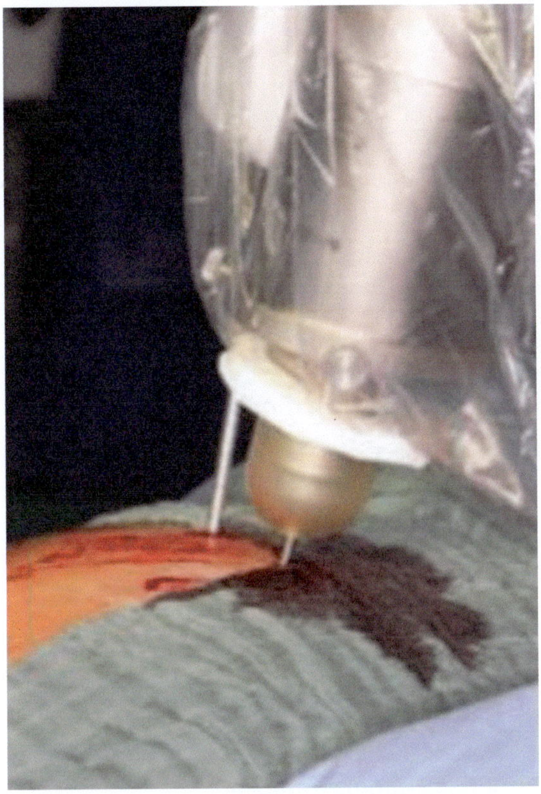

Fig. 12.9 Applicator positioned in the metallic sleeve for IORT (8 Gy at 5 mm distance from the applicator surface)

patients in whom such bending occurs, there are no negative effects for the patients.

No severe intra- or postoperative complications were seen. In particular, no procedure-related neurological dysfunction occurred. In some patients, asymptomatic paravertebral cement leakage was observed.

Median follow-up duration was 4.5 months (range, 1–10 months). The 4-month overall survival rate for all 18 patients was 80 %, and the 6-month overall survival rate was 67 %.

A clinical evaluation of pain experienced preoperatively and 1 day and 6 weeks postoperatively was available for 11 patients. Median VAS back pain decreased from 5/10 preoperatively to 2.5/10 on the first postoperative day and to 0/10 6 weeks after kypho-IORT (Fig. 12.11). This outcome was accompanied by a clear reduction in pain medication (67 % of cases preoperatively vs. 30 % postoperatively).

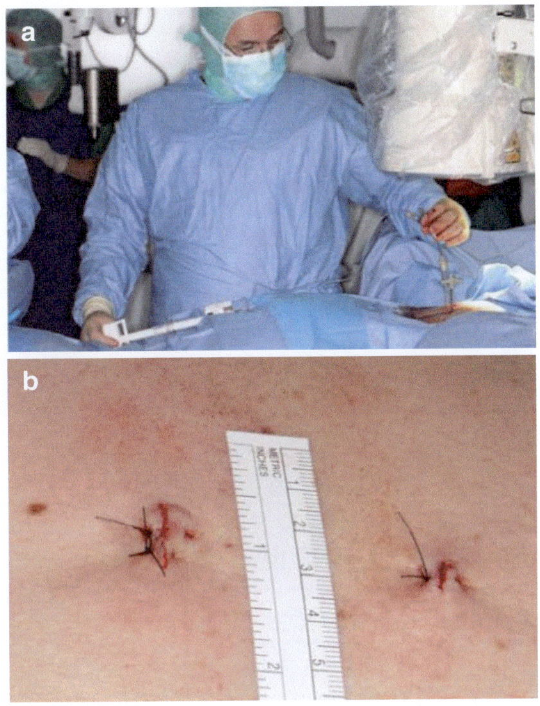

Fig. 12.10 (**a**) Cement injection after inflation and deflation of the kyphoplasty balloon; (**b**) wound after closing

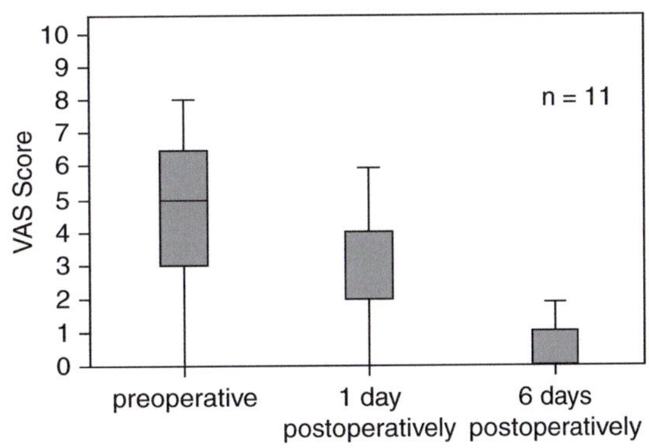

Fig. 12.11 Visual analogue scale (*VAS*) score of back pain preoperatively and 1 day and 6 weeks after kypho-IORT

Serial imaging studies (CT, MRI) were available for 15 of the 18 patients. Stable disease within the irradiated vertebral body was seen in 14 (93 %) patients (Fig. 12.12), while local progressive disease was seen in only one (7 %), 6 weeks after kypho-IORT. This patient underwent re-operation and postoperative EBRT 10 months after kypho-IORT due to progressive pain and neurological

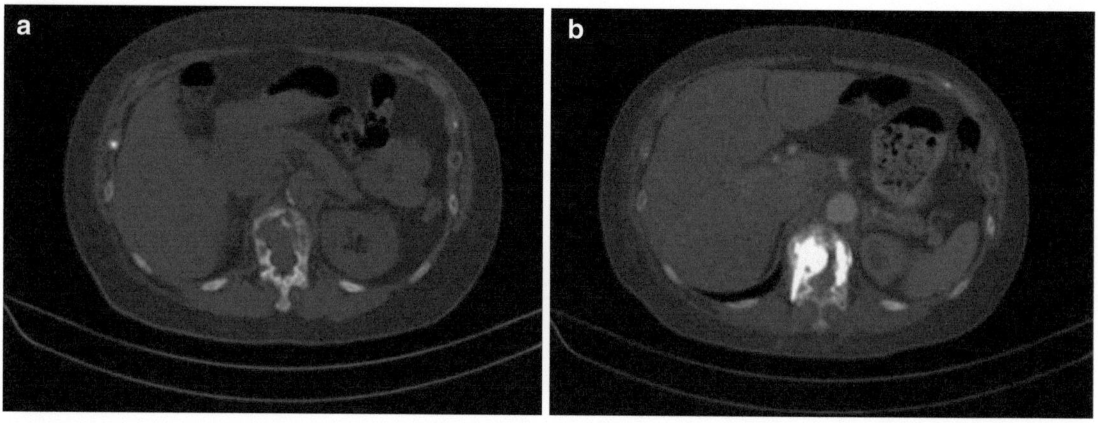

Fig. 12.12 (**a**) Preoperative axial CT showing an osteolytic metastasis in the 1st lumbar vertebra; (**b**) axial CT 6 weeks after kypho-IORT

dysfunction. Of the 15 patients (73 %), 11 developed progressive visceral and further bone metastases (Reis et al. 2012).

12.3.4 Dose Escalation Study – Study Design

After the pilot phase and approval from the local ethics committee and the Federal Office for Radiation Protection, we have started a dose escalation study. This study is a prospective phase II study to establish the maximum tolerable dose (MTD). Therefore three dose escalation groups are planned:

- 8 Gy at 5 mm distance from the applicator surface
- 8 Gy at 8 mm distance from the applicator surface
- 8 Gy at 10 mm distance from the applicator surface

Overall, 18 patients will be enrolled, i.e. three to six per dose group. If no MTD criteria (dysfunction of wound healing, infections, osteoradionecrosis, nerve and spinal cord damage, pathological fracture within 90 days) appear in the lowest dose group of three patients, the next three patients will be treated in second highest dose group. If any patient meets MTD criteria, we shall again treat three patients in the same dose group. If we do not observe the MTD criteria in any of these further patients, we shall move to the next dose step. If we experience MTD criteria in a second patient, we shall return to the lower dose group. In this dose group we shall treat six patients.

Inclusion criteria are:

- Age ≥50 years
- Presence of oligometastases
- Presence of visceral metastases allowed
- Histologically or imaging proven spinal metastases below the third vertebra (max. Ø: 2 cm)
- Karnofsky index ≥60 %
- Written informed consent
- Contraceptive method (female patients of reproductive potential)

Exclusion criteria are:

- Prior radiation to the vertebra
- Intercurrent diseases (e.g. infections), coagulopathy
- Unsuitability for general anaesthesia
- Contraindications to MRI or CT scans
- Pregnancy/lactation

Endpoints are:

- Compatibility/side-effects of IORT using defined MTD criteria
- Effectiveness defined by CT or MRI and/or clinical relapses/progression and pain

12.4 Intravaginal X-ray Brachytherapy

12.4.1 Background and Physical Aspects

The vaginal cuff is the most common site of locoregional failure after hysterectomy in patients with endometrial cancer. To prevent recurrences, patients are commonly treated with postsurgical endovaginal brachytherapy. Vaginal brachytherapy is usually performed with ^{192}Ir high-dose-rate (HDR) afterloading. Disadvantages of ^{192}Ir HDR afterloading are the high energy, which imposes complex radiation protection requirements, and the high cost arising from the four source changes that are necessary annually because of the limited half-life of ^{192}Ir. Because of the low-energy X-ray source associated with the INTRABEAM system, the radiation shielding requirements for this electronic brachytherapy are much less than for ^{192}Ir HDR afterloading. Furthermore, use of the INTRABEAM is relatively inexpensive, because in contrast to ^{192}Ir HDR afterloading only one permanent source is needed. The difference in the relative biological effectiveness (RBE) of the HDR technique and the low-energy X-rays of the INTRABEAM system also has to be mentioned: due to the increased linear energy transfer, low-energy X-rays have an increased RBE compared with high-energy photons (Herskind et al. 2005).

In order to use the INTRABEAM for intravaginal X-ray brachytherapy, the spherical dose distribution of the INTRABEAM must be transformed into a cylindrical one. Therefore a cylindrical applicator has been developed for stepwise axial motion of the radiation source along a longitudinal axis. To create a homogeneous dose distribution, Schneider et al. (2009) moved the source of the INTRABEAM system (3–5 steps within a distance of 17–23 mm) along the cylindrical vaginal applicator. The axial shift was established by a stepping mechanism, which was mounted on a table support. The total dose/dose distribution was determined using film dosimetry (Gafchromic EBT) in a "solid water" phantom. Comparison of results with a ^{192}Ir HDR afterloading plan showed a similar dose distribution.

12.4.2 Clinical Use

To enable clinical use of the INTRABEAM system for endovaginal brachytherapy, four cylindrical applicators (INTRABEAM Gyn Applicator) with different diameters (2, 2.5, 3 and 3.5 cm) were designed (Fig. 12.13) as well as a special table attachment with leg rests similar to a gynaecological examination chair on which the patient lies in the supine position (Fig. 12.14). To protect the sensitive source of the INTRABEAM system, a second inner detonator tube (INTRABEAM Gyn Probe Guard) is used (Fig. 12.13). The applicators are connected to the table attachment with a metal base plate. For achievement of exact distances between different dwell points, specially manufactured distance rings (INTRABEAM Gyn Dwell Stepper) are available (width: 20, 37 and 54 mm) (Fig. 12.13). A CT scan is performed for treatment planning with an adequate applicator in place.

More than 20 patients have been treated with endovaginal brachytherapy using the INTRABEAM system. To cite an example: one of the patients was a 73-year-old woman with a histologically confirmed endometrial cancer (adenocarcinoma, G2), diagnosed in April 2012. The patient underwent a laparoscopic hysterectomy and adnexectomy. The tumour stage was pT1b pN0 cM0, R0. The tumour was positive for both oestrogen and progesterone receptors. According to the guidelines, patients with endometrial cancer with tumour stage FIGO IB (G2 and G3) should receive intravaginal brachytherapy to reduce the risk of recurrence at the vaginal stump. For calculation of the dose distribution in the aforementioned patient, a planning CT was performed with an adequate applicator in

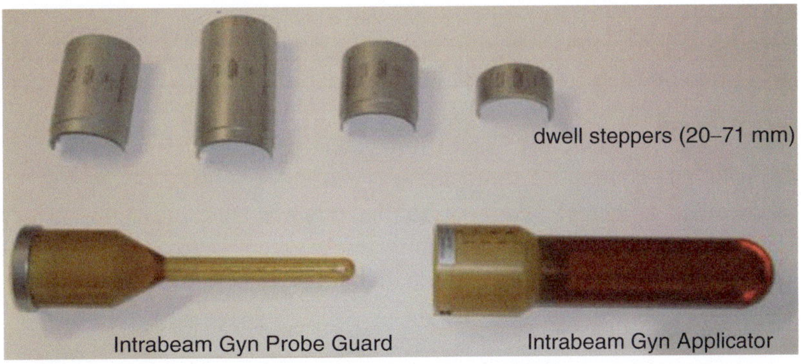

Fig. 12.13 *Top*: INTRABEAM dwell steppers (20–71 mm); *bottom*: INTRABEAM Gyn Probe Guard and INTRABEAM Gyn Applicator (Ø 35 mm) for intravaginal X-ray brachytherapy

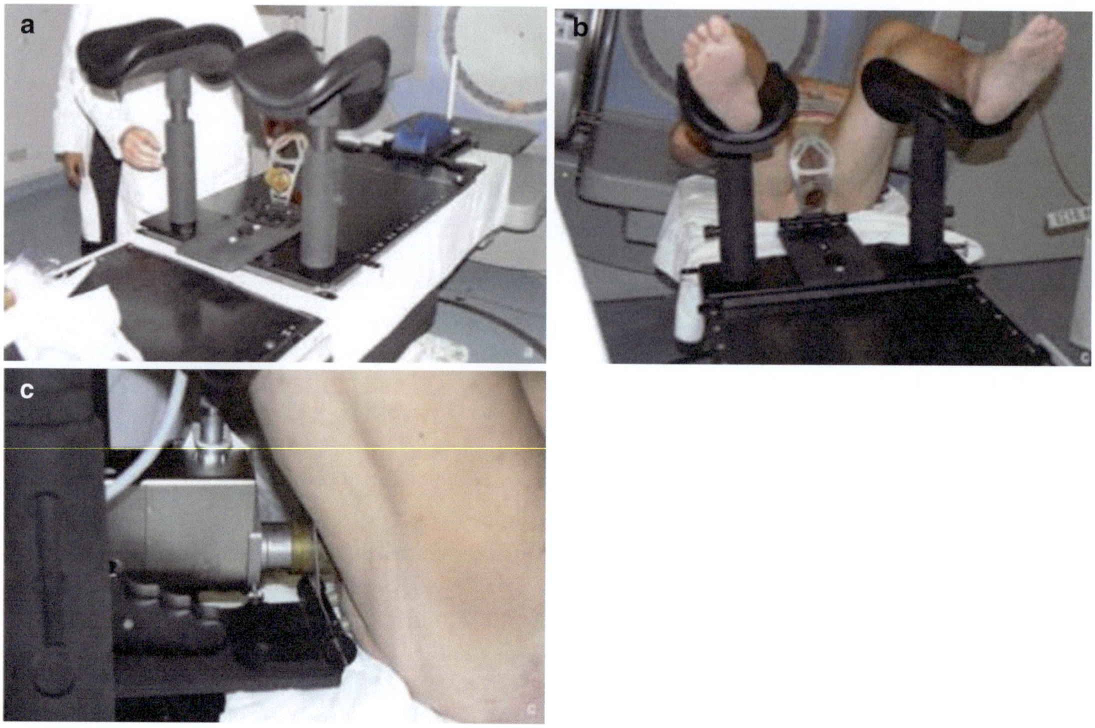

Fig. 12.14 (**a**) Special table attachment with leg rests similar to a gynaecological examination chair; (**b**, **c**) patient in the treatment position

place. In this case an applicator with a diameter of 3 cm was used; the length of the vaginal stump was 10 cm. Applicator insertion was done with the patient in the supine position on the special table attachment. After insertion of the drift tube of the INTRABEAM system into the applicator protected by the Gyn Probe Guard, an additional CT scan directly before every brachytherapy treatment ensured the proper position of the applicator and the correct position of the radiation source within the applicator (Fig. 12.15). The patient received a dose of 4×4 Gy (16 Gy), once weekly. Every fraction delivered 4 Gy (RBE corrected) to a 5 mm tissue depth using three dwell positions with an overall treatment time of 13.1 min per fraction (first dwell position, 5.1 min; second dwell position, 3.06 min; third dwell position, 4.54 min). The treatment was performed in a planning CT room and was generally well tolerated. Under treatment neither medical complications such as acute toxicity nor severe technical problems occurred. At the final medical examination, no therapy-related skin toxicity was seen. No dysuria, radiation-related proctitis or vaginal bleeding was observed.

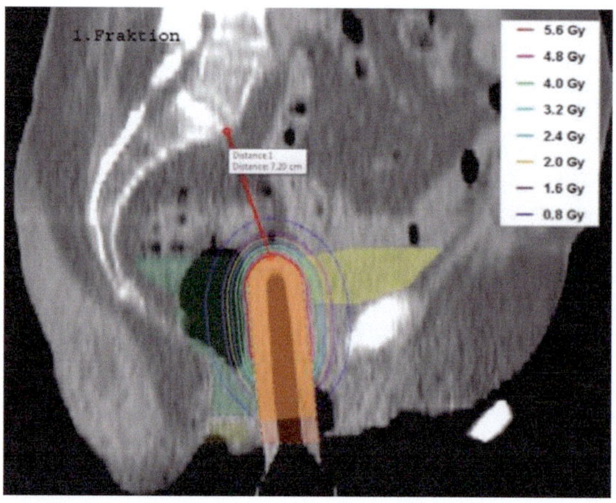

Fig. 12.15 CT scan before brachytherapy treatment with the calculated dose distribution to ensure proper position of the applicator and the radiation source within the applicator

The first follow-up was done 6 weeks after treatment. The patient reported slightly increased stool frequency (3–4/day) and grade 1 incontinence (CTCAE version 3.0). Gynaecological examination and vaginal ultrasound showed no pathological findings or signs of recurrence. The condition of the patient was good (Karnofsky index 90 %). The treatment was tolerated very well, without severe acute toxicity.

Conclusion

Delivery of irradiation during surgical resections as part of a multimodal or single treatment enables a high dose to be delivered to the tumour bed while excluding dose-limiting sensitive structures. Despite improved therapies such as combined radio-chemotherapy regimens and newer radiation therapies [intensity modulated radiotherapy (IMRT), image-guided radiotherapy (IGRT)], high rates of local failure occur in patients with locally advanced rectal cancer, sarcomas, gynaecological tumours and other malignancies. IORT seems to provide an additional benefit in terms of local recurrence rate and overall survival for both primary and recurrent tumours.

Given the availability of applicators of newer design, the use of the INTRABEAM device for IORT in clinical practice will likely grow, with increasing integration into the treatment of other malignancies like vertebral metastases (kypho-IORT) or endometrial cancer (intravaginal X-ray brachytherapy).

References

Boland PJ, Lane JM, Sundaresan N (1982) Metastatic disease of the spine. Clin Orthop Relat Res 169: 95–102

Ferenschild FT, Vermaas M, Nuyttens JJ, Graveland WJ, Marinelli AW, van der Sijp JR et al (2006) Value of intraoperative radiotherapy for locally advanced rectal cancer. Dis Colon Rectum 49:1257–1265

Garfin SR, Yuan HA, Reiley MA (2001) New technologies in spine: kyphoplasty and vertebroplasty for the treatment of painful osteoporotic compression fractures. Spine 26:1511–1515

Gerszten PC, Mendel E, Yamada Y (2009) Radiotherapy and radiosurgery for metastatic spine disease: what are the options, indications, and outcomes? Spine 34: 578–592

Gilbert RW, Kim JH, Posner JB (1978) Epidural spinal cord compression from metastatic tumor: diagnosis and treatment. Ann Neurol 3:40–51

Haddock MG, Gunderson LL, Nelson H, Cha SS, Devine RM, Dozois RR, Wolff BG (2001) Intraoperative irradiation for locally recurrent colorectal cancer in previously irradiated patients. Int J Radiat Oncol Biol Phys 49:1267–1274

Hage WD, Aboulafia AJ, Aboulafia DM (2000) Incidence, location and diagnostic evaluation of metastatic bone disease. Orthop Clin North Am 3:515–528

Halpin RJ, Bendok BR, Liu JC (2004) Minimally invasive treatments for spinal metastases: vertebroplasty, kyphoplasty and radiofrequency ablation. J Support Oncol 2:339–351

Harrington KD (1986) Metastatic disease of the spine. J Bone Joint Surg Am 68:1110–1115

Herskind C, Steil V, Kraus-Tiefenbacher U, Wenz F (2005) Radiobiological aspects of intraoperative radiotherapy (IORT) with isotropic low-energy X rays for early-stage breast cancer. Radiat Res 163:208–215

Janjan NA (1997) Radiation for bone metastases: conventional techniques and the role of systemic radiopharmaceuticals. Cancer 80:1628–1645

Lehnert T, Schwarzbach M, Willeke F, Treiber M, Hinz U, Wannenmacher MM et al (2000) Intraoperative radiotherapy for primary and locally recurrent soft tissue sarcoma: morbidity and long-term prognosis. Eur J Surg Oncol 26:S21–S24

McDermott FT, Hughes ES, Pihl E, Johnson WR, Price AB (1985) Local recurrence after potentially curative resection for rectal cancer in a series of 1008 patients. Br J Surg 75:34–37

Moulding HD, Elder JB, Lis E, Lovelock DM, Zhang Z, Yamada Y, Bilsky MH (2010) Local disease control after decompressive surgery and adjuvant high-dose single-fraction radiosurgery for spine metastases. J Neurosurg Spine 13:87–93

Reis T, Schneider F, Welzel G, Schmidt R, Obertacke U, Wenz F (2012) Intraoperative radiotherapy during kyphoplasty for vertebral metastases (Kypho-IORT): first clinical results. Tumori 98:434–440

Rosenberg SA, Tepper J, Glatstein E, Costa J, Baker A, Brennan M et al (1982) The treatment of soft-tissue sarcomas of the extremities: prospective randomized evaluations of (1) limb-sparing surgery plus radiation therapy compared with amputation and (2) the role of adjuvant chemotherapy. Ann Surg 196: 305–315

Schneider F, Fuchs H, Lorenz F, Steil V, Ziglio F, Kraus-Tiefenbacher U et al (2009) A novel device for intravaginal electronic brachytherapy. Int J Radiat Oncol Biol Phys 74:1298–1305

Schneider F, Greineck F, Clausen S, Mai S, Obertacke U, Reis T, Wenz F (2011) Development of a novel method for intraoperative radiotherapy during kyphoplasty for spinal metastases (Kypho-IORT). Int J Radiat Oncol Biol Phys 15(81):1114–1119

Sindelar WF, Kinsella TJ, Chen PW, DeLaney TF, Tepper JE, Rosenberg SA et al (1993) Intraoperative radiotherapy in retroperitoneal sarcomas. Final results of a prospective, randomized, clinical trial. Arch Surg 128:402–410

Smith JW, Vielvoye GJ, Goslings BM (2000) Embolization for vertebral metastases of follicular thyroid carcinoma. J Clin Endocrinol Metab 85:989–997

Suzuki K, Gunderson LL, Devine RM, Weaver AL, Dozois RR, Ilstrup DM et al (1995) Intraoperative irradiation after palliative surgery for locally recurrent rectal cancer. Cancer 75:939–952

Valentini V, Morganti AG, Gambacorta MA, Mohiuddin M, Doglietto GB, Coco C et al (2006) Preoperative hyperfractionated chemoradiation for locally recurrent rectal cancer in patients previously irradiated to the pelvis: a multicentric phase II study. Int J Radiat Oncol Biol Phys 64:1129–1139

van der Linden YM, Steenland E, van Houwelingen HC, Post WJ, Oei B, Marijnen CA, Leer JW (2006) Dutch Bone Metastasis Study Group. Patients with a favourable prognosis are equally palliated with single and multiple fraction radiotherapy: results on survival in the Dutch Bone Metastasis Study. Radiother Oncol 78:245–253

Welch JP, Donaldson GA (1978) Detection and treatment of recurrent cancer of the colon and rectum. Am J Surg 135:505–508

Wong DA, Fornasier L, MacNab I (1990) Spinal metastasis: the obvious, the occult, and the imposters. Spine 15:1–4

Intraoperative Photon Radiosurgery in Patients with Malignant Brain Tumours

13

Sam Eljamel

13.1 Introduction

Malignant brain tumours (MBTs) comprise primary malignant tumours (PMTs) and metastatic tumours (METs). MBTs are responsible for 3 % of all cancer deaths worldwide and are the second most common cause of cancer death in young people. They carry a very dismal prognosis, typically representing a death sentence that may be deferred by up to merely 36 weeks inspite of treatment (Obwegeser et al. 1995; Eljamel 2004). PMTs represent 40 % of all primary brain tumours, and glioblastoma multiforme (GBM) is the commonest type (Stupp 2007). Although progress has been made in the pathophysiology of GBMs, overall survival remains very poor and individual prediction of clinical outcome remains an elusive goal. Despite extensive clinical trials, the median survival of patients with GBM is still 12–14 months, with fewer than 26 % surviving for 2 years. In a series of 279 patients, only five (1.8 %) survived for 3 years (Lamborn et al. 2004). Multimodality therapeutic approaches would be necessary to improve this dismal outcome.

The joint tumour section of the American Association of Neurological Surgeons/Congress of Neurological Surgeons produced guidelines for the management of GBMs (Scott et al. 1998). The guidelines recommend maximum safe surgical resection, followed by 60 Gy of radiotherapy to the enhancing lesion, encompassing a 2-cm cuff around the lesion. The guidelines also recommend concurrent chemoradiation using Temozolomide and BCNU (Gliadel) in those who undergo craniotomy. Temozolomide offers a 2-year survival rate of merely 26 %, with median survival of 14.6 months and progression-free survival of 7.2 months (Olsen and Ryken 2008), while Gliadel offers survival of 13.9 months (Olsen and Ryken 2008). The poor outcome of these tumours is due to local invasion and local relapse. Eighty percent recur locally within 2 cm of the resection margin and patients often succumb to local recurrence, emphasising that a more aggressive local therapy is still awaited. However, complete radical surgical excision is hindered by the significant amount of tumour that is invisible to the surgeon even with the aid of the surgical microscope; indeed, its complete identification at surgery is an impossible task. Most of these tumours have invaded the brain widely by the time they manifest clinically, making a wider excision margin out of the question.

On the other side of the coin, METs are much more common (Vecht et al. 1990). They have an incidence of 12/100,000 per year and 15–40 % of systemic cancers metastasise to brain. The most frequent sources are lung tumours (40–50 %), breast cancers (15–25 %)

S. Eljamel, MBBCh, MD, FRCSIr, FRCSEd, FRCS(SN), ACS/ALS
Centre for Neurosciences,
Ninewells Hospital and Medical School,
Dundee DD1 9SY, Scotland, UK
emial: m.s.eljamel@dundee.ac.uk,
sameljamel@doctors.net.uk

M. Keshtgar et al. (eds.), *Targeted Intraoperative Radiotherapy in Oncology*,
DOI 10.1007/978-3-642-39821-6_13, © Springer-Verlag Berlin Heidelberg 2014

and melanoma (5–20 %) (Vecht et al. 1990). The frequency of METs appears to be rising as a result of improved brain imaging and more effective treatment of primary cancers (Klos and O'Neill 2004; Chang et al. 2007). Common clinical features of METs are similar to those of PMTs, i.e. headache, neurological deficit and seizures.

If METs remain untreated, they are rapidly fatal. Surgery is indicated for solitary metastases in patients with a good performance status, and when the primary cancer is under control (Mehta et al. 2003). However, eradication of METs is not always possible owing to inability to resect the tumour en masse with a cuff of normal brain tissue, and adjuvant therapies are often used, e.g. whole brain radiotherapy, stereotactic radiosurgery, interstitial radiotherapy and chemotherapy.

Overall, therefore, aggressive local multimodality therapy holds the key in the successful treatment of MBTs, and the Photon Radiosurgery System (PRS) provides a means to deliver local interstitial radiotherapy at the same time as surgery.

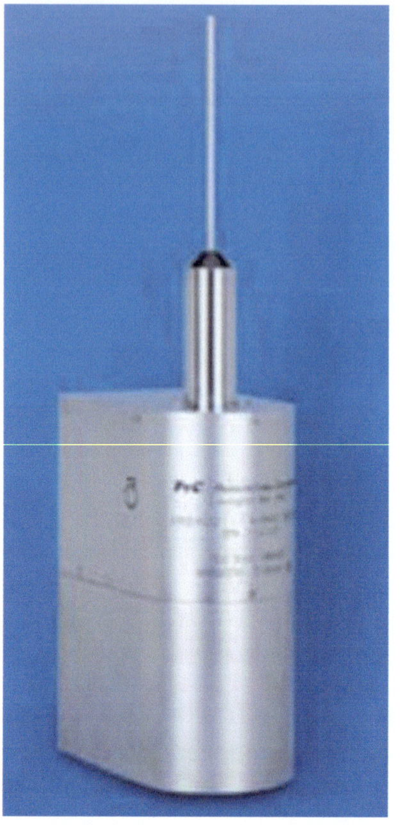

Fig. 13.1 Photograph of the PRS designed to fit the CRW frame

13.2 Use of PRS in the Treatment of Brain Tumours

13.2.1 Rationale

The PRS was initially designed for use in MBTs using the Cosman-Roberts-Wells (CRW) stereotactic frame. That is why the PRS probe is 3 mm wide and 160 mm long: this permits placement of the active tip in the centre of the CRW arc. The unit weighs 3.6 lb. The shape and diameter of the probe neck is designed to fit the CRW frame (Figs. 13.1 and 13.2).

The basic principles of the design were intended to enable neurosurgeons to obtain a biopsy using the CRW frame followed by interstitial stereotactic intraoperative radiosurgery (IORS) at the same sitting. After the early neurosurgical experience, it was realised that a wider applicator was essential to enable PRS use during open surgical resection (Fig. 13.3).

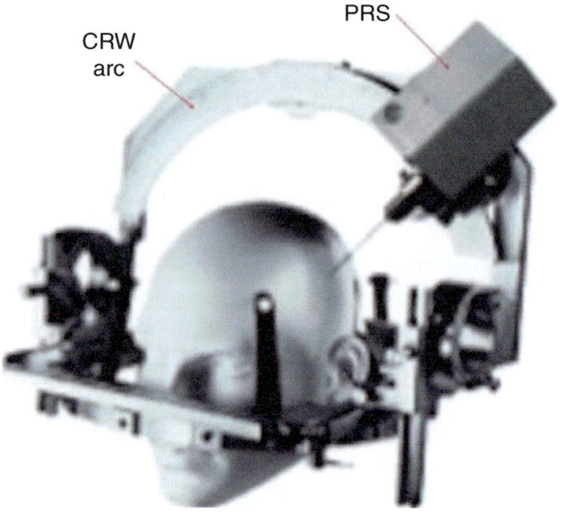

Fig. 13.2 Schematic drawing demonstrating the PRS in the CRW frame

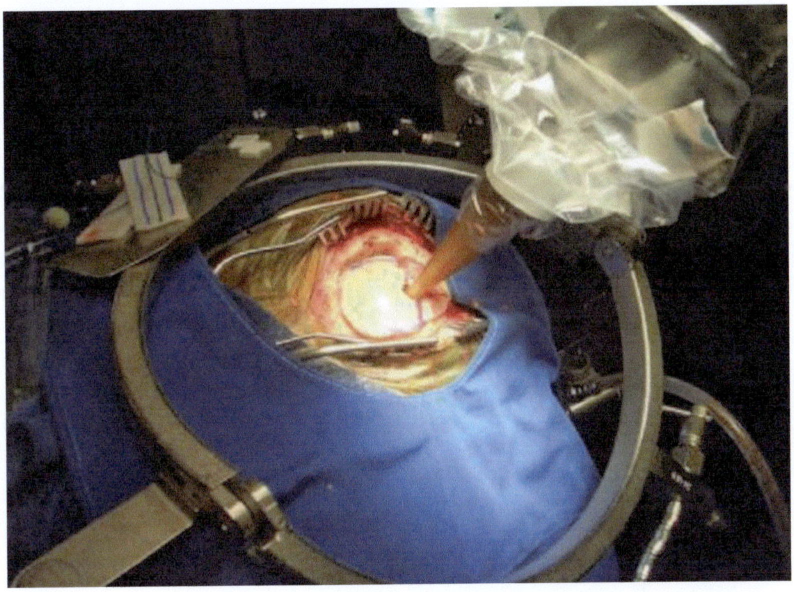

Fig. 13.3 Intraoperative photograph of the PRS with an applicator in place. Note that the bone flap was replaced to reduce radiation

13.2.2 Clinical Experience

Overall, 151 patients with MBTs have been treated using the PRS, including 14 children. The adult population has included 61 PMTs and 64 METs with a female to male ratio of 1.1 and a mean age of 56 years. Of the 64 METs, 51 have been solitary; the mean dose has been 15 Gy and the mean treatment time, 20 min (Fig. 13.4). The side-effects in these patients have been seizures in 1.8 %, cerebral oedema in 2.4 % and unrelated complications in 0.8 %, with zero mortality and zero neurological morbidity. The findings of particular studies are discussed in more detail below, under "Results".

13.2.3 Dosimetry

The PRS produces a radiation field similar to that of a conventional high-dose interstitial brachytherapy source, but with controllable intensity and peak energies (Dinsmore et al. 1996). The X-ray beam behaves essentially as a point isotropic source (current of 40 Amp and voltage of 30–50 kV), giving 15 Gy/min at a distance of 10 mm. Because the photons produced by the PRS are low energy, the X-rays produced are attenuated rapidly within the brain and a dose decline rate of $1/r^3$ is obtained, rather than the $1/r^2$ seen for standard higher energy radioactive isotopes. The resultant 30 % dose reduction per millimetre of brain tissue creates an extremely steep dose fall-off, and background exposure to personnel more than 2 m from the probe upon insertion is approximately 0.05–0.1 mSv/h. Therefore no special shielding of the patient or healthcare personnel is required (Beatty et al. 1996; McDermott et al. 1996) (Fig. 13.5).

13.2.4 Treatment Technique

As mentioned above, the PRS is designed for use with the CRW, and initial experience has been acquired using the CRW frame (Integra, New Jersey, USA). After fixation of the frame ring to the patient's head, the CT localiser is fixed to the frame ring and a stereotactic CT scan with contrast is obtained through the tumour. The antero-posterior, lateral and vertical dimensions of the tumour are determined and target coordinates are calculated for the centre of the tumour. A standard stereotactic biopsy is then performed through a burr hole and specimens are submitted for frozen section analysis. If intraoperative pathology confirms the diagnosis of MBT, the irradiation treatment can be instituted

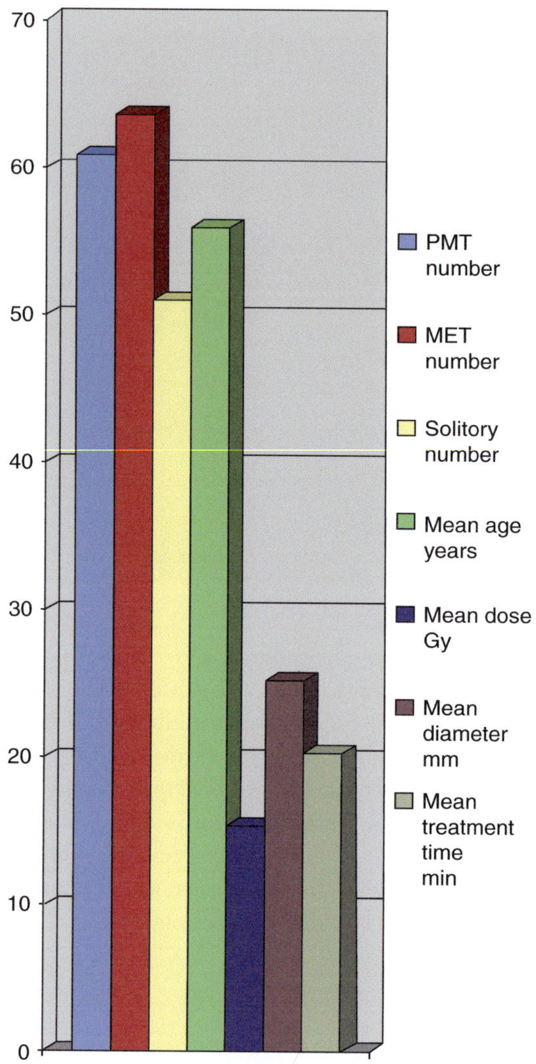

Fig. 13.4 Clinical features of patients with brain tumours treated by the PRS

immediately. First, the biopsy needle tract is dilated to accommodate the probe tip using a graduated series of dilators. The PRS device is then mounted on the arc of the frame (Fig. 13.2) and advanced along the biopsy tract to the target. In the case of open surgical resection, the appropriate PRS applicator is attached to the PRS probe after the PRS has been fixed to the Intrabeam (Zeiss, Germany) (Fig. 13.6).

In general, MBTs 3 cm or less in diameter are prescribed 15–18 Gy, while lesions greater than 3 cm in diameter are prescribed 10–12 Gy. The exact tumour dimensions obtained from the contrast-enhanced brain scan are combined with dose/depth and isodose curves of the PRS to determine the optimal radiation treatment plan. The probe tip position, beam voltage and current are used to calculate the duration of treatment required to administer the prescribed dose to the periphery of the tumour with a 2-mm margin. With all components connected to the control unit, the prescribed voltage and current parameters are selected, and the timer is set to the calculated treatment time. The device is activated by starting the timer and automatically terminates after completion of the selected treatment time. The treatment is monitored throughout the treatment. The PRS probe is then removed, and the incision is closed as usual.

13.2.5 Results

Twenty-seven patients were treated in Harvard (MA, USA), including 25 with METs (16 men, mean age 56 years) of which 12 were solitary (Cosgrove et al. 2012). The primary source of METs was lung cancer in 16, melanoma in six, renal cell carcinoma in two and Merkel cell carcinoma in one. Mean diameter was 16.8 mm (range 4–30 mm). A single dose of radiation between 10 and 20 Gy (mean 15.8 Gy) was administered in all cases, with an average treatment time of 19.5 min (range 4–75). Fourteen patients with METs had received prior whole brain radiotherapy, while the remainder received 30 Gy in 10 fractions within 2 weeks of PRS therapy. All patients tolerated the treatment well and most were discharged home the day after treatment. The mean follow-up was 7 months. Two patients (7.4 %) experienced isolated seizures, two (7.4 %) developed brain oedema that resolved on steroids and one (3.7 %) developed a subdural haematoma 3 months after treatment on the opposite side. There were no deaths, infections or serious neurological morbidity. Local control (defined as stabilisation or reduction of tumour size) was obtained in 19 (73 %). Tumour progression was observed at 3 months post-PRS treatment in five patients, at 6 months in one and at

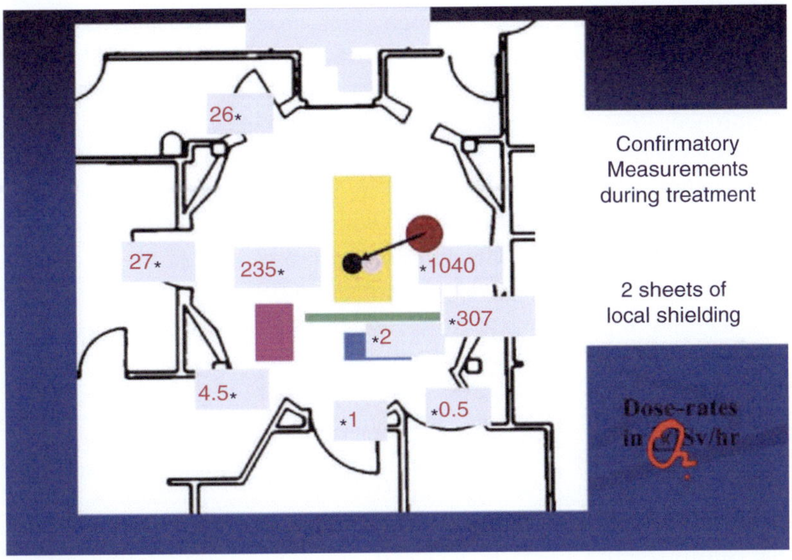

Fig. 13.5 Theatre (OR) setup to reduce radiation risk

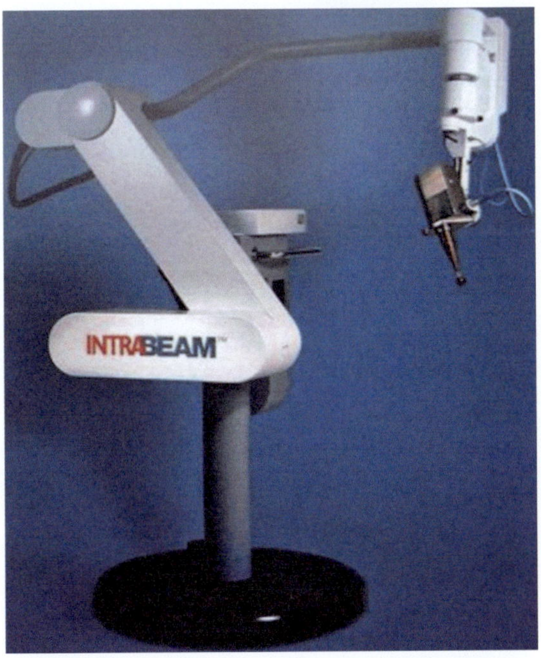

Fig. 13.6 Photograph of the PRS in the Intrabeam

10 months in one. Surgical resection was performed in two patients with enlarging tumours at 4 and 10 months post-PRS treatment and pathological analysis demonstrated central necrosis along with a thin rim of viable tumour around the periphery of the lesion. Two patients had a post-mortem examination: one patient with malignant melanoma who died 12 months after treatment, with documented absence of tumour cells in the treated lesion, and one with adenocarcinoma of lung who died 20 months after treatment and demonstrated no tumour cells in the treated frontal lesion. At last follow-up, 19 patients with cerebral metastases had died: 13 from systemic disease, five from distant cerebral metastases and one after percutaneous gastrostomy for recurrent aspiration pneumonia. Local control of the treated tumours was documented in all five patients who died from progressive CNS metastases and in nine of those who died from systemic disease, while local failure was evident in the others. Six patients with cerebral metastases are alive and well. Median survival was 13 months.

Fifty-four patients were treated in Ninewells Hospital and Medical School, Dundee, Scotland, including 42 with PMTs and ten with METs. Their mean age was 56.2 years and 30 were females. The mean KPS was 80, the mean IORS dose was 11.5 Gy and the mean applicator diameter was 2.5 cm. The mean duration of IORS therapy was 20 min. The mean survival of patients with PMTs was 58.2 weeks while for those with METs it was 35 weeks. None of the patients with METs had local recurrence. Time to tumour recurrence of GBM in this series was 6 months without fluorescence-guided resection (FGR) and 8 months with FGR. Patients were randomised prospectively between high-dose (12–15 Gy) and low-dose (8–10 Gy) IORS. There were no significant differences in time to tumour recurrence, overall survival or side-effects between the two groups.

Twenty-one patients were treated in Vicenza General Hospital, Italy, including 17 with PMTs and four with METs. Their mean age was 56 years and 12 were females. The mean KPS was 71 and 13 had had previous whole brain radiotherapy. The median dose was 15 Gy, the mean applicator diameter was 3 cm and the median treatment time was 35 min. Sixteen patients (76 %) were still alive at the time of last follow-up (7 months) (Volpin et al. 2011).

Fourteen children were treated with 10 Gy in the Northwestern University, Chicago, including 13 with ependymomas. They were followed up for 16 months. Three patients (21 %) developed radionecrosis. Eight (57 %) had local control of the tumour (Kalapurakal et al. 2006).

Thirty-five patients with histologically diagnosed METs were treated with a single fraction of IORS (median, 18 Gy) in Freiberg, Germany. Clinical and radiological evaluations were performed at 2-, 6- and 12-week intervals postoperatively and every 3 months thereafter. Survival, local control and distant and overall brain freedom from disease progression were calculated using the Kaplan-Meier method. The median survival was 7.37 months and the actuarial survival rates at 6 and 12 months were 60.0 and 34.3 %, respectively. Acute complications in six patients (17 %) were associated with shorter survival. Local tumour control rates at the initial and last follow-up were 82 and 50 %. Eighteen patients (53 %) developed distant brain metastases after treatment. At 1 year, the local control rate and the distant and overall brain freedom from progression were 33.0, 43.3 and 14.7 %, respectively. Shorter local tumour control was observed following PRS treatment of recurrent tumour and when tumour configuration was irregular (Pantazis et al. 2009).

Conclusions

Interstitial intraoperative radiosurgery using the PRS offers an immediate, safe and potentially cost-effective treatment for patients with solitary, small, spherical MBTs. MBTs of <3 cm in diameter can be safely prescribed 15–18 Gy and those over 3 cm in diameter can be safely treated with 12–15 Gy. The ideal shape of MBTs for PRS therapy is spherical, and the ideal dose includes a 2-mm cuff around the lesion.

References

Beatty J, Biggs PJ, Gall KP et al (1996) A new miniature x-ray device for interstitial radiosurgery: dosimetry. Med Phys 23:53–62

Chang EL, Wefel JS, Maor MH, Hassenbusch SJ 3rd, Mahajan A, Lang FF et al (2007) A pilot study of neurocognitive function in patients with one to three new brain metastases initially treated with stereotactic radiosurgery alone. Neurosurgery 60:277–283

Cosgrove R, Abdelaziz O, Zervas NT (2012) Interstitial radiosurgery: the photon radiosurgical system. http://neurosurgery.mgh.harvard.edu/functional/prsdevic.htm

Dinsmore M, Hart KJ, Sliski AP, Smith DO, Nomikos PM, Dalterio MJ et al (1996) A new miniature x-ray source for interstitial radiosurgery: device description. Med Phys 23:45–52

Eljamel S (2004) Photodynamic assisted surgical resection and treatment of malignant brain tumors; technique, technology and clinical application. Photodiag Photodyn Ther 1:93–98

Kalapurakal JA, Goldman S, Stellpflug W, Curran J, Sathiaseelan V, Marymont MH, Tomita T (2006) Phase I study of intraoperative radiotherapy with photon radiosurgery system in children with recurrent brain tumors: preliminary report of first dose level (10 Gy). Int J Radiat Oncol Biol Phys 65:800–808

Klos KJ, O'Neill BP (2004) Brain metastases. Neurologist 10:31–46

Lamborn KR, Chang SM, Prados MD (2004) Prognostic factors for survival of patients with glioblastoma: recursive partitioning analysis. Neuro Oncol 6:227–235

McDermott MW, Cosgrove GR, Larson DA, Sneed PK, Gutin PH (1996) Interstitial brachytherapy for intracranial metastases. Neurosurg Clin N Am 7:485–495

Mehta MP, Rodrigus P, Terhaard CH, Rao A, Suh J, Roa W et al (2003) Survival and neurologic outcomes in a randomized trial of motexafin gadolinium and whole-brain radiation therapy in brain metastases. J Clin Oncol 21:2529–2536

Obwegeser A, Ortler M, Seiwald M, Ulme H, Kostron H (1995) Therapy of glioblastoma multiforme, a cumulative experience of 10 years. Acta Neurochir (Wien) 137:29–33

Olsen JJ, Ryken T (2008) Guidelines for the treatment of newly diagnosed glioblastoma: introduction. J Neuro Oncol 89:255–258

Pantazis G, Trippel M, Birg W, Ostertag CB, Nikkhah G (2009) Stereotactic interstitial radiosurgery system for metastatic brain tumours: a prospective single-centre clinical trial. Int J Radiat Oncol Biol Phys 75:1392–1400

Scott JN, Rewcastle NB, Brasher PM, Fulton D, Hagen NA, MacKinnon JA et al (1998) Long-term glioblastoma multiforme survivors: a population-based study. Can J Neurol Sci 25:197–201

Stupp R (2007) Malignant gliomas: ESMO clinical recommendations for diagnosis, treatment and follow up. Ann Oncol 18(Suppl 2):60–70

Vecht CJ, Avezaat CJ, van Putten WL, Eijkenboom WM, Stefanko SZ (1990) The influence of the extent of surgery on the neurological function and survival in malignant glioma. A retrospective analysis in 243 patients. J Neurol Neurosurg Psychiatry 53:466–471

Volpin L, Zanusso M, Cora S, Santangelo V, Della Monica P (2011) Intrabeam system for intraoperative radiotherapy (IORT) and malignant brain tumours. In: Proceedings of the first intrabeam workshop, Freiberg, November, 2011

14 Intraoperative Radiotherapy with Low-Energy Photons in Rectal Cancer Recurrence

Magdalena Skórzewska and Wojciech P. Polkowski

14.1 Introduction

Despite the significant progress in treatment of patients with colorectal cancer (CRC) over recent decades, local recurrence (LR) continues to pose a significant therapeutic challenge. LR is one of the most common forms of relapse after conventional treatment of CRC. LR significantly worsens the prognosis and constitutes one of the major causes of CRC treatment failure. Long-term local control and survival rates vary from 41 to 77 % and from 1 to 50 %, respectively, with the most favourable results in patients with positive prognostic factors (Pezner et al. 2002). Reported median survival in patients with LR is 11–15 months and the 5-year survival rate is less than 5 % (Haddock et al. 2011). Loco-regional relapse is associated with high mortality, and a positive circumferential margin in primary tumour resection is proven to be directly associated with a high LR rate (Kang et al. 2010). Advanced relapse, often infiltrating adjacent bony structures and pelvic organs, prevents the execution of salvage radical surgery (Lopez-Kostner et al. 2001). In rectal cancer the LR risk among patients who have undergone surgical treatment only is reported to be from 19 to 30 % (Lopez-Kostner et al. 2001; Dubois et al. 2011). This risk is significantly reduced to 2.5–16 % if surgery is supplemented with radiotherapy (preoperative or postoperative) (Dubois et al. 2011; Moriya 2006). When total mesorectal excision is performed after preoperative radiotherapy, LR risk can be decreased to 4.6 % (Dubois et al. 2011). Prevention of LR depends primarily on meticulous surgical technique with achievement of clear (>2 mm) circumferential resection margins. Treatment with curative intent depends on radical resection with microscopically uninvolved margins (R0), as a negative resection margin is the strongest prognostic factor. Obtaining R0 resection is extremely important and has a direct impact on long-term survival and local control of disease with acceptable quality of life (Lopez-Kostner et al. 2001; Wiggers et al. 2003).

Preoperative external beam radiation therapy (EBRT), if used in combination with 5-fluorouracil-based chemotherapy, facilitates resectability by downstaging of the tumour volume (Moriya 2006; Wydmanski et al. 2005). However, this effect may be missed by non-radical, poor quality surgery (Moriya 2006; Wiggers et al. 2003; Nagtegaal and Quirke 2008). Chemoradiation improves median survival from 8 months in untreated patients with LR to 14 months (Moriya 2006). Compared with a postoperative regimen, preoperative radiochemotherapy has a more beneficial effect and increases the complete excision rate in patients with locally advanced rectal cancer (Kang et al. 2010). Comparison between two radiotherapy

M. Skórzewska (✉) • W.P. Polkowski
Department of Surgical Oncology,
Medical University of Lublin,
SPSK nr 1 ul. Staszica 11,
20-081 Lublin, Poland
e-mail: i_boog@o2.pl;
wojciech.polkowski@am.lublin.pl

M. Keshtgar et al. (eds.), *Targeted Intraoperative Radiotherapy in Oncology*,
DOI 10.1007/978-3-642-39821-6_14, © Springer-Verlag Berlin Heidelberg 2014

protocols combined with surgery has shown a greater than twofold increase in 5-year survival rates (12–25 %) after resection supplemented with intraoperative radiation therapy (IORT) as compared with post-surgical EBRT (5–10 %) (Moore et al. 2004).

When LR occurs after primary treatment of advanced rectal carcinoma with preoperative radiotherapy and surgery, treatment options are limited to (extensive) surgery alone, as re-irradiation with EBRT is controversial, although strongly advocated by some very specialised groups (Haddock et al. 2011; Moriya 2006; Treiber et al. 2004; Dresen et al. 2008). There are two common scenarios in radical multimodality treatment of LR. Patients without a history of previous irradiation should follow a regimen of surgical resection with optional IORT with preoperative EBRT, 50.4 Gy in 28 fractions, with concomitant fluoropyrimidine. Multiple studies have proven that re-irradiation is associated with acceptable toxicity. For previously irradiated patients, EBRT, 30 Gy in 15–17 fractions, followed immediately by resection and optional IORT, should be considered. When IORT is added to fractionated EBRT, the total duration of radiation can be shortened by 1–2 weeks (Haddock et al. 2011; Wydmanski et al. 2005). Combination of an EBRT dose of 30 Gy with 12.5 Gy intraoperative electron-beam radiation therapy is considered to be equivalent to 62 Gy, and cases with a positive circumferential margin after resection should be treated with a dose higher than 60 Gy (Haddock et al. 2011; Kang et al. 2010). Nonetheless, IORT should never be considered as a substitute for R0 resection as it does not compensate for poor (non-radical) surgery (Haddock et al. 2011).

14.2 Technical Considerations

The first documented use of IORT for CRC was by Japanese groups in the 1960s (Mathis et al. 2009). IORT enables direct tumour visualisation with the ability to displace or shield surrounding normal tissues from the irradiated volume, thus potentially reducing morbidity (Nag et al. 1999). There are three basic techniques of IORT: intraoperative electron-beam radiation therapy (IOERT), intraoperative high-dose-rate brachytherapy (IOHDR) and intraoperative X-ray radiation therapy (IOXRT) (Wydmanski et al. 2005). The energy of the IORT ranges from 30- to 50-keV photons (orthovoltage) in the INTRABEAM® Photon Radiosurgery System (PRS) to 4–25 MeV (megavoltage) with electron beam linear accelerators. IORT provides irradiation to the volume of the tumour cavity directly after excision to achieve oncological sterilisation of the surgically defined area (Moriya 2006; Treiber et al. 2004). Radiobiologically IOERT and IOHDR differ from IOXRT as the dose distribution provided by linear accelerators is more homogeneous within the target. The surface dosage is proportional to the energy of electrons, ranging from 75 % for 6 MeV to almost 100 % for 18 MeV; therefore depth control is more accurate with the electron beam (Wydmanski et al. 2005; Mathis et al. 2009). When resection margins are narrow or involved by tumour cells, IORT can be used to give a boost dose to the tumour bed at the time of surgery, under direct visual control (Moriya 2006; Wydmanski et al. 2005; Treiber et al. 2004; Dresen et al. 2008). The surgeon and the radiotherapist assess the target volume for IORT. Intraoperative irradiation is considered to be a safe procedure and the only disadvantage may be limited intraoperative pathological confirmation of LR. Standard depth to a dose calculation is 5 or 10 mm (Wydmanski et al. 2005). IORT is administered during an operation as a single boost dose. The focal point of interest is post-resection areas at highest risk of LR. The procedure is performed with special shielding or displacement from the treatment area of dose-sensitive organs, such as the small intestine and ureters. The biological effectiveness of IORT is equivalent to an additional 30–40 Gy of fractionated EBRT (Mathis et al. 2009; Kusters et al. 2010). IORT has a higher therapeutic index than EBRT because the boost is precisely administered to structures at risk and normal, healthy tissues are spared (Mathis et al. 2009).

The most frequent side-effects of IORT are peripheral neuropathy and ureteric stricture.

Neuropathy is primarily related to the IORT dose and occurs if doses are greater than or equal to 15 Gy, while ureteral obstruction is more common at doses exceeding 12 Gy (Kang et al. 2010; Mathis et al. 2009). However, these complications are infrequent and not life-threatening, and for this reason the ureter is considered a "dose-sensitive" rather than a "dose-limiting" structure (Mathis et al. 2009).

In the authors' experience, the operation and IORT delivery are performed in a regular operating theatre. After the tumour has been resected, both the radiation oncologist and the surgeon select the appropriate applicator size to fit the tumour bed (Fig. 14.1), which determines the dosage. The applicator is then positioned in the area of the abdomen or in the pelvis. During irradiation the surgical staff leave the operating theatre. The operative field is secured with sterile sheets, with an applicator on the INTRABEAM arm, placed in the surgical bed (Figs. 14.2 and 14.3). After IORT, the applicator is removed and the final stage of the operation is conducted. The dose is determined by the radiation oncologist, depending on the amount of residual disease after maximal tumour excision. The dose, prescribed to the surface of the applicator, is administered according to the following scheme: 10 Gy in patients with negative circumferential margins, 12.5 Gy for close or microscopically positive circumferential margins, and 15–17.5 Gy for non-radical resection.

14.3 Results

IORT is thought to supplement surgery, resulting in improved local control of disease. To date very few studies have been conducted using orthovoltage IOXRT. Instead, most trials have been based on IOERT. Assimilation of the necessary equipment in non-modified operating theatres is, however, not possible. IOERT requires stringent radiation protection measures and the operating theatre needs to comply with the conditions of a radiotherapy bunker because the radiation energy is much higher and the penetration of radiation, greater. Radiotherapy using the INTRABEAM PRS based on kilovoltage photons allows the use of IOXRT within the existing premises of the operating theatre due to the low penetration of radiation. Since the radiation dose is frequently limited by the tolerance of surrounding tissues, INTRABEAM enables escalation of the dosage without affecting adjacent organs (Treiber et al. 2004; Dresen et al. 2008).

While there are few publications on the use of the INTRABEAM system in CRC, the Cleveland

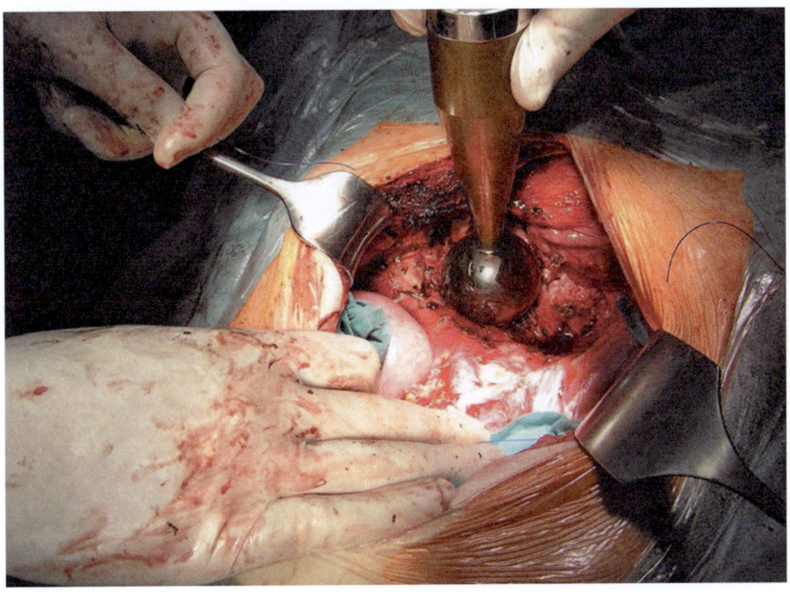

Fig. 14.1 Visualisation of the surgical bed. The surgeon checks the fit of the applicator to the dimensions of the tumour cavity

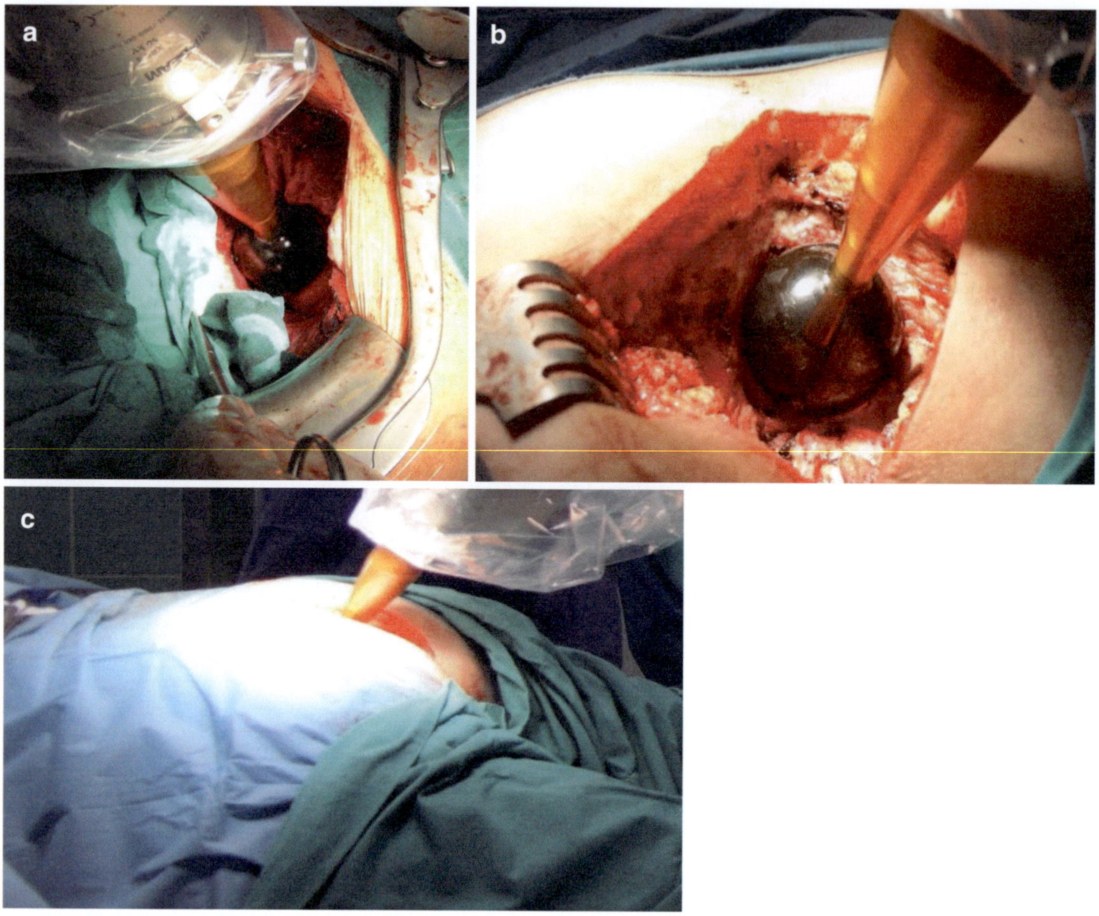

Fig. 14.2 The applicator on an arm of the INTRABEAM PRS 500 is placed in the tumour cavity: (**a**) via laparotomy; (**b**, **c**) via a sacro-perineal approach

radiotherapy group has longstanding experience (Guo et al. 2012). At the European Society of Surgical Oncology congress in 2010, S. Guo presented the preliminary results of 10 years' experience with the use of orthovoltage IORT in highly selected patients with primary advanced and recurrent CRC. These results have been published recently (Guo et al. 2012). In the recurrence study group, median survival was 32 months with a median follow-up of 22 months. Addition of orthovoltage IORT to surgery in patients with locally recurrent rectal cancer resulted in an overall 3-year survival of 43 %. Median hospitalisation time after surgery was 7 days (range 2–59 days). These results were similar to those obtained in other U.S. centres where IOERT equipment is used. Studies from the Mayo Clinic demonstrated a median survival of 36 months and a 3-year overall survival of 43 % (Guo et al. 2012) (Fig. 14.4). This contrasts with a median survival of 19 months with palliative surgery alone (Garcia-Aguilar et al. 2001).

In the Department of Surgical Oncology of the Medical University of Lublin, between 2006 and 2011, 79 patients with recurrent CRC underwent surgical treatment. Surgery supplemented with IORT using the PRS system was performed in 22 cases of locally recurrent rectal cancer. Twelve women and ten men were treated; the median age of the entire group was 66 years (range 26–77 years). The median duration of IORT was 17 min (range 6–47 min). The types of surgical

Fig. 14.3 Ongoing intraoperative radiation. The operating field is secured with sterile surgical sheets

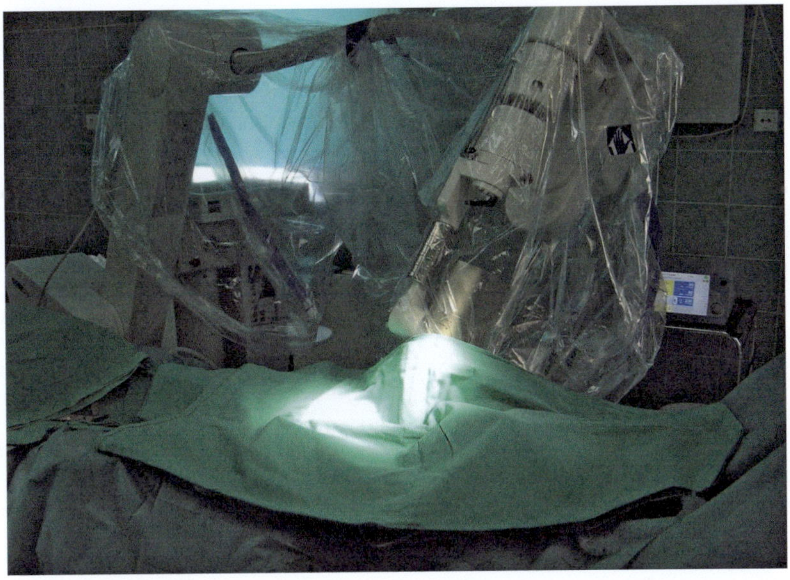

Fig. 14.4 Results of a retrospective phase I/II study on CRC at the Cleveland Clinic, Ohio (Guo et al. 2012)

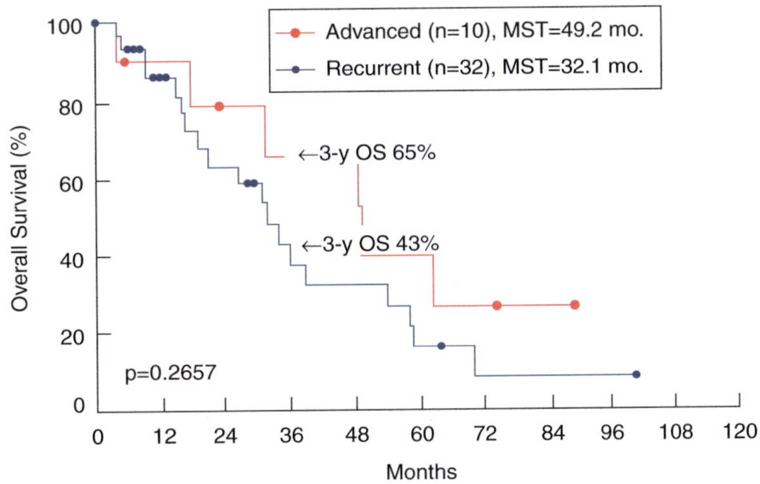

procedure performed were as follows: 13 transabdominal resections of the tumour, six transanal resections (transanal microsurgical tumour excision), two abdominosacral amputations of the rectum and one sacrectomy. In 13 cases (59 %), extended multivisceral resections had to be done due to extensive spread of the tumour and involvement of other organs. There were no postoperative complications that might be purely attributable to the use of IORT. In particular, no cases of ureteric stenosis were detected during the postoperative course. None of the patients died during postoperative hospitalisation. In four (18 %) patients, re-operations were necessary, in two cases because of the intestinal obstruction, in one because of the presence of a fistula (anastomotic dehiscence) and in one due to intraperitoneal bleeding. The median postoperative hospital stay was 7 days (range 2–23 days). One patient who received IORT died early after surgery (90-day mortality, 4.5 %) owing to exacerbation of chronic renal failure during the postoperative period. The median follow-up time is 11 months (range 1–53 months), which is too short for late outcome evaluation.

Conclusions

Since there are only scattered data on the use of IORT in recurrent CRC patients, IORT cannot be considered standard treatment and should still be regarded as an experimental treatment option (Wydmanski et al. 2005). It seems that IORT performed after surgical resection is a safe and feasible procedure with a good therapeutic index that can improve treatment results and significantly increase local tumour control. The use of IORT as an adjunct to surgical resection does not prolong hospitalisation. Thorough follow-up should be conducted (with the use of tumour markers, endoscopy and modern metabolic imaging) to identify LR in the earliest stage, and R0 resection remains the baseline in accomplishing satisfying long-term survival rates.

14.4 Take Home Message

Orthovoltage IORT after surgical resection is a safe and feasible procedure that improves local tumour control of recurrent colorectal carcinoma. The INTRABEAM PRS 500 is a versatile system which may be used with various surgical approaches, such as laparotomy or the sacral (perineal) or even transanal approach. IORT is an adjunct to surgical resection but does not compensate for non-radical surgery in loco-regionally advanced cases.

References

Dresen RC, Gosens MJ, Martijn H, Nieuwenhuijzen GA, Creemers GJ, Daniels-Gooszen AW et al (2008) Radical resection after IORT-containing multimodality treatment is the most important determinant for outcome in patients treated for locally recurrent rectal cancer. Ann Surg Oncol 15:1937–1947

Dubois JB, Bussieres E, Richaud P, Rouanet P, Becouarn Y, Mathoulin-Pélissier S et al (2011) Intra-operative radiotherapy of rectal cancer: results of the French multi-institutional randomized study. Radiother Oncol 98:298–303

Garcia-Aguilar J, Cromwell JW, Marra C, Lee SH, Madoff RD, Rothenberger DA (2001) Treatment of locally recurrent rectal cancer. Dis Colon Rectum 44:1743–1748

Guo S, Reddy CA, Kolar M, Woody N, Mahadevan A, Deibel FC et al (2012) Intraoperative radiation therapy (IORT) with the photon radiosurgery system (PRS) in locally advanced and recurrent rectal cancer: retrospective review of the Cleveland Clinic experience. Radiat Oncol 7:110

Haddock MG, Miller RC, Nelson H, Pemberton JH, Dozois EJ, Alberts SR, Gunderson LL (2011) Combined modality therapy including intraoperative electron irradiation for locally recurrent colorectal cancer. Int J Radiat Oncol Biol Phys 79: 143–150

Kang MK, Kim MS, Kim JH (2010) Intraoperative radiotherapy for locally advanced rectal cancer. J Korean Soc Coloproctol 26:274–278

Kusters M, Valentini V, Calvo FA, Krempien R, Nieuwenhuijzen GA, Martijn H et al (2010) Results of European pooled analysis of IORT-containing multimodality treatment for locally advanced rectal cancer: adjuvant chemotherapy prevents local recurrence rather than distant metastases. Ann Oncol 21:1279–1284

Lopez-Kostner F, Fazio VW, Vignali A, Rybicki LA, Lavery IC (2001) Locally recurrent rectal cancer: predictors and success of salvage surgery. Dis Colon Rectum 44:173–178

Mathis KL, Nelson H, Pemberton JH (2009) Can unresectable colorectal cancer be cured? Adv Surg 43:211–219

Moore HG, Shoup M, Riedel E, Minsky BD, Alektiar KM, Ercolani M et al (2004) Colorectal cancer pelvic recurrences: determinants of resectability. Dis Colon Rectum 47:1599–1606

Moriya Y (2006) Treatment strategy for locally recurrent rectal cancer. Jpn J Clin Oncol 36:127–131

Nag S, Martinez-Monge R, Martin EW (1999) Intraoperative electron beam radiotherapy in recurrent colorectal carcinoma. J Surg Oncol 72:66–71

Nagtegaal ID, Quirke P (2008) What is the role for the circumferential margin in the modern treatment of rectal cancer? Clin Oncol 26:303–312

Pezner RD, Chu DZ, Ellenhorn JD (2002) Intraoperative radiation therapy for patients with recurrent rectal and sigmoid colon cancer in previously irradiated fields. Radiother Oncol 64:47–52

Treiber M, Lehnert T, Oertel S, Krempien R, Bischof M, Buechler M et al (2004) Intraoperative radiotherapy – special focus: recurrent rectal carcinoma. Front Radiat Ther Oncol 38:52–56

Wiggers T, Mannaerts GH, Marinelli AW, Martijn H, Rutten HJ (2003) Surgery for locally recurrent rectal cancer. Colorectal Dis 5:504–507

Wydmanski J, Miszczyk L, Suwiński R, Bogusław M, Andrzej O, Bekman A et al (2005) A new method of targeted intraoperative radiotherapy using the orthovoltage photon radiosurgery system. Nowotwory J Oncol 55:320–323

Case Reports 15

Katharine Pigott, Frederik Wenz, Mohammed Keshtgar, Sam Eljamel, Wojciech P. Polkowski, Tina Reis, Yasser Abo-Madyan, and Michael Ehmann

15.1 Case 1: Old Age at Presentation

A 93-year-old woman reported a 1-month history of left nipple irritation and of a lump in the left breast. On examination she had a 5 mm by 10 mm mass in the left lower inner quadrant. Mammogram (M5) demonstrated a 21-mm mass, while ultrasound (U5) revealed a 19-mm lesion of the left lower inner quadrant. Core biopsy showed grade 1 invasive ductal carcinoma. The lesion was oestrogen receptor positive with a Quick score of 8, progesterone receptor positive with a Quick score of 8 and HER2 negative.

The patient had a past medical history of Dukes B carcinoma treated with partial colectomy in 1979. She also had hypertension, osteoporosis and polymyalgia rheumatica. She lived alone and had a home help coming in once a day to assist with washing and dressing in the morning. She also had help with shopping and cleaning.

She underwent wide local excision and sentinel lymph node biopsy with off-trial intraoperative radiotherapy (IORT). Histology confirmed a 17-mm grade 1 invasive ductal carcinoma with clear margins. The lesion was oestrogen receptor positive with a Quick score of 8, progesterone receptor positive with a Quick score of 8 and HER2 negative. Two lymph nodes were clear of tumour.

This 93-year-old woman was given IORT to spare her the burden of 15 fractions of adjuvant whole breast radiotherapy. She was medically fit enough for surgery and despite her age, she wanted active treatment of the malignancy and was offered

K. Pigott (✉)
Department of Radiation Oncology, Royal Free London Foundation NHS Trust, Pond Street, Hampstead NW3 2QG, UK
e-mail: katharinehpigott@hotmail.com

F. Wenz • T. Reis • M. Ehmann
Department of Radiation Oncology, University Medical Center Mannheim, University of Heidelberg, Theodor-Kutzer-Ufer 1-3, D-68167 Mannheim, Germany
e-mail: frederik.wenz@medma.uni-heidelberg.de, frederik.wenz@umm.de, http://www.umm.de; tina.reis@umm.de; michael.ehmann@umm.de

M. Keshtgar, BSc, FRCSI, FRCS (Gen), PhD
Division of Surgery and Interventional Sciences, Department of Breast Surgery, University College London Medical School, Royal Free London Foundation NHS Trust, Pond Street, Hampstead NW3 2QG, UK
e-mail: m.keshtgar@ucl.ac.uk

S. Eljamel, MBBCh, MD, FRCSIr, FRCSEd, FRCS(SN)
Centre for Neurosciences, Ninewells Hospital and Medical School, Dundee DD1 9SY, Scotland, UK

W.P. Polkowski
Department of Surgical Oncology, Medical University of Lublin, SPSK nr 1 ul. Staszica 11, 20-081 Lublin, Poland
e-mail: wojciech.polkowski@am.lublin.pl

Y. Abo-Madyan
Department of Radiation Oncology, University Medical Centre Mannheim, University of Heidelberg, Theodor-Kutzer-Ufer 1-3, D-68167 Mannheim, Germany

Department of Clinical Oncology and Nuclear Medicine (NEMROCK), Faculty of Medicine, Cairo University, Cairo, Egypt
e-mail: yasser.abomadyan@umm.de, http://www.umm.de

M. Keshtgar et al. (eds.), *Targeted Intraoperative Radiotherapy in Oncology*, DOI 10.1007/978-3-642-39821-6_15, © Springer-Verlag Berlin Heidelberg 2014 wide local excision of the tumour and local radiotherapy or mastectomy. She was, however, anxious about the logistical difficulties of coming to daily hospital appointments over a 3-week period as she lived alone and had no personal means of transport. Furthermore, she did not want a mastectomy. Therefore, after multidisciplinary team (MDT) discussion, she was offered IORT radiotherapy to reduce the physical and social problems associated with her treatment. It is slightly contentious, however, as to whether, at 93 years old, this patient should have been given any adjuvant radiotherapy at all, as her lifetime risk of local recurrence with this low-risk tumour is very small.

15.1.1 Discussion

A number of studies have examined the role of radiotherapy in patients with low-risk breast cancer and these have on the whole found the risk of recurrence to be low when radiotherapy is omitted. The NSABP B21 trial (Wolmark et al. 2000) randomised patients to receive tamoxifen, tamoxifen plus radiotherapy or radiotherapy plus placebo. The ipsilateral recurrence rate in the tamoxifen-alone arm was 11.9 % compared to 5.7 % in the radiotherapy-alone arm. However, this trial was not conducted specifically in the elderly.

In contrast the CALGB/RTOG/ECOG trial (Hughes et al. 2004) of lumpectomy and adjuvant tamoxifen with or without breast radiotherapy in women 70 years and older revealed a very low recurrence rate in the tamoxifen-alone arm (1.3 %), compared to 0 % in the tamoxifen and radiotherapy arm. It is of interest that only 1 of the 39 deaths seen was due to breast cancer, suggesting that co-morbidity rather than breast cancer becomes the major cause of death in patients over the age of 70.

15.2 Case 2: Connective Tissue Disease

A 62-year-old woman presented with a lump in her left breast and complained of a history of pain in the left nipple. On clinical examination she had a discrete 30 mm by 30 mm lesion in the upper outer quadrant of the left breast. Ultrasound of the left breast confirmed a 27 mm by 14 mm hypo-echoic lesion (U5) in the upper outer quadrant. The axilla was clear. Mammogram demonstrated increased breast density (M4) and an MRI scan showed a 17-mm unifocal tumour. A core biopsy of the breast mass was performed and reported as a grade 1 invasive ductal carcinoma that was oestrogen receptor positive with a Quick score of 8, progesterone receptor positive with a Quick score of 8 and HER2 negative.

This patient had a significant past medical history and suffered from scleroderma and Raynaud's syndrome. She was discussed at the MDT and in view of her history of scleroderma it was recommended that she should either have a mastectomy and sentinel node biopsy, thus avoiding the need for radiotherapy, or wide local excision, sentinel node biopsy and off-trial IORT. She opted for the latter and received a dose of 6 Gy prescribed to 1 cm from the applicator.

Her case was discussed again in the MDT and the final histology was a grade 2 invasive ductal carcinoma, 15 mm in size, with all margins clear without involvement of any of the three sentinel lymph nodes. Adjuvant hormone treatment in the form of Arimidex for 5 years was recommended by the MDT.

15.2.1 Discussion

It is a commonly held notion that collagen vascular diseases such as rheumatoid arthritis, scleroderma, Raynaud's syndrome, lupus erythematosus, Sjögren's syndrome and polymyositis are absolute contraindications to radiotherapy since the effects on normal tissue are more marked, with a higher incidence of acute and late radiation toxicity. Published results remain controversial. Several studies claim that it is safe to give high-dose radiation in these patients, although scleroderma appears to have a higher incidence of complications than other collagen vascular diseases. This being the case, in patients with scleroderma radiotherapy tends to be avoided and mastectomy recommended instead of wide local excision. In patients with low-risk breast cancer, as in this case, IORT may offer patients the chance of breast-conserving surgery.

15.3 Case 3: Patient in Whom External Beam Radiotherapy Is Technically Impossible

A 68-year-old woman was referred from the breast screening unit with a left breast cancer diagnosed on routine screening. She had had no previous breast problems and had no risk factors for breast cancer apart from using HRT for 7 years. On examination she had some nodularity in the upper outer quadrant of the left breast.

Her mammogram demonstrated a 15-mm pleomorphic calcification in the upper outer quadrant (M3), and the lesion was also observed on ultrasound (U2). Core biopsy confirmed a grade 2 invasive ductal carcinoma with associated high-grade ductal carcinoma in situ. The lesion was oestrogen receptor positive with a Quick score of 8, progesterone receptor positive with a Quick score of 8 and HER2 negative.

This woman had severe Parkinson's disease with a very marked tremor such that it would have been impossible for her to remain still for external beam radiotherapy (EBRT). She was discussed in our MDT meeting and the treatment recommendation was mastectomy or wide local excision with off-trial IORT. The patient was not keen on mastectomy and wanted to proceed with breast-conserving surgery and IORT. She was made aware that the histology would be reviewed after the wide local excision and sentinel node biopsy and that, if it was felt the IORT was inadequate treatment because of up-staging of the tumour, then a mastectomy would be recommended.

Post-surgical histology confirmed a 10-mm grade 3 ductal carcinoma with high-grade DCIS. All margins were clear and the tumour receptor status was oestrogen receptor positive with a Quick score of 8, progesterone receptor positive with a Quick score of 8 and HER2 negative. Two sentinel lymph nodes were clear. She was again discussed by the MDT and Arimidex for 5 years was recommended.

15.3.1 Discussion

There are a number of situations in which it is technically difficult to deliver standard EBRT to the breast, such as the case above. Other situations encountered in our practice include a frozen shoulder where the arm would have been in the radiation field. Another example is early-onset dementia, where there is concern that the patient would move during treatment. In this selected group of cases for which EBRT is contraindicated or difficult, IORT is a viable option provided it does not compromise the likelihood of local tumour control and survival (Keshtgar et al. 2011). In patients with high-risk breast cancer, mastectomy has to remain the gold standard.

15.4 Case 4: Pacemaker and IORT

An 83-year-old female presented with a 2-week history of self-detected lump in the upper outer quadrant of the left breast. Clinically there was a 15-mm suspicious lump in the left breast. Mammography did not reveal any abnormality (R1) while ultrasound scan findings were consistent with the diagnosis of breast cancer (U5). Clinical and ultrasound examination of the axilla was unremarkable. Core biopsy of the lesion confirmed the diagnosis of invasive ductal carcinoma.

Past medical history of note was that a cardiac pacemaker had been inserted in 1996 for persistent sinus bradycardia and this was replaced in 2003 with a St Jude Medical dual-chamber pacemaker. The pacemaker was programmed to VVIR 70 ppm and the hysteresis rate was programmed to 60 ppm; the pacemaker was programmed to single chamber mode due to atrial lead failure. The dominant rhythm was atrial fibrillation with intermittent ventricular pacing. The pacemaker was sensing and pacing appropriately. The patient's heart rate varied between 60 and 107 bpm. The patient had been self caring and recent transthoracic echocardiography showed a normal ejection fraction and left ventricular size. Clinically the pacemaker was located in a subcutaneous tissue pocket in the upper pole of the left breast 9 cm from the primary tumour (Figs. 15.1, 15.2).

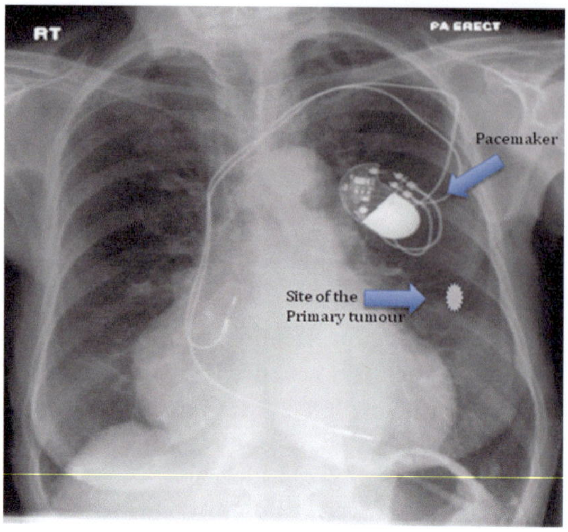

Fig. 15.1 Chest x-ray of the patient showing the pacemaker in situ and the approximate position of the breast cancer

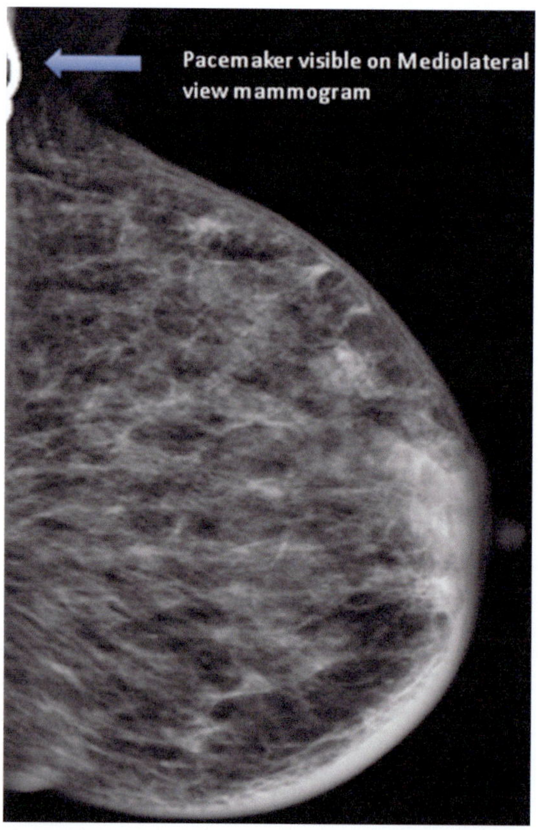

Fig. 15.2 Mammogram (mediolateral view) showing the pacemaker. The breast cancer was mammographically occult

After discussion at the MDT meeting, we recommended wide local excision and sentinel node biopsy, and in view of the size of the tumour and the presence of the pacemaker, it was also decided to offer the patient IORT using the TARGIT technique.

Prior to surgery, the details of the pacemaker device were obtained from the implanting hospital, and the distance from the tumour to the device measured at an assessment session. During surgery, after harvesting the sentinel node and wide local excision, IORT using the INTRABEAM device (50 kV) was performed. A 3-cm-diameter applicator was used, delivering approximately 20 Gy at the surface of the breast tissue in direct contact with the applicator, and 6 Gy at 1 cm from the surface, for the duration of 26 min. During the surgery a packet of thermoluminescent dosimeters (TLD) was placed on the edge of the device closest to the X-ray source and the distance between the applicator shaft of the INTRABEAM and the pacemaker was recorded. The measured reading was converted to dose using a batch calibration value corrected for supralinearity. The average reading of the TLD packet was 0.08 Gy.

The patient tolerated the procedure very well; there was no malfunction of the pacemaker during the surgery and IORT and the patient was discharged home the following day. Pacemaker function was tested by a cardiology technician before and after treatment.

Histology confirmed a 14-mm grade 2 invasive ductal carcinoma which was node negative and oestrogen receptor positive with a Quick score of 8, progesterone receptor positive with a Quick score of 8 and HER2 negative. She was advised an aromatase inhibitor as adjuvant treatment.

15.4.1 Discussion

The position of this patient's pacemaker was such that it would have been in the tangential whole breast radiotherapy fields and would have thus received the full dose. There is a risk that ionising irradiation can interfere with modern

CMOS (complementary metal oxide semiconductor) equipped cardiac pacemakers (Hudson et al. 2001), resulting in their failure. The option with this patient was to reposition the pacemaker and give standard EBRT or to treat the tumour bed with IORT, allowing the dose to the pacemaker to be kept low.

In 1994, the American Association of Physicists in Medicine (AAPM) stated that a cardiac pacemaker can fail at radiotherapy (RT) doses as low as 10 Gy and even 2 Gy could lead to significant functional changes (Marbach et al. 1994). This resulted in the "AAPM guideline for pacemakers in radiation oncology", which suggested that the dose at the pacemaker should be limited to 2.0 Gy (Marbach et al. 1994).

Nowadays, modern pacemakers are equipped with CMOS circuitry and RAM (random access memory). These electronic elements facilitate programming of devices (e.g. holding the current information about frequency threshold, modes of pacing and sensing) and improve reliability and energy consumption. Nevertheless, an increase in IR sensitivity has been described as well. Several cases have been reported where the threshold programming was deleted or the devices failed at low doses (overview at Hudson et al. 2001). On the other hand, no manufacturer has quoted a safe minimum radiation dose.

At present, very little is known about direct and scatter irradiation effects, especially concerning the newer pacemakers equipped with modern CMOS. Manufacturers provide estimates for their pacemaker models regarding to which dose a device can be irradiated (St. Jude 20–30 Gy (Rhythm Management Division 2005), Medtronic 5 Gy (CRDM Technical Services 2008), Guidant n.n. (European Technical Services 2004)) The wide range of manufacturer-stated acceptable radiotherapy doses and in vitro data generated since the 1994 AAPM guideline for radiotherapy (Marbach et al. 1994), showing that PM can fail at any dose (Mouton et al. 2002), represent the fragile situation at which radiotherapy operates in regard to modern CMOS-equipped pacemakers.

Therefore, at least for EBRT, in cases where the pacemaker would be close to treatment fields, adjustments (encompassing modification of the radiotherapy field size and shape, moving the pacemaker surgically out of the field, withholding radiotherapy from the patient or considering IORT if appropriate) to the treatment planning procedure might become necessary.

15.5 Case 5: Randomisation into the TARGIT-A Trial

A 69-year-old woman attended for routine breast screening and was found on mammography to have a 22-mm spiculated mass with microcalcification in the left upper outer quadrant (M5). Ultrasound revealed a hypoechoic lesion with normal lymph nodes (U5). A core biopsy diagnosed a grade 2 ductal carcinoma that was oestrogen receptor positive (Quick score 8), progesterone receptor positive (Quick score 8) and HER2 negative (B5). MRI scan showed a unifocal, unicentric mass 16 mm in size with type II enhancement and no lymphadenopathy.

Her case was discussed in the MDT meeting and a recommendation for wire-guided localisation of the lesion was made prior to wide local excision and sentinel node sampling. The patient met the criteria for entry into the TARGIT trial. This was discussed with her prior to surgery and she agreed to participate in the trial and was randomised to the IORT arm. At the time of surgery a dose of 6 Gy at 1 cm from the applicator surface was delivered. OSNA testing of the sentinel node was positive and the surgeon therefore went ahead with an axillary clearance.

Following the surgery her case was again discussed at the multidisciplinary meeting. The final histology confirmed the presence of a 17-mm grade 3 ductal carcinoma with associated DCIS; all margins were clear and 3 out of 11 lymph nodes were positive. The MDT meeting therefore recommended staging with bone scan and CT of the chest, abdomen and pelvis, followed, if clear, by chemotherapy, radiation treatment to the whole breast and endocrine treatment.

15.5.1 Discussion

At initial presentation, imaging and biopsy suggested we were dealing with a low-risk breast cancer. It was therefore reasonable to offer the patient entry into the TARGIT trial, which compares IORT with standard radiotherapy consisting of whole breast irradiation followed by a boost to the tumour site (Vaidya et al. 2010). However, following surgery this lady was found to be node positive and therefore at higher risk for both local and systemic recurrence. This being the case, the above recommendation was made in order to try and reduce the risk of recurrence. Results from the TARGIT trial revealed that following IORT about 15 % of patients went on to receive whole breast irradiation because of upstaging of the disease. This patient had 40.05 Gy in 15 fractions to the left breast.

15.6 Case 6: Previous Radiotherapy in the Treatment Area

A 63-year-old lady presented with a lump in her right breast. On examination she had a 10-mm lump in the upper outer quadrant of the right breast. Mammogram and ultrasound findings were diagnostic of breast cancer (M5, U5). Core biopsy revealed a grade 1 invasive ductal carcinoma that was oestrogen receptor positive (Quick score 8), progesterone receptor positive (Quick score 8) and HER2 negative.

She had been treated 12 years earlier for non-Hodgkin's lymphoma centred on the left neck. She initially received CHOP × 6, ESHAP × 2 mini beam but a year later developed resistant diffuse B cell lymphoma which was a presumed transformation from follicular lymphoma. She went on to have full-dose BEAM with autologous bone marrow transplant followed by radiotherapy to the mediastinum and neck.

She was discussed in the MDT meeting and the recommendation was for mastectomy because the right breast would have received a significant radiation dose from the mediastinal radiation fields employed 12 years earlier for the treatment of her lymphoma. However, the patient was adamant that she wished to undergo breast-conserving surgery. IORT off-trial was offered to her on the understanding that if she was found to have high-risk disease following the wide local excision and sentinel lymph node sampling, mastectomy would have to be considered.

She underwent right wire-guided wide local excision and sentinel node sampling with IORT. At the time of surgery a dose of 6 Gy at 1 cm from the applicator surface was delivered. The histology confirmed a 14.4-mm grade 1 invasive ductal carcinoma with clear margins but an incidental finding of follicular lymphoma in the sentinel node. The MDT recommended Arimidex for 5 years and referral to the haematologist with regard to her follicular cell lymphoma.

15.6.1 Discussion

Radiation-induced secondary malignancies can occur many years after patients have received treatment. They commonly occur within the radiation field. There is a growing amount of data for patients who receive chemotherapy and radiotherapy for Hodgkin's disease, where an increase in second solid tumours has been observed, especially cancers of the lung, breast, thyroid, bone/soft tissue, stomach, oesophagus, colon and rectum, uterine cervix, head and neck, and mesothelioma. These tumours occur primarily after radiation therapy or with combined modality treatment, and approximately 75 % occur within radiation ports. At a 15-year follow-up, the risk of second solid tumours is approximately 13 %.

In a case control study of 106 patients who developed breast cancer after therapy for Hodgkin's disease, cumulative absolute risks for developing breast cancer were calculated as a function of radiation therapy dose and the use of chemotherapy. With a 30-year follow-up, cumulative absolute risks of breast cancer with exposure to radiation range from 8.5 to 39.6 %, depending on the age at diagnosis. The younger the age at treatment, the higher is the incidence.

There are a number of patients in whom standard breast radiotherapy cannot be delivered because of previous radiotherapy in that area for other malignancies such as lymphoma and oesophageal and lung cancer. In these cases the standard recommendation would be mastectomy, thus avoiding radiotherapy. In patients with low-risk breast cancer, IORT at the time of surgery offers the chance of undergoing breast-conserving surgery.

15.7 Case 7: Inclusion into Kypho-IORT Dose Escalation Study

A 60-year-old female patient with osseous metastasizing breast cancer under tamoxifen, trastuzumab and denosumab presented with newly diagnosed progressive metastases of the 9th and 10th thoracic vertebrae (Fig. 15.3). The remaining osseous metastases were stable or regressive. There were no visceral or lymphatic metastases. On clinical examination the patient had a Karnofsky Index of 100 %, without any back pain. The patient had a strong therapy wish.

The initial diagnosis of a receptor-positive invasive ductal carcinoma [pT1c pN3a (12/15) L1 V0 R0 M1] of the left breast was made in May 2011. After breast-conserving surgery with axillary dissection, the patient received whole-breast radiotherapy including the axillary lymph nodes with boost (50 + 16 Gy) followed by systemic therapy using trastuzumab, Aromasin and

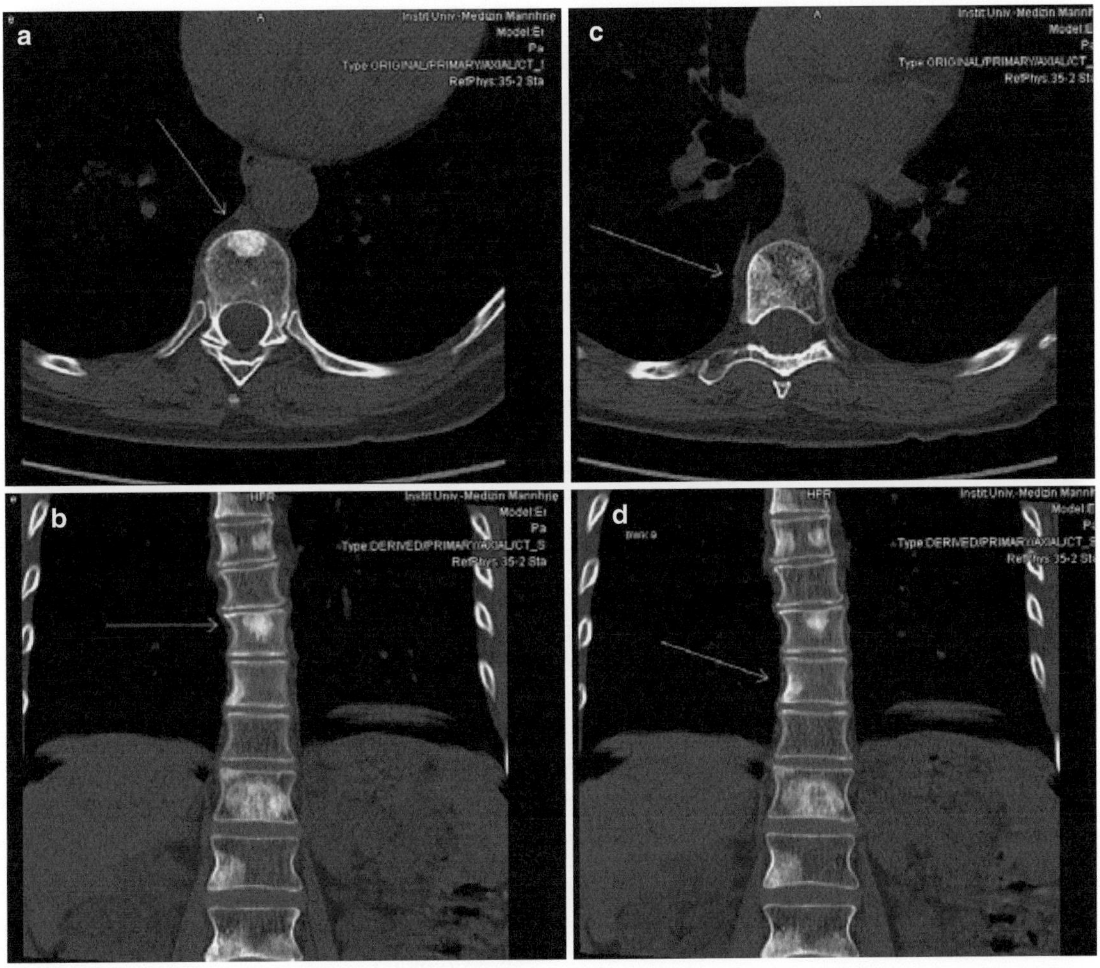

Fig. 15.3 Postoperative follow-up T1-weighted MRI demonstrating enhancement in the operative site with compensatory dilatation of the left occipital horn of the lateral ventricle

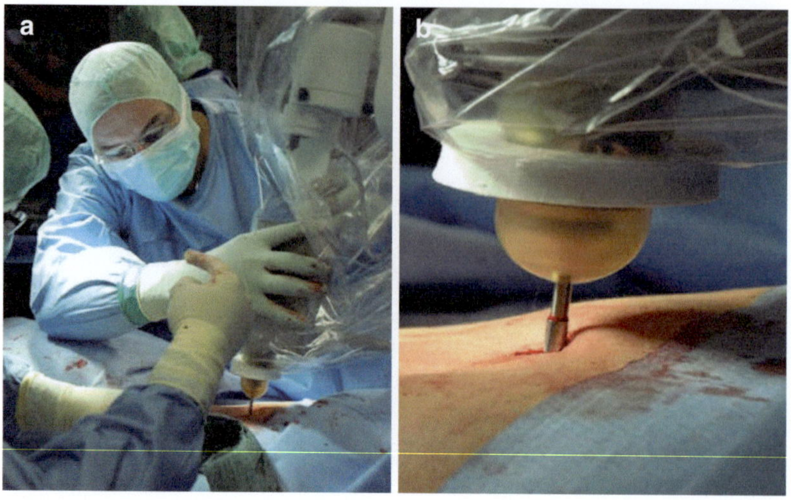

Fig. 15.4 Results of the PET/CT scan performed in April 2006. (**a**) PET scan; (**b**) fused axial PET-CT. FDG-avid disease is seen within the upper mediastinal nodes

bisphosphonates. Simultaneous to the whole breast radiotherapy, the patient received a palliative irradiation of the right hip (40/2 Gy). The first progressive osseous metastases were diagnosed in June 2012 during routine follow-up and palliative irradiation of C3-T1, T5-T8 and T11-L4 (30/3 Gy) was initiated. Moreover, endocrine therapy was switched from Aromasin to tamoxifen, and denosumab was started instead of bisphosphonates.

After discussion of her case with the orthopaedic surgeons, we recommended a Kypho-IORT of the 9th and 10th thoracic vertebrae. The patient met the criteria for entry into the Kypho-IORT dose escalation study. This was discussed with her prior to surgery and she agreed to participate in the trial. During balloon kyphoplasty a dose of 8 Gy at 10 mm from the applicator surface was delivered (Fig. 15.4). After completion of the radiation therapy, kyphoplasty was concluded in accordance with standard procedure.

The patient tolerated the procedure very well and there were no intra- or postoperative complications. She was discharged home the following day.

15.7.1 Discussion

Optimal dose fraction schedule or optimal standard dose for the treatment of vertebral metastases has not been established and is consistently discussed (Souchon et al. 2009). Especially, there is increasing interest in minimally invasive techniques, such as kyphoplasty, combined with other physical methods to achieve synergistic therapeutic effects. Recently published trials show good results for pain relief and local tumour control in patients with spinal metastases treated with kyphoplasty combined with intravertebral administration of samarium-153 or interstitial implantation of iodine-125 seeds (Ashamalla et al. 2009; Yang et al. 2009). Another possibility is intravertebral radiofrequency ablation in addition to surgical procedures (Van der Linden et al. 2007). However, the cytotoxic effect of radiofrequency ablation is still not well documented.

Using the INTRABEAM system for Kypho-IORT allows the application of single high-dose radiotherapy in the centre of the metastases during balloon kyphoplasty. This novel approach is a technically feasible, minimally invasive procedure without severe side-effects that provides immediate pain relief and achieves structural stability (Schneider et al. 2009; Schmidt et al. 2012; Reis et al. 2012). Moreover, using this X-ray-based approach, the risk of open radionuclides can be avoided.

Compared to fractionated therapy regimens, this single-step procedure shortens treatment time and may become a valuable treatment option in the palliative setting.

15.8 Case 8: Intraoperative Radiotherapy (IORT) in Brain Tumour

A 67-year-old female presented with speech difficulty of several weeks' duration. Previously she had undergone pulmonary lobectomy for lung cancer, and she had subsequently had no local recurrence for more than 4 years. Examination confirmed that she was right handed and had nominal dysphasia. There were no other signs.

Her MRI demonstrated a lesion in the grey-white matter interface with significant oedema. The lesion enhanced with contrast and was surrounded by small cysts (Fig. 15.5).

The lesion was totally removed using image-guided surgery technology, followed by IORT. The surgery was able to remove the solid component easily but to remove the cystic wall would almost certainly have increased the neurological deficit. Therefore IORT was recommended. She received 15 Gy.

The patient made an excellent postoperative recovery. Her nominal dysphasia improved significantly. The histopathology confirmed metastatic brain cancer of lung origin. She was followed up regularly in the joint neuro-oncology clinic, clinically and radiologically.

Her postoperative MRI scan 11 months after surgery and IORT demonstrated no evidence of recurrence (Fig. 15.6).

Twenty-one months after surgery, MRI demonstrated changes at the treatment site, which took up contrast (Fig. 15.7). This was explored and the histology confirmed that this was radionecrosis rather than recurrence. Radionecrosis can occur after IORT in brain but we observed it only in this case after treating 56 patients with doses varying from 8 to 15 Gy. She continued under clinical and radiological surveillance, and 5 years after treatment she still had not developed any recurrence.

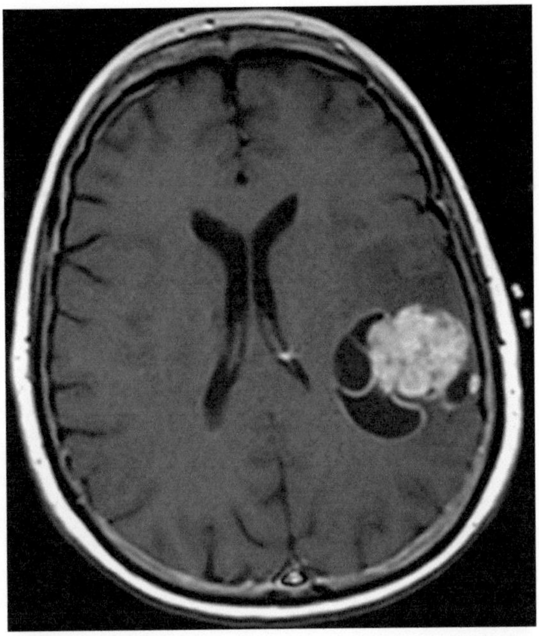

Fig. 15.5 Axial T1-weighted MRI with contrast demonstrating an enhancing lesion in the grey-white matter interface with small cysts around it

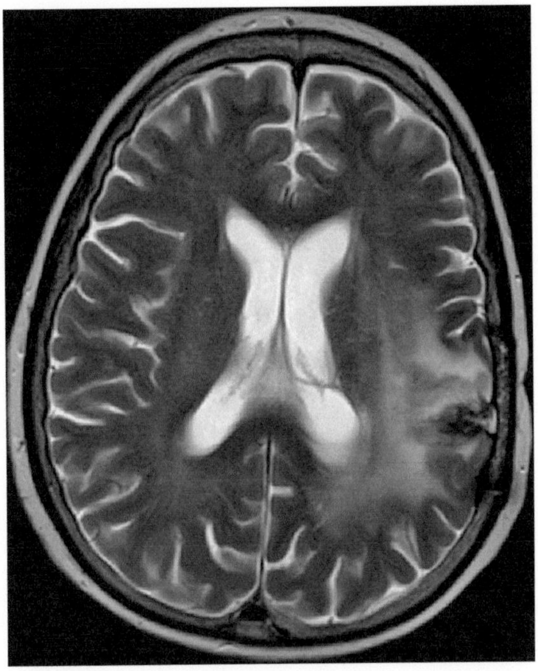

Fig. 15.6 T2-weighted axial MRI demonstrating the location of craniotomy for excision of metastatic lung cancer in the brain 11 months after surgery and IORT

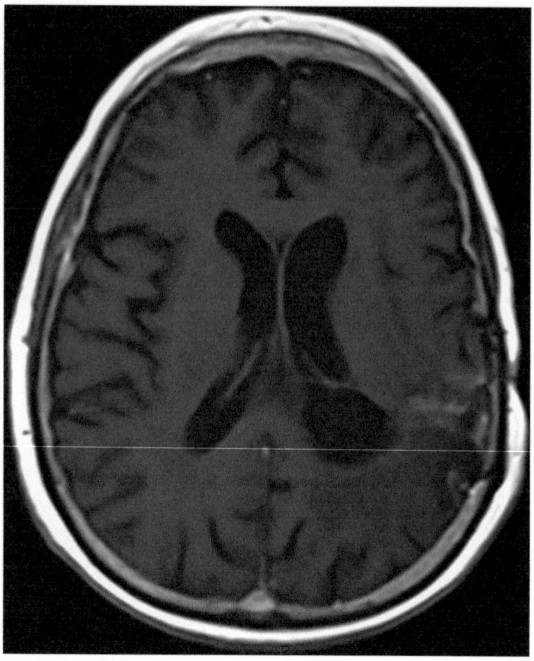

Fig. 15.7 Postoperative follow-up T1-weighted MRI demonstrating enhancement in the operative site with compensatory dilatation of the left occipital horn of the lateral ventricle

15.9 Case 9: Intra-operative Radiotherapy in Rectal Cancer

A 66-year-old white, female patient was initially operated on for rectal cancer in August 2001. An exophytic lesion was located 14 cm from the anal verge. Surgical treatment of the primary tumour comprised anterior resection of the rectum extended with cholecystectomy due to cholelithiasis. A poorly differentiated (G3) ulcerative adenocarcinoma of the rectum with tubular and papillary components and 3 × 2 cm in size was identified at pathology. The tumour was staged according to the 7th edition of the TNM classification system (2010) as pT3N0Mx, since out of six lymph nodes removed, all were reactive, stage III. The gallbladder had features of chronic cholecystitis. The patient subsequently proceeded to receive adjuvant chemoradiotherapy. EBRT was performed with a ^{60}Co unit, using the four-field technique. The patient was treated to a total dose of 52 Gy, delivered in 6 weeks at 2 Gy per fraction. A concomitant boost of 6 Gy was given in the last week of pelvic radiotherapy. The patient received concurrent Mayo regimen chemotherapy (5-fluorouracil bolus 425 mg/m^2/day + folinic acid 20 mg/m^2/day × 5 days every 28 days).

After completion of adjuvant therapy, the patient started follow-up. In October 2004 an elevated level of serum CEA was found. CT results were inconclusive, but revealed a mass 5 cm in diameter in the pelvis, adjacent to rectal tissue, suspected to correspond to local recurrence. The patient was not re-irradiated using EBRT but instead underwent exploratory laparotomy, performed in the Department of Surgical Oncology of the Medical University of Lublin (38 months after primary surgery), which did not confirm the presence of local relapse. Since that time the patient has remained in follow-up. On control CT examination in November 2005, four enlarged lymph nodes (to 10 mm) in the upper mediastinum and at the sides of the common iliac artery were seen. A further PET scan (April 2006) suggested proliferative processes in mediastinal lymph nodes (Fig. 15.8). Subsequent CT studies disclosed further enlargement of lymph nodes in the mediastinum (to 15–17 mm), with a retroperitoneal 3-cm tumour adherent to the uterine wall. Increases in CEA level (from 2.7 to 6.3 ng/ml) and CA 19–9 (from 24.6 to 55.5 U/ml) were observed, with no macroscopic lesions on colonoscopy.

In July 2007 the patient was re-admitted to the Department of Surgical Oncology with a diagnosis of recurrent rectal cancer, 83 months after primary surgery. She did not present symptoms of the disease, such as pain and bowel dysfunction, and therefore was categorised as S0 according to the Suzuki classification. Resection of local rectal cancer recurrence was extended with supravaginal hysterectomy with bilateral adnexectomy. A tumour 4 cm in diameter was found in the corner between the uterus and the right fallopian tube. After excision, intraoperative histopathological examination was performed, which confirmed the presence of neoplastic tissue with extensive necrosis, without evidence of infiltration of the rectum. Due to suspicion of close or

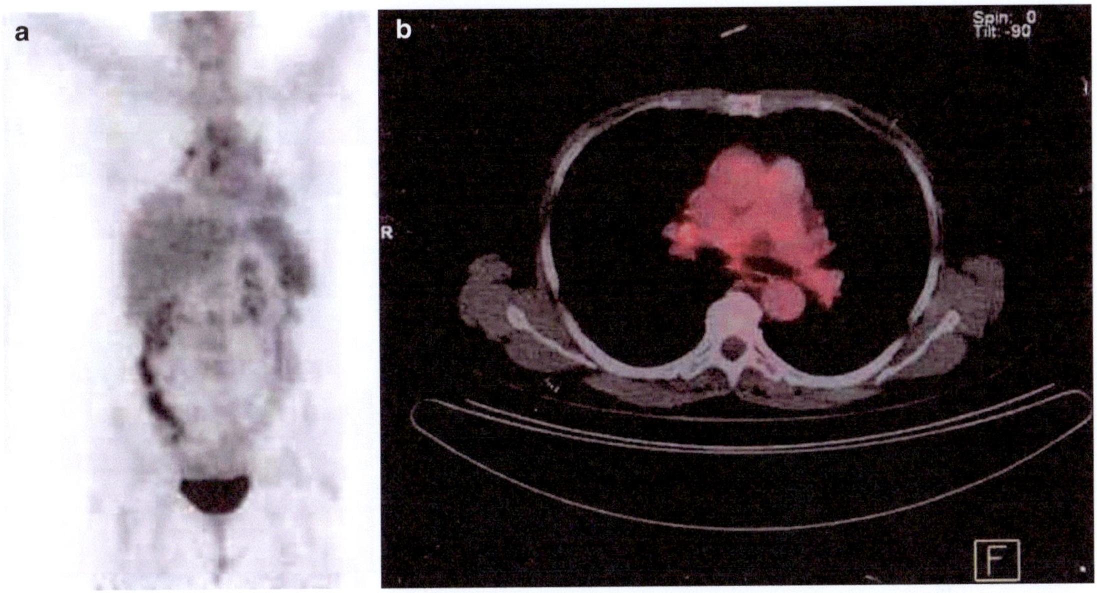

Fig. 15.8 Results of the PET/CT scan performed in April 2006. (**a**) PET scan; (**b**) fused axial PET-CT. FDG-avid disease is seen within the upper mediastinal nodes

Fig. 15.9 Visualisation of the tumour bed after excision

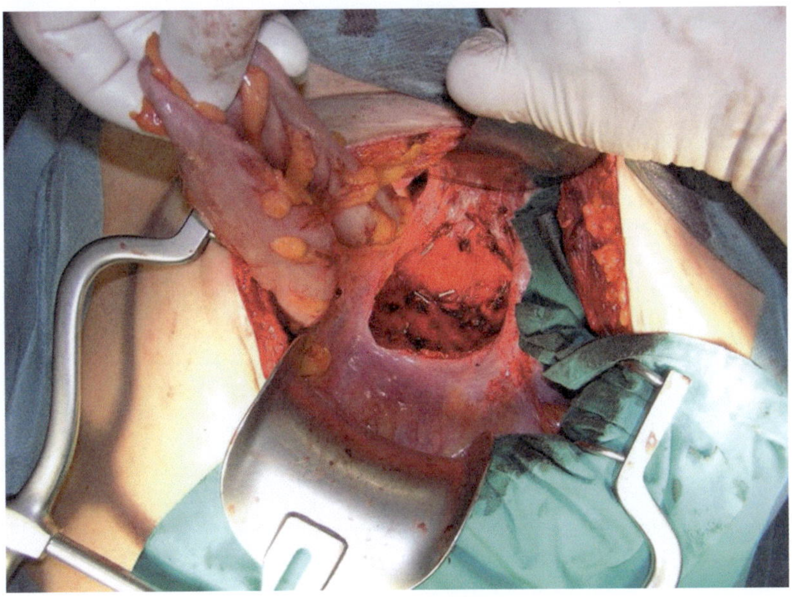

positive margins, IORT was performed using the INTRABEAM PRS 500 (Figs. 15.9, 15.10, and 15.11). The applicator size used was 5 cm. The prescribed dose was 12.5 Gy to the surface of the applicator, and the irradiation time was 33 min. The postoperative period was uneventful and the hospital stay was 6 days. The postoperative pathological report did not reveal neoplastic infiltration of the uterine wall and adjacent structures. Tumour marker levels declined significantly in the postoperative period, CEA falling to 2.9 ng/ml and CA 19–9 to 16.3 U/ml. The patient qualified for and received adjuvant systemic therapy from August to October 2007, comprising five

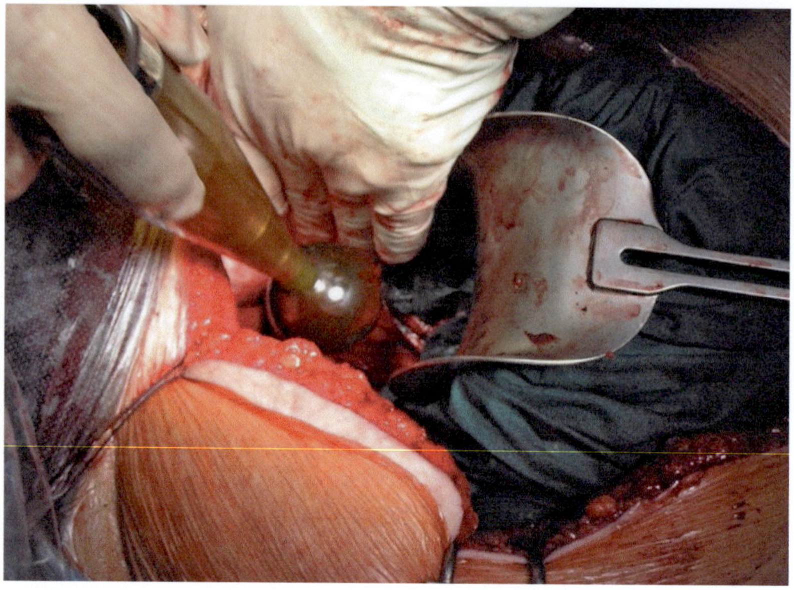

Fig. 15.10 Fitting the applicator (Ø 5 cm) to the tumour bed

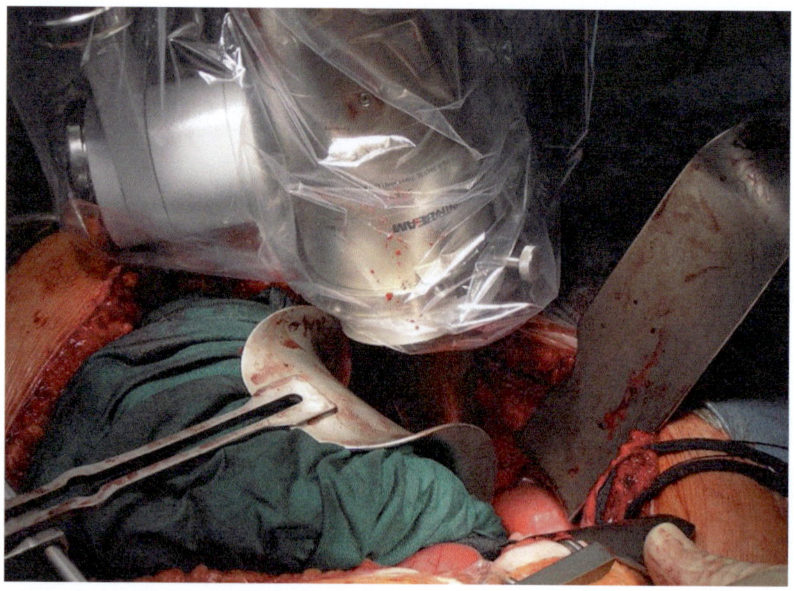

Fig. 15.11 INTRABEAM arm with applicator placed in the tumour bed

cycles of the CLF regimen (irinotecan, 5-fluorouracil, leucovorin) with bevacizumab in weekly administrations.

A control CT study in March 2008 revealed further enlargement in mediastinal lymph nodes without features of local re-relapse in the pelvis. The next line of chemotherapy was administered, the patient receiving six cycles of FOLFOX-type (oxaliplatin, 5-fluorouracil, leucovorin) chemotherapy. Following completion of treatment, the patient has remained in follow-up since April 2008. She is alive 65 months after surgery for local recurrence. The last follow-up was in November 2012, with no symptoms of disease as well as negative laboratory and imaging study results.

15.10 Intraoperative Radiotherapy for Recurrent Head and Neck Cancer Using a Mobile 50 Kilovoltage Mini-accelerator: A Case Report

In April 1987, at the age of 40 years, a white Caucasian male patient with history of tobacco exposure of 48 pack years (till 1987) and moderate alcohol abuse (till 1990) was referred to our radiation oncology clinic after surgical management of a superficially ulcerating, moderately differentiated non-keratinizing invasive squamous cell carcinoma (SCC) of the floor of the mouth, mixed with an in-situ component. The surgery consisted of local excision and bilateral supraomohyoid lymphadenectomy. With a TNM-stage of T2 N2 M0, the patient received his adjuvant irradiation up to a dose of 60 Gy over 11 weeks (alternating right and left sides every second day with significant delays) from May till July-1987 using a Cobalt 60 Teletherapy machine. A 2-D plan was used to cover the volume including both sides of the neck and the oral cavity/oropharyngeal region.

Two years later (in 1989) the patient suffered local and neck node relapse which was treated surgically by wide excision of the floor of the mouth and left sided neck dissection.

In July 1992, a second diagnosis of stage I anaplastic non-Hodgkin's Lymphoma of the right upper cervical lymph nodes was made. Treatment with chemotherapy (4xCHEOP) was given followed by irradiation of the right upper neck region at the angle of the mandible using 12 MeV Electrons up to a dose of 40/2.5 Gy over 2.5 weeks till February 1993. Since then, no further evidence of Lymphoma was observed till today.

In January 2011, a second poorly differentiated SCC infiltrating from the right side of the tongue to the base of the tongue was diagnosed. After complete tumor resection and right sided neck dissection, with a TNM-stage of T4a N0 M0 L0 V0 R0, due to fear of further morbidity and side effects, the patient was closely monitored without and adjuvant treatment. However, 21 months later, a local recurrence in the deep muscles of the right tongue infiltrating the floor of the mouth and tonsillar pillars was discovered. Clinical examination and FDG-PET scan revealed

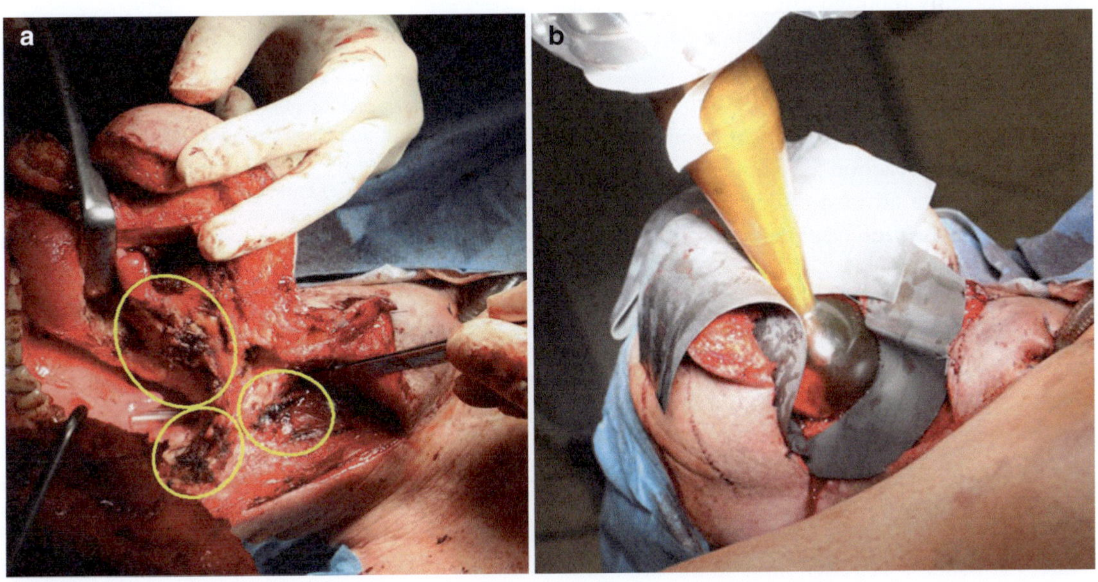

Fig. 15.12 (**a**) Tumor bed directly after resection, surfaces to be treated at the right tongue, floor of mouth and tonsillar pillar are marked in *yellow*. (**b**) Applicator in position with ruberred tungsten foil fixed to protect tissue surfaces not to be treated

only localized disease. In October 2012, the patient underwent tumor resection with partial tongue/floor of mouth resection and partial pharyngectomy. Intraoperatively, a single dose of 8 Gy prescribed in 5 mm depth (equivalent to 14.8 Gy surface dose) was simultaneously applied to all surfaces of the tumor bed using the 5 cm spherical applicator of the Intrabeam system over 33 min (Fig. 15.12). This was followed by reconstruction of the operative bed and defect coverage with a pectoralis major flap. Histological examination revealed complete tumor resection (R0).

The postoperative period went smoothly. Four weeks after surgery the patient was discharged from the hospital with no documented complications. Wound healing was complete. After 5.5 weeks from surgery and IORT, re-EBRT using IMRT was started to the right oral cavity, floor of mouth and oropharynx including lymph node levels 1–3. A dose of 50.4/1.8 Gy was reached with no evidence of grade 3 or 4 acute radiation side effects.

15.10.1 Discussion

A series of 16 patients with SCC of the oral cavity was recently reported after a combined treatment of KV-IORT with Intrabeam (range 5–7.5 Gy at 5 mm depth, surface dose 7.8–12.7 Gy) followed by 50 Gy EBRT. The group reported no increase in acute mucosal reaction. Early mucosal reaction did not exceed RTOG grade 3. No late adverse effects were observed. Local tumor control was reported in all cases (Rutkowski et al. 2000).

The decision to irradiate the head and neck region for a third time is not an easy one. First, nearby organs at risk (spinal cord, skin, connective tissue and mandible) has to show adequate vitality and lack of late effects from previous treatments that would indicate possible tolerance to further treatment. Second, doses equivalent to at least 60 Gy should be technically achievable. Here, the benefits of IORT include the high precision of tumor bed localization, delivery of a more biologically effective high single dose to the tumor bed that would reduce if not eradicate any microscopic tumor residual in the region with the highest risk for recurrence. Wound healing was not an issue helped by the fact that the muscle flap was not exposed to the IORT treatment dose. In contrast, if an EBRT-Boost was planned, the tumor bed would have been very difficult to localize probably leading to definition of a larger volume to avoid a geographic miss increasing the risk of loss of flap and wound dehiscence.

Conclusion

KV-IORT in the head and neck region seems to be safely applicable even in situations after multiple surgeries and re-irradiation.

References

Ashamalla H, Cardoso E, Macedon M, Guirguis A, Weng L, Ali S et al (2009) Phase I trial of vertebral intracavitary cement and samarium (VICS): novel technique for treatment of painful vertebral metastasis. Int J Radiat Oncol Biol Phys 75:836–842

Chen AM, Obedian E, Haffty BG (2001) Breast-conserving therapy in the setting of collagen vascular disease. Cancer J 7:480–491

CRDM Technical Services (2008) Therapeutic radiation. Medtronic Incorporated, Mounds View

European Technical Services (2004) Impact of therapeutic radiation and guidant ICD/CRT-p/pacing systems review. Guidant Corp, St. Paul, pp 1–6

Hancock SL, Hoppe RT (1996) Long-term complications of treatment and causes of mortality after Hodgkin's disease. Semin Radiat Oncol 6:225–242

Hudson F et al (2010) Effect of radiation therapy on the latest generation of pacemakers and implantable cardioverter defibrillators: a systematic review. J Med Imaging Radiat Oncol 54(1):53–61

Hughes KS, Schnaper LA, Berry D, Cirrincione C, McCormick B, Shank B (2004) Lumpectomy plus tamoxifen with or without irradiation in women age 70 or older with early breast cancer. N Engl J Med 351:971–977

Keshtgar MR, Vaidya JS, Tobias JS, Wenz F, Joseph D, Stacey C et al (2011) Targeted intraoperative radiotherapy for breast cancer in patients in whom external beam radiotherapy is not possible. J Radiat Oncol Biol Phys 80:31–38

Marbach JR et al (1994) Management of radiation oncology patients with implanted cardiac pacemakers: report of AAPM Task Group No. 34. American Association of Physicists in Medicine. Med Phys 21(1):85–90

Mouton J et al (2002) Influence of high-energy photon beam irradiation on pacemaker operation. Phys Med Biol 47(16):2879–2893

Reis T, Schneider F, Welzel G, Schmidt R, Bludau F, Obertacke U, Wenz F (2012) Intraoperative radiotherapy during kyphoplasty for vertebral metastases (Kypho IORT): first clinical results. Tumori 98:434–440

Rhythm Management Division (2005) Radiation. St. Jude Medical, Sylmar

Rutkowski T et al (2010) Intraoperative radiotherapy (IORT) with low-energy photons as a boost in patients with early-stage oral cancer with the indications for postoperative radiotherapy: treatment feasibility and preliminary results. Strahlenther Onkol 186(9): 496–501

Swerdlow AJ, Douglas AJ, Hudson GV, Hudson BV, Bennett MH, MacLennan KA (1992) Risk of second primary cancers after Hodgkin's disease by type of treatment: analysis of 2846 patients in the British National Lymphoma Investigation. BMJ 304:1137–114

Schmidt R, Wenz F, Reis T, Janik K, Bludau F, Obertacke U (2012) Kyphoplasty and intra-operative radiotherapy, combination of kyphoplasty and intra-operative radiation for spinal metastases: technical feasibility of a novel approach. Int Orthop 36:1255–1260

Schneider F, Greineck F, Clausen S, Mai S, Obertacke U, Reis T, Wenz F (2011) Development of a novel method for intraoperative radiotherapy during kyphoplasty for spinal metastases (Kypho-IORT). Int J Radiat Oncol Biol Phys 81:1114–1119

Souchon R, Wenz F, Sedlmayer F, Budach W, Dunst J, Feyer P et al (2009) DEGRO practice guidelines for palliative radiotherapy of metastatic breast cancer: bone metastases and metastatic spinal cord compression (MSCC). Strahlenther Onkol 185:417–424

Travis LB, Hill D, Dores GM, Gospodarowicz M, van Leeuwen FE, Holowaty E et al (2005) Cumulative absolute breast cancer risk for young women treated for Hodgkin lymphoma. J Natl Cancer Inst 97:1428–1437

Vaidya JS, Joseph DJ, Tobias JS, Bulsara M, Wenz F, Saunders C et al (2010) Targeted intraoperative radiotherapy versus whole breast radiotherapy for breast cancer (TARGIT-A trial): an international, prospective, randomised, non-inferiority, randomised, non-inferiority phase 3 trial. Lancet 376:91–102

Wo J, Taghian A (2007) Radiotherapy in setting of collagen vascular disease. Int J Radiat Oncol Biol Phys 69:1347–1353

Wolmark N, Dignam J, Margolese R, Wickerham DL, Fisher B (2000) The role of radiotherapy and tamoxifen in the management of node negative invasive breast cancer <1.0 cm treated with lumpectomy: preliminary results of NSABP protocol B-21. Proc Am Soc Clin Oncol 19:70a, Abstract 271

Van der Linden E, Kroft LJ, Dijkstra PD (2007) Treatment of vertebral tumor with posterior wall defect using image-guided radiofrequency ablation combined with vertebroplasty: preliminary results in 12 patients. J Vasc Interv Radiol 18:741–747

Yang Z, Yang D, Xie L, Sun Y, Huang Y, Sun H et al (2009) Treatment of metastatic spinal tumours by percutaneous vertebroplasty versus percutaneous vertebroplasty combined with interstitial implantation of 125I seeds. Acta Radiol 50:1142–1148

Intra Operative Radiotherapy in Developing Countries: Experience with TARGIT from University of Dammam, Saudi Arabia

16

Maha Abdel Hadi and Mohammed Keshtgar

Over recent decades the number of new cases of breast cancer diagnosed worldwide has risen dramatically, from about 640,000 in 1980 to 1.6 million in 2010. What is striking is that most of these 1.6 million new cases of breast cancer (51 %) occurred in developing countries (Forouzanfar et al. 2011). This increasing incidence of breast cancer in developing countries raised the level of apprehension among the affected communities.

Breast cancer accounts for 13–35 % of all female cancers, and in developing Arab countries is diagnosed a decade earlier younger than in industrialised nations (El Saghir et al. 2007). In Saudi Arabia, data from the Saudi National Cancer Registry for 2005 show that breast cancer accounted for 25.4 % of all newly diagnosed female malignancies and that it is characterised by young age and advanced disease at initial presentation. The trend towards an increased incidence of breast cancer and a young age at presentation are reflected in our data from the King Fahd Hospital, University of Dammam (Figs. 16.1 and 16.2).

Among women in Arab communities, great cultural value is placed on body image. Anxiety about cancer detection and fear of breast loss consequently lead women to resist seeking help: breast cancer represents a cultural stigma to be dealt with in utmost secrecy. Women prefer to be silent sufferers who tolerate considerable distress before ultimately presenting with relatively advanced disease (Abdel Hadi 2000; Ravichandran et al. 2011).

The fact that strategies aimed at early detection have generally not succeeded over the years is attributable to the fact that the surgical options have not altered. Mastectomy tends to be offered to patients regardless of disease stage, and is reportedly used in as many as 80 % of cases (Ibrahim et al. 2005), in sharp contrast to figures from the Western world. Nevertheless, limited local campaigns aimed at raising awareness have shown a positive impact on early presentation, leading to a lower stage at diagnosis and making breast-conserving surgery a real possibility (Abdel Hadi 2000).

The scarcity of radiotherapy facilities in developing countries further compounds the problem. It has been reported that there are only 205 radiation therapy centres, 256 radiation oncologists and 1,216 radiation technologists in all Arab countries, as compared with 2,734, 2,683 and 4,518, respectively, in the USA, which has an

M. Abdel Hadi (✉)
Department of Surgery,
University of Dammam,
Dammam, Saudi Arabia
e-mail: abdelhadi_m@hotmail.com

M. Keshtgar, BSc, FRCSI, FRCS (Gen), PhD
Division of Surgery and Interventional Sciences,
Department of Breast Surgery, University College
London Medical School, Royal Free London
Foundation NHS Trust, Pond Street,
Hampstead NW3 2QG, UK
e-mail: m.keshtgar@ucl.ac.uk

M. Keshtgar et al. (eds.), *Targeted Intraoperative Radiotherapy in Oncology*,
DOI 10.1007/978-3-642-39821-6_16, © Springer-Verlag Berlin Heidelberg 2014

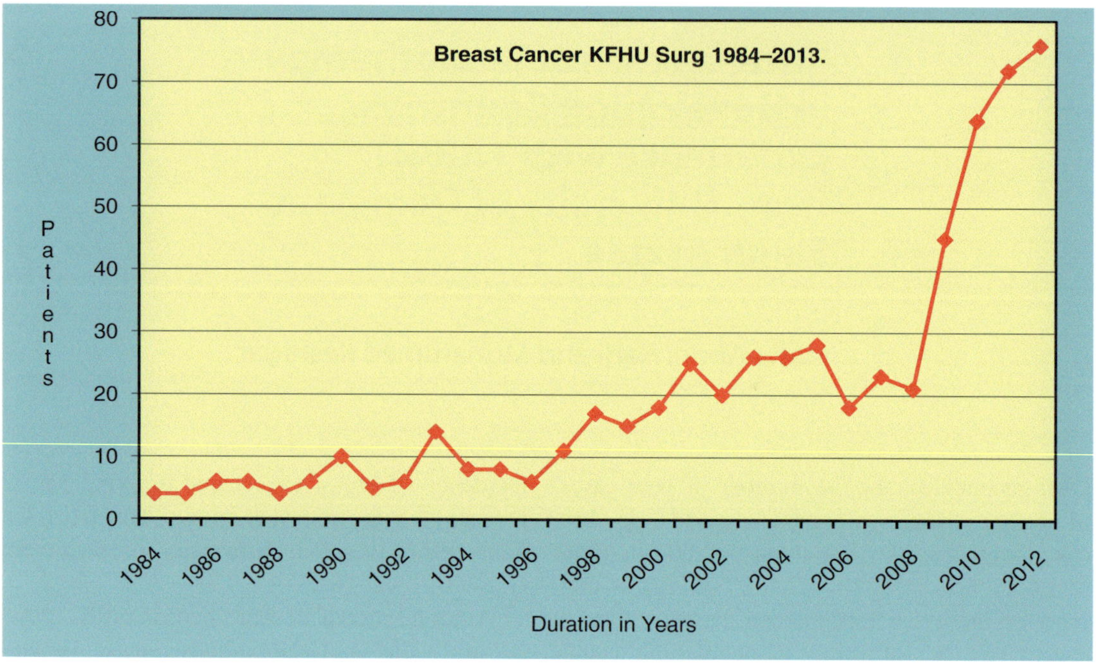

Fig. 16.1 Increase in the number of breast cancer patients at the King Fahd Hospital, University of Dammam

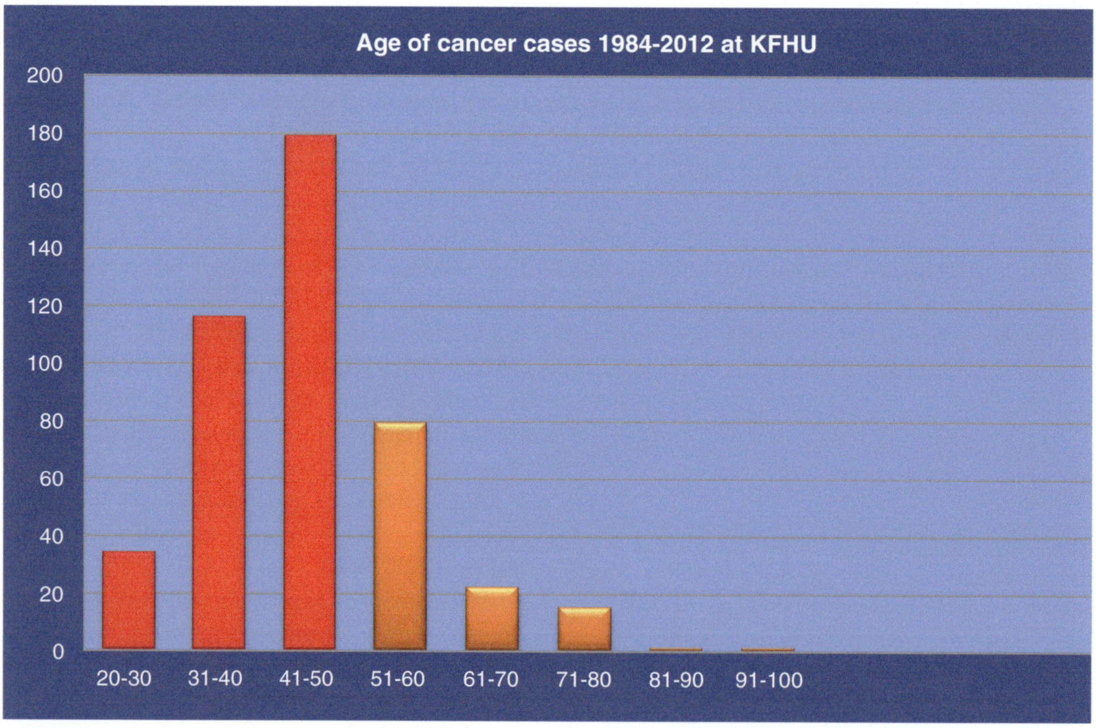

Fig. 16.2 Age distribution of breast cancer patients at the King Fahd Hospital, University of Dammam: 36 % of patients are below the age of 40 years

equivalent population of about 300 million (El Saghir et al. 2007; http://www-naweb-iaea.org/nahu/dirac/query3.asp 2013). Furthermore, the radiation centres tend to be located in major cities and may be a considerable distance from the patient's place of residence; the patient is then likely to be dependent on her male partner for travel arrangements. This, along with the fact that radiotherapy is often delivered over a protracted period of 3–4 weeks, results in disruption and non-compliance.

Due to the above limitations, it may not always be feasible to offer breast-conserving surgery followed by external beam radiotherapy. Intraoperative radiotherapy (IORT) is a major breakthrough in the treatment of breast cancer and represents an appealing option for our patients as it provides appropriate treatment for breast cancer in a single hospital visit.

The introduction of IORT at our institution nevertheless faced initial resistance the multidisciplinary team. This was soom overcame by a review of the scientific evidence and analysis of the data from the TARGIT randomised trial as well as the data from the TARGIT boost trial. We also presented a business case to the administration, which was looked upon positively.

We have been pleasantly surprised by the readiness of our culturally conservative patients to accept this new treatment modality, and their willingness to participate in the programme reflects their desperation to access breast-preserving options. Increased awareness about the availability of this innovative therapy has resulted in a steady increase in patients presenting with earlier disease.

This positive response from the community resulted in the founding of a scientific chair funded by the National Commercial Bank to support the IORT project for breast cancer treatment in the Eastern Province of Saudi Arabia.

Communication with pioneers in the field at University College London has supported the project by way of the provision of expertise and structured training through the TARGIT Academy. This has involved attendance of a core team of surgical and clinical oncologists and a radiation physicist at a 2-day training course in London, followed by proctored training by one of the experts in Dammam.

Once this process had been initiated, resistance slowly dissipated and the treatment modality was adopted, encouraging other centres to explore this therapeutic option as well.

As there are a small number of patients with early breast cancer in our centre, the use of IORT as a single fraction is limited. It can, however, be more extensively utilised as boost therapy during wide local excision in patients who have received neoadjuvant chemotherapy, which is then followed by whole breast external beam radiation therapy (EBRT). The reported results of wide local excision and boost combined with EBRT have been favourable, with a low local recurrence rate, and this accordingly is an attractive option for our current setup. The accurate placement of applicators in the tumour bed and the immediacy of the treatment, which has a favourable effect on the tumour microenvironment, are key to the success of this therapy (Vaidya et al. 2006; Keshtgar et al. 2011).

16.1 Local Experience at the King Fahd Hospital

From the practical point of view, the ease of adopting IORT using mobile radiation equipment (INTRABEAM®) in unmodified operating rooms without special radiation protection measures has been an intriguing experience for the team.

It became very clear from the outset that a very limited number of patients would be suitable for IORT alone, according to the TARGIT-A criteria for patient selection. In the first 18 months after the introduction of IORT, 3,447 patients presented with various breast complaints, of whom only 108 (3 %) were diagnosed with breast cancer.

Based on the selection criteria, of these 108 patients only seventeen (15 %) were suitable for treatment with IORT. All of these patients were diagnosed with invasive ductal carcinoma with a tumour size on imaging of 1.3–3.7 cm. Tumour characteristics are summarised in Table 16.1. Special emphasis was paid to those patients with unfavorable characteristics such as; nodal involvements, positive margins or lymphovascular

Table 16.1 Summary of data for the seven patients suitable for breast-conserving surgery and IORT, plus the management plan

#	MR#	AGE	DIAGNOSIS	IMG SIZE	PATH SIZE	NEO-ADJ	TUMOR GRADE	MARGIN STATUS	NODAL STATUS	LYMPHO - VAS INVASION	APPLICATOR SIZE	APP. TIME	RX
1	69994	55	IDC	2.2x1.9	3.0X3.0	-ve	III	-ve	0\19	-ve	5.0	39:02	IORT+ EBR
2	80215	69	IDC	2.4x1.3	3.0X2.3	-ve	III	-ve	1\12	+ve	4.5	31:19	IORT+ EBR
3	1238645	47	IDC	2.4x1.6	2.5X0.5	-ve	II	-ve	0\23	-ve	5.0	39:12	IORT
4	74427	68	IDC	3.7X1.7	4.0X4.5	-ve	III	-ve	2\5	-ve	5.0	39:18	IORT+ EBR
5	357815	38	IDC	1.3x1	2.0x1.5	-ve	II	-ve	0\19	-ve	3.5	20:27	IORT
6	852271	42	IDC	1.4x0.8	1.5x0.5	-ve	II	+ve	0\7	-ve	3.0	23:57	IORT+ EBR
7	561711	50	IDC	2.3x1.3	1.8x1.5	-ve	II	-ve	0\7	+ve	4.0	25:39	IORT+ EBR
8	413348	48	IDC	2.9x3.3	2.5x2.0	+ve	II	-ve	0\11	+ve	3.0	23:58	IORT+ EBR
9	136838	57	IDC	1.3X0.9	1.3x1.0	-ve	i	-ve	0\16	-ve	2.5	17:40	IORT
10	920996	49	IDC	2.5x2.8	3.0x5.0	-ve	I	-ve	0\11	-ve	4.0	24:04	IORT+EBR
11	294426	74	IDC	3.0x3.5	2.2x2.2	-ve	II	-ve	4\14	-ve	3.5	18:00	IORT
12	1275777	57	IDC	2.4X1.7	2.8X1.4	-ve	III	-ve	2\11	+ve	3.00	22:22	IORT+EBR
13	1277608	31	IDC	1.1X0.8	1.0X1.0	-ve	I	-ve	0/2 SN	-ve	2.5	17;33	IORT
14	1284425	54	IDC	1.1x0.9	1.0x0.8	-ve	II	-ve	1/18	-ve	3.0	21 :01	IORT
15	1269832	49	IDC	1.1x1.1	0.5x0.5	+ve	II	+ve	1\17	-ve	5.0	34:52	IORT+EBR
16	1285777	48	IDC	2.2x2.5	2.5x2.5	-ve	II	-ve	0\3 SN	-ve	5.0	34:00	IORT
17	634100	51	IDC	1.3x1.0	2.0x2.0	-ve	II	-ve	1\13	-ve	4.0	22:45	IORT

IDC Intraductal carcinoma, *IORT* intraoperative radiotherapy, *EBRT* external beam radiation therapy

invasion. To our surprise, these only comprised for 9 out of the 17 patients (52 %), which were treated with additional EBRT (omitting the the boost).

These results were very encouraging with 8 (48 %) were treated with exclusive IORT. These results with certainly promote and support early detection programs in our communities.

Our earlier notion to employ this advanced technology as a boost therapy has certainly been influenced by our modest encouraging results. Using IORT as an exclusive modality or as a boost had changed our perspectives in the management of advanced of breast cancer.

The fact remains, establishment of effective early detection programs cannot be overemphasized. Currently, the main use of IORT in developing countries will remain for a while, as a boost therapy after the initial wide excision. (Vaidya et al. 2011).

In our early experience, the short comprehensive training course combined with guidance from experts in the field has aided in:

- Alleviating radiation concerns
- Preparing the operating theatre setup
- Understanding the equipment
- Providing safety measures
- Documenting operating theatre details
- Implementing suitable patient selection criteria
- Documenting accurate clinical and radiation data
- Follow-up

16.2 Concluding Remarks

Our initial experience in setting up a targeted IORT program in our region has been very positive. We have proven that establishing this technology in our part of the world is feasible, with both patients and staff reporting high levels of satisfaction. We can safely speculate that given the fact that patients present with more advanced disease in developing countries, the main use of this technology in the near future will remain the replacement of the radiotherapy boost at the time of surgery, with postoperative EBRT to the whole breast. However, with increased awareness hopefully more patients will present with early disease, allowing IORT to be used as sole treatment.

Although our experience with IORT is relatively brief, we have received positive feedback from both staff and patients. It has proven a valuable piece of equipment that can be adopted in our regular hospital setup as it:

1. Promotes early detection strategies
2. Eliminates the fear of mastectomy
3. Promotes more surgical options
4. Avoids the sequelae of mastectomy
5. Provides comprehensive treatment options
6. Shortens the radiotherapy treatment time by eliminating the boost
7. Decreases the burden on the scarce radiotherapy centres
8. Avoids the problem of non-compliance
9. Reduces the morbidity associated with mastectomy reconstructive surgery

16.3 Take Home Message

In an era of advancing technology and financial constraints, it is almost impossible to erect and maintain radiotherapy facilities in every city. IORT is an ideal treatment modality which is expected to encourage women to present earlier with their disease, thereby aiding in cutting costs and reducing the burden on healthcare services in the long term.

16.4 References

Abdel HM (2000) Breast cancer awareness among health-care professionals. Ann Saudi Med 20:135–136

El Saghir NS, Khalil MK, Eid T, El Kinge AR, Charafeddine M, Geara F et al (2007) Trends in epidemiology and management of breast cancer in developing Arab countries: a literature and registry analysis. Int J Surg 5:225–233

Forouzanfar MH, Foreman KJ, Delossantos AM, Lozano R, Lopez AD, Murray CJ, Naghavi M (2011) Breast and cervical cancer in 187 countries between 1980 and 2010: a systematic analysis. Lancet 378: 1461–1484

Ibrahim EM, Ezzat AA, Rahal MM, Raja MM, Ajarim DS (2005) Adjuvant chemotherapy in 780 patients with early breast cancer: 10-year data from Saudi Arabia. Med Oncol 22:343–352

Keshtgar MR, Vaidya JS, Tobias JS, Wenz F, Joseph D, Stacey C et al (2011) Targeted intraoperative radiotherapy for breast cancer in patients in whom external beam radiation is not possible. Int J Radiat Oncol Biol Phys 80:31–38

Ravichandran K, Al-Hamdan NA, Mohamed G (2011) Knowledge, attitude, and behavior among Saudis toward cancer preventive practice. J Fam Commun Med 18:135–142

Vaidya JS, Baum M, Tobias JS, Massarut S, Wenz F, Murphy O et al (2006) Targeted intraoperative radiotherapy (TARGIT) yields very low recurrence rates when given as a boost. Int J Radiat Oncol Biol Phys 66:1335–1338

Vaidya JS, Baum M, Tobias JS, Wenz F, Massarut S, Keshtgar M et al (2011) Long-term results of targeted intraoperative radiotherapy (Targit) boost during breast-conserving surgery. Int J Radiat Oncol Biol Phys 81:1091–1097

Treating Patients with TARGIT

17

Norman R. Williams and Claire Reynolds

17.1 Background to the TARGIT Studies

Whole breast external beam radiotherapy is a safe and effective treatment, but despite the advances that have been achieved over the years, there are a number of areas where further improvements might be made. First, there is an undesirable delivery of radiation to normal tissues such as the skin, heart, ribs and lungs. The radiotherapy is delivered as daily fractions spread over several weeks, which entails daily visits to the radiotherapy centre. There is a delay between surgery and radiotherapy, which can be several months if chemotherapy is given. Finally, there is a risk of "geographic miss" of the tumour bed, particularly if cosmetic reconstruction has been performed. The TARGIT technique directly addresses these concerns, as the radiotherapy is delivered from within the breast only to the tumour bed, under direct visualisation at the time of surgery, in a single fraction.

N.R. Williams, BSc, PhD, MICR, CSci (✉)
Clinical Trials Group, Division of Surgery and Interventional Science, Faculty of Medical Sciences, University College London, Charles Bell House, 67-73 Riding House Street, London W1W 7EJ, UK
e-mail: norman.williams@ucl.ac.uk

C. Reynolds
Department of Radiotherapy, Royal Free London Foundation Trust, Pond Street, Hampstead, London NW3 2QG, UK
e-mail: clairehourihane@nhs.net

17.2 TARGIT-A Trial

The international multicentre TARGIT trial (ISRCTN34086741) was designed to determine non-inferiority between the TARGIT technique [intraoperative radiotherapy with INTRABEAM (Carl Zeiss Meditec, Germany)] and conventional external beam radiotherapy (EBRT) in women with early breast cancer. IORT is given as a single dose of 20 Gy at the surface of the applicator (equivalent to 6 Gy at 1 cm) delivered directly to the tumour bed. The primary outcome measure is local relapse within the treated breast; secondary endpoints are site of relapse within the breast, relapse-free and overall survival, and local toxicity/morbidity (TARGIT A Trial on the HTA website.). Evidence for the efficacy and safety of this novel approach has, since March 2000, been gathered through a randomised controlled trial (Vaidya et al. 2010) which has recently completed accrual. Results are presented elsewhere in this book.

17.3 TARGIT-B Trial

TARGIT-B (for boost, ISRCTN43138042) is a multicentre randomised controlled trial designed to determine whether the replacement by IORT of the EBRT boost is superior in outcome to conventional EBRT plus an external boost (TARGIT B Trial on the HTA website). All patients will receive EBRT to the whole breast. The study began accrual in june 2013.

M. Keshtgar et al. (eds.), *Targeted Intraoperative Radiotherapy in Oncology*,
DOI 10.1007/978-3-642-39821-6_17,

The target population is patients with breast cancer who have a high risk of local recurrence. Specifically, patients should be either younger than 46 or, if older, need to have pathological features that confer a high risk of local recurrence of breast cancer, such as lymphovascular invasion, gross nodal involvement (not micrometastasis), more than one tumour in the breast but still suitable for breast-conserving surgery through a single specimen, ER negative, grade 3 histology or positive margins at first excision.

The trial is based on a phase II study of 300 patients recently updated with long-term data (Vaidya et al. 2011), together with a mathematical model of TARGIT that suggests that it could be superior to conventional radiotherapy (Enderling et al. 2007); in addition, translational research has found evidence that treatment with TARGIT alters the molecular composition and biological activity of wound fluid in the tumour bed, which impairs the surgical trauma-stimulated proliferation and invasiveness of cultured breast cancer cells (Belletti et al. 2008).

Patient assessments will be by clinical examination (every 6 months for the first 3 years, then annually to 10 years) and annual mammography (up to 5 years, then according to local practice). The primary outcome is local recurrence. The secondary outcomes are: site of relapse in the breast, overall survival and local toxicity (assessed by RTOG and LENT SOMA criteria).

The trial will include an assessment of quality of life (using FACT B+4 and EQ5D). There will also be assessments of financial costs to patients since boost treatment with EBRT is likely to require additional time and travel.

17.4 TARGIT-D Trial

TARGIT-D (for DCIS) will be a multicentre randomised controlled trial designed to determine whether TARGIT is a safe and effective alternative to whole breast EBRT for the treatment of small, focal DCIS typically found during mammographic breast cancer screening. A start date for this study is not yet known.

17.5 TARGIT-E Study

TARGIT-E (for Elderly) is a single-arm trial on use of TARGIT in elderly patients being run in Mannheim by Professor Frederik Wenz. The protocol is based on the international TARGIT-A study. The purpose is to investigate the efficacy of a single intraoperative radiotherapy treatment within elderly low-risk patients (≥70 years, cT1, cN0, cM0, invasive ductal carcinoma) which is followed by EBRT only when adverse risk factors are present (TARGIT E on the ClinicalTrials.gov website).

17.6 TARGIT-US

TARGIT-US (for United States) is a Phase IV Registry Trial being run in the USA through the University of California, San Francisco to study the efficacy and toxicity of breast radiotherapy given intraoperatively as a single dose after breast-conserving surgery, with or without whole breast radiation as indicated by pathological risk factors, in women with early stage breast cancer (TARGIT US on the ClinicalTrials.gov website).

17.7 TARGIT-R

TARGIT-R (for Registry, http://www.controlled-trials.com/ISRCTN91179875) will be an open registry study with very wide inclusion criteria, enabling clinicians to treat patients with the TARGIT technique provided they have the support of their institution and colleagues. Data collection will be as per the existing TARGIT-A trial and is ideal for centres involved in this trial who wish to continue to treat patients now that randomisations have ceased. The study is expected to open in 2013.

17.8 Patient Selection and Information

All of the TARGIT studies aim to provide high-quality safety and efficacy data so that evidence-based medicine can determine future clinical practice. In addition, selection of suitable patients and discussion of treatment options must also be led by evidence.

17.9 Patient Inclusion Criteria

The rationale for patient selection for IORT is primarily based on the fact that the risk of relapse for patients with localised breast cancer is dependent on age as older patients are considered at lower risk than younger patients, who may have more aggressive disease. Therefore patients selected for TARGIT are usually older than 45 years of age, but this may be altered to fit local criteria within the treating centre.

Table 17.1 shows the main inclusion and exclusion criteria when reviewing patients who may be suitable for TARGIT alone (low-risk patients).

All patients should undergo a triple assessment (mammography, ultrasound and histopathology) and the results should be discussed in a multidisciplinary team meeting (comprising breast surgeons, medical and clinical oncologists, radiologists, histopathologists, etc.). These experts work collaboratively and within their scope of practice in order for the most appropriate decision to be made regarding the best possible treatment for the patient before selecting the patient for TARGIT.

The above criteria for patient selection are taken from the eligibility criteria for the TARGIT-A trial, but it should be noted that both the American Society for Radiation Oncology (ASTRO) (Smith et al. 2009) and the European Society for Therapeutic Radiology and Oncology (ESTRO) (Polgár et al. 2010) have released guidelines (Table 17.2) for the selection of patients for accelerated partial breast irradiation (APBI) outside the context of a clinical trial. It is important to note that these guidelines are based upon all trials and methods of APBI, which are similar (but not identical) to TARGIT. They conclude that there appears to be a group of patients in whom the use of PBI could be deemed safe as the sole method of radiotherapy treatment but for some modalities there is limited recurrence and survival data.

Table 17.1 TARGIT-alone eligibility criteria

Inclusion criteria	Exclusion criteria
Age ≥45[a] years	No informed consent
T1–2 (≤2.0[a] cm; mammography, ultrasound)	Non-compliance
cN0 (examination, ultrasound)	Age <45[a] years
Histopathology: ductal-invasive	Tumour size >2.0[a] cm
Unifocal	cN+ Multifocal lesions Lobular or non-invasive Metastases

[a]Or according to local criteria

17.10 What to Tell the Patient

Once the patient has been selected, she is seen by the breast surgeon, who will discuss the results of the triple assessment and give the diagnosis and treatment options, one of which may be wide local excision of the tumour immediately followed by TARGIT. Patients should be informed that there is still a chance they will go on to need EBRT if certain high-risk factors are present which were not previously identified. These factors include positive margins at excision, lobular carcinoma, lymphovascular invasion and node positivity. In the TARGIT-A trial, approximately 15 % of patients will require subsequent EBRT to the whole breast, though no boost to the tumour bed is given as the IORT treatment is considered as the boost in these cases.

Table 17.2 Comparison of ASTRO and ESTRO guidelines with TARGIT-alone eligibility criteria

Organisation/trial	Age (years)	Tumour size (cm)	Histopathology	Exclusion criteria
ASTRO	≥60	≤2	Ductal invasive or other favourable subtypes	cN1, R+, L1, EIC, mf, HR negative
ESTRO	>50	≤3	Ductal invasive or other favourable subtypes	cN1, R+, L1, EIC, mf
TARGIT-A	>45	≤2	Ductal invasive	L1, R+, cN+, mf, EIC

EIC Extensive intraductal component, *HR* hormone receptors, *L* lymphovascular invasion, *mf* multifocal lesions, *N* involved nodes, *R* resection margin

Patients should also be told that TARGIT has low toxicity, good cosmetic outcome and low local recurrence rates.

17.11 The Patient Pathway

While the patient pathway will vary between different hospital sites that offer TARGIT as well as between different countries, the basic format should be similar and formulated before offering the service (Fig. 17.1).

Once patients have been identified as suitable for the procedure, they are seen by the breast surgery team to inform them of their diagnosis and explain the treatment options. A second consultation is sometimes necessary for patients to be consented and randomised, if participating in a trial, and for the surgery date to be agreed and booked.

Following this consultation the patient will be referred to the clinical oncologist for a further discussion on the role of TARGIT. Under UK regulations the clinical oncologist acts as the practitioner for the IORT procedure and must therefore justify the exposure of radiation given. The clinical oncologist will discuss the IORT option with the patient, and the clinical oncologist must then complete the radiotherapy prescription card, which will be a permanent record of the patient's radiotherapy treatment.

17.12 TARGIT Follow-Up Assessments

TARGIT follow-up assessments are listed in Table 17.3. These will vary according to local practice.

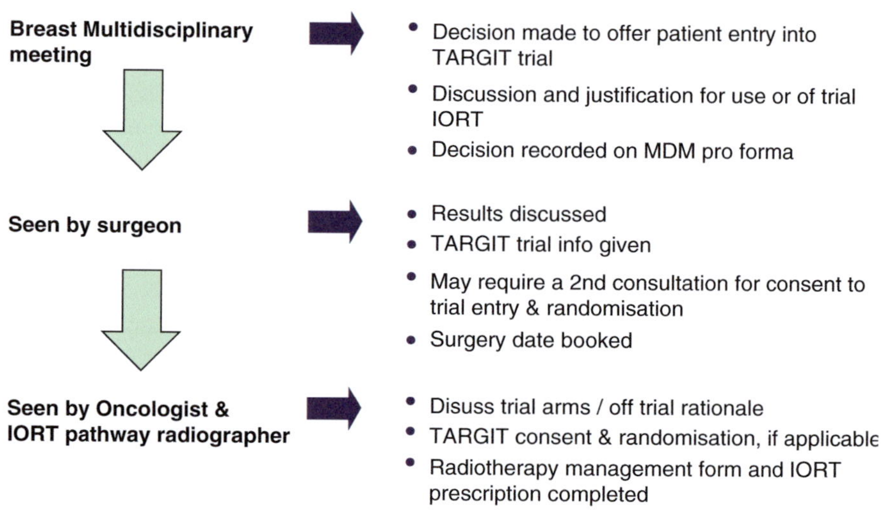

Fig. 17.1 TARGIT patient pathway

Table 17.3 TARGIT follow-up assessments

Toxicity	Relapse
RTOG or LENT SOMA or other	Medical check-up
Fibrosis, telangiectasia, oedema, retraction, ulcertation, lymphoedema, heperpigmentation, pain	Mammography
Standardised photo	Ultrasound
	Quality of life
	QLQ-C30
	QLQ-BR23

References

Belletti B, Vaidya JS, D'Andrea S, Entschladen F, Roncadin M, Lovat F et al (2008) Targeted intraoperative radiotherapy impairs the stimulation of breast cancer cell proliferation and invasion caused by surgical wounding. Clin Cancer Res 14:1325–1332

TARGIT E on the ClinicalTrials.gov website. http://clinicaltrials.gov/ct2/show/NCT01299987

TARGIT US on the ClinicalTrials.gov website. http://clinicaltrials.gov/ct2/show/NCT01570998

Enderling H, Chaplain MA, Anderson AR, Vaidya JS (2007) A mathematical model of breast cancer development, local treatment and recurrence. J Theor Biol 246:245–259

TARGIT B Trial on the HTA website. http://www.hta.ac.uk/2946

TARGIT A Trial on the HTA website. http://www.hta.ac.uk/project/1981

Polgár C, Van Limbergen E, Pötter R, Kovács G, Polo A, Lyczek J et al (2010) Patient selection for accelerated partial breast irradiation (APBI) after breast-conserving surgery: Recommendations of the Groups Européen de Curiethérapie-European Society for Therapeutic Radiology and Oncology (GEC-ESTRO) Breast Cancer Working Group based on clinical evidence (2009). Radiother Oncol 94:264–273

Smith BD, Arthur DW, Buchholz TA, Haffty BG, Hahn CA, Hardenburgh PH et al (2009) Accelerated partial breast irradiation consensus statement from the American Society for Radiation Oncology (ASTRO). Int J Radiat Oncol Biol Phys 74:987–1001

Vaidya JS, Joseph DJ, Tobias JS, Bulsara M, Wenz F, Saunders C et al (2010) Targeted intraoperative radiotherapy versus whole breast radiotherapy for breast cancer (TARGIT-A trial): an international, prospective, randomised, non-inferiority phase 3 trial. Lancet 376:91–102

Vaidya JS, Baum M, Tobias JS, Wenz F, Massarut S, Keshtgar M et al (2011) Long-term results of targeted intraoperative radiotherapy (Targit) boost during breast-conserving surgery. Int J Radiat Oncol Biol Phys 81:1091–1097

18 Patient Selection and Information

Claire Reynolds and Elena Sperk

18.1 Introduction

Breast cancer is the most common cancer in women worldwide, but more than 89 % of women diagnosed with breast cancer are alive at 5 years following diagnosis (Parkin et al. 2008). For women suitable to undergo breast-conserving surgery (BCS), postoperative radiotherapy is recommended in order to reduce the rate of local recurrence (National Institute for Clinical Excellence 2002; Hughes et al. 2004). The change in treatment delivery from mastectomy to breast-conserving treatment has provided a solution that is equivalent in terms of treatment outcome but also offers improved cosmesis and reduced morbidity for the patient.

It has, however, been reported that only 10–80 % of patients who are eligible for BCS undergo it for a variety of reasons, including access to radiotherapy facilities (Njeh et al. 2010). For this reason there has been a wish to identify a group of patients who may not benefit from radiotherapy following BCS but as yet no subset has been identified.

C. Reynolds (✉)
Department of Radiotherapy,
Royal Free London Foundation Trust,
Pond Street, Hampstead, London NW3 2QG, UK
e-mail: clairehourihane@nhs.net

E. Sperk
Department of Radiation Oncology,
University Medical Centre Mannheim, University of Heidelberg, Theodor-Kutzer-Ufer 1-3, D-68167,
Mannheim, Germany
e-mail: elena.sperk@umm.de

It has been estimated that approximately 85 % of recurrences within the treated breast occur in the index quadrant despite findings that two-thirds of mastectomy specimens show microscopic tumours disseminated throughout the breast (Vaidya et al. 2004). Therefore radiotherapy to the whole breast may be over-treatment for some patients and investigations into the use of partial breast irradiation have evolved, focussing on options such as the Mammosite balloon technique, brachytherapy with catheters and intraoperative radiotherapy with electrons or X-rays.

18.2 Intraoperative Radiotherapy

Intraoperative radiotherapy (IORT) is one method of delivering partial breast irradiation (PBI) and has increased rapidly in popularity, mainly in Europe. It is currently being investigated through the international TARGIT trial (Vaidya et al. 2010).

This method of treating the tumour bed is very desirable as the radiotherapy is given at the time of surgery and there is therefore no delay in starting treatment. Additionally, there is no geographical miss as the treatment volume can be clearly identified during surgery and immediately after removal of the tumour. It also means that patients who do not have ready access to radiotherapy facilities can be spared the multiple journeys for fractionated external beam radiotherapy (EBRT), thus saving up to 6 weeks of treatment. A concomitant benefit is the creation of space on very

M. Keshtgar et al. (eds.), *Targeted Intraoperative Radiotherapy in Oncology*,
DOI 10.1007/978-3-642-39821-6_18, © Springer-Verlag Berlin Heidelberg 2014

busy linear accelerators within radiotherapy departments.

IORT is not always given as part of the TARGIT trial as cases have been identified in which the patient may not fall into the inclusion criteria for the trial but would benefit from this treatment, for example as an advanced boost. However, it is important to consider that IORT has a limited target and treatment volume. The spherical applicators for treatment range in size from 1.5 to 5 cm in 0.5-cm increments. This means that patients identified as suitable for IORT should have a tumour that is ≤3.5 cm (or otherwise defined by the local protocol) in order that enough normal tissue can be removed with the tumour during the wide local excision.

The use of the INTRABEAM system is discussed in another chapter.

18.3 Patient Inclusion Criteria

The rationale for patient selection for IORT is based on the fact that the risk of relapse for patients with localised breast cancer is dependent on age, and older patients are considered at lower risk than younger patients, who may have more aggressive disease. These identified low-risk patients have a smaller risk for both relapses and metastases. Therefore patient selection for IORT is based on the age of the patient being older than 45 years. However, this may be altered to fit local criteria within the treating centre. Table 18.1 shows the main inclusion and exclusion criteria when reviewing patients who may be suitable for IORT.

PBI should only be used in those patients who have an invasive ductal carcinoma (or other favourable subtype) as lobular carcinoma is more likely to present as multifocal and multicentric disease and as Anwar et al. (2010) found that almost 30 % of patients who underwent BCS for lobular carcinoma required further surgery as excised tumours had positive margins. All patients should undergo a triple assessment (mammography, ultrasound and histopathology) and the results should be discussed before selecting the patient for IORT. This allows for a more comprehensive view of the tumour in determining the appropriateness of the treatment for the patient.

Table 18.1 Main inclusion and exclusion criteria for IORT

Inclusion criteria	Exclusion criteria
Age ≥45 years[a]	No informed consent
T1-2 (≤3.5 cm[a]; mammography, ultrasound)	Non-compliance
cN0 (examination, ultrasound)	Age <45 years[a]
Histopathology: ductal-invasive	Tumour size >3.5 cm
Unifocal	cN+
	Multifocal lesions
	Lobular or non-invasive
	Metastases

[a]Or according to local criteria

While these criteria for patient selection are taken from the TARGIT-A trial, both the American Society for Radiation Oncology (ASTRO) (Smith et al. 2009) and the European Society for Therapeutic Radiology and Oncology (ESTRO) (Polgár et al. 2010) have released guidelines (Table 18.2) for the selection of patients for accelerated partial breast irradiation (APBI) outside the context of a clinical trial. It is important to note that these guidelines are based upon all trials and methods of APBI, of which IORT is a subset. They conclude that there appears to be a group of patients in whom the use of PBI could be deemed safe as the sole method of radiotherapy treatment but for some modalities there are limited recurrence and survival data.

The TARGIT-A trial, which evaluates IORT as PBI, reported in 2010 (Vaidya et al. 2010) in *The Lancet*, low local recurrence rates (1 %) at a median follow-up of 4 years. These results are very encouraging though it is recognised that longer follow-up of these patients is needed.

Delegates at the 12th International Breast Cancer Conference in March 2011 were asked to vote on the use of IORT as a replacement for whole breast EBRT and the use of IORT as a replacement for the EBRT boost to the tumour

Table 18.2 Selection criteria for PBI/APBI

Organisation/trial	Age (years)	Tumour size (cm)	Histopathology	Exclusion criteria
ASTRO	≥60	≤2	Ductal invasive or other favourable subtypes	cN1, R+, L1, EIC, MF, HR negative
ESTRO	>50	≤3	Ductal invasive or other favourable subtypes	cN1, R+, L1, EIC, MF
TARGIT-A	>45	≤2	Ductal invasive	L1, R+, cN+, MF, EIC

L Lymphovascular invasion, *R* resection margin, *EIC* extensive intraductal component, *MF* multifocal lesions; *N* involved nodes, *HR* hormone receptor

bed. The vote was in favour of the use of IORT in both of these situations.

18.4 The Role of the Multidisciplinary Team

As previously stated, all patients should undergo a triple assessment to confirm the diagnosis of invasive breast cancer. The results of these investigations should then be discussed in a forum of clinical experts (e.g. breast surgeons, medical and clinical oncologists, radiologists, histopathologists). These experts work collaboratively and within their scope of practice in order to achieve the most appropriate decision regarding the best possible treatment for the patient. This forum also flags up patients who are suitable to enter the TARGIT-A trial, based upon the inclusion criteria. However, it is also required to justify the use of IORT outside the context of the trial as some patients may not fit the inclusion criteria but are deemed suitable for IORT when the guidelines from both ASTRO and ESTRO are taken into consideration.

18.5 The TARGIT-A Trial

The TARGIT-A trial aims to demonstrate the non-inferiority of IORT to the tumour bed compared with EBRT to the whole breast following wide local excision. The inclusion and exclusion criteria have been discussed previously and here we will discuss the course of events after the patient has been selected based on the trial inclusion criteria.

Once the patient has been selected she is seen by the breast surgeon, who will discuss the results of the triple assessment and give the diagnosis and treatment options, one of which will be IORT, following wide local excision of the tumour. If the patient is happy to enter the trial, once all the patient information has been digested, then informed consent is obtained and the patient is randomised via the trial centre.

Patients are randomised to either surgery plus a single dose of IORT with INTRABEAM (TARGIT group A) or surgery plus EBRT (EBRT group B) (Fig. 18.1). If patients draw group A then they are informed that there is still a chance they will go on to need EBRT if the final histology result demonstrates certain previously unknown factors indicating that the patient is higher risk than originally thought. These factors include unsuspected lobular carcinoma, lymphovascular invasion and positive margins at excision. It has been estimated that approximately 15 % of patients in group A will go on to need EBRT to the whole breast, though no boost to the tumour bed is given since the IORT is considered as the boost in these cases. If patients draw group B then they will receive a dose of 40–50 Gy in 15–25 fractions with or without a breast boost to the tumour bed of 10–16 Gy in 5–8 fractions.

18.6 What to Tell the Patient

If patients are selected as appropriate candidates for the TARGIT-A trial then it is important that the patient is aware that the decision on which treatment they will receive is not made by the surgeon or oncologist but by a computer in order to ensure that there are an equivalent number of patients in each arm, as this is a randomised trial. While this can be hard for patients to accept, they all appreciate that it is in the nature of entering a clinical trial.

The short treatment time of IORT, which adds between 20 and 50 min to the time of surgery, depending on the size of the applicator chosen, is an important consideration for patients, as is the shortened delay between surgery and further treatment. Also, if the patient goes on to need EBRT then the course is shorter by 5–8 treatments owing to the IORT substituting for the tumour bed boost. IORT has also demonstrated low toxicity, good cosmesis and low local recurrence rates (Fig. 18.2). While patients are selected in whom IORT would be suitable as the only necessary radiotherapy treatment, they can be reassured that a second treatment with breast-conserving surgery and EBRT is possible if the final histology result does not reflect that of the original core biopsy, on which the decision to offer IORT was based. This course of treatment is also an option if there are positive margins after the first surgery.

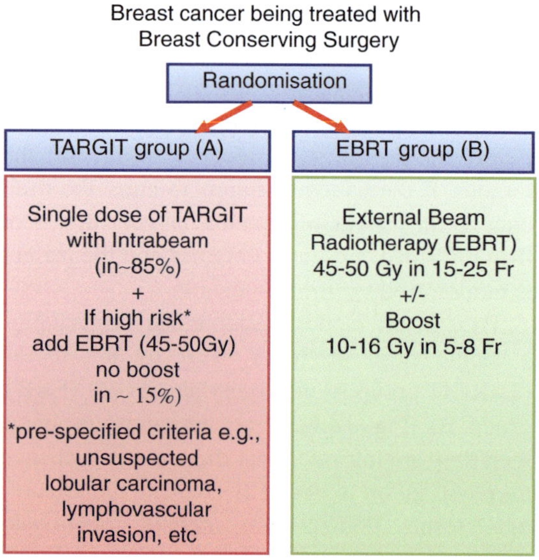

Fig. 18.1 Randomisation in the TARGIT-A trial

18.7 The Patient Pathway

While the patient pathway will vary between different hospital sites that offer IORT, as well as between different countries, the basic format should be similar and formulated before offering the service (Fig. 18.3).

All patients are discussed at the breast multidisciplinary meeting (MDM), which is attended by

Fig. 18.2 The advantages of IORT

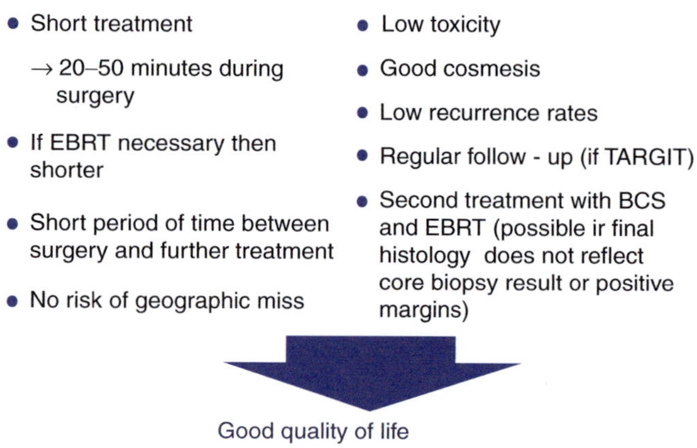

many staff groups, including breast surgeons, medical and clinical oncologists, histopathologists, radiologists, breast care nurses and members of the IORT team from the radiotherapy department. Within this forum, results of the investigations that the patient has undergone (imaging and histopathology) are discussed and a consensus agreement is reached by all parties as to the most suitable course of action. In this way, criteria for the TARGIT trial can be evaluated along with seeking justification for off-trial IORT patients using the guidelines published by ASTRO and ESTRO. If patients fulfil the inclusion criteria for the TARGIT-A trial or are suitable for IORT in an off-trial setting, then the patient will be offered IORT. This decision is recorded on the MDM pro forma and kept as part of the patient's medical records to demonstrate the management plan being offered.

Once patients have been identified as suitable for the procedure, they are seen by the breast surgery team to inform them of their diagnosis and explain the treatment options. At this stage the patient can be offered the patient information sheet (PIS) for the TARGIT trial in order to make an informed decision. Off-trial patients can also be offered the PIS as the information contained within can help with their decision-making process and gives them the opportunity to formulate questions regarding the management plan. A second consultation is sometimes necessary for acquisition of patient consent, for randomisation of patients (if part of the trial) and for the surgery date to be agreed and booked.

Following this consultation, the patient will be referred to the clinical oncologist for a further discussion on the role of IORT. Under UK regulations [IR(ME)R] the clinical oncologist acts as the practitioner for the IORT procedure and must therefore justify the exposure of radiation given. The clinical oncologist will discuss with the patient the IORT option, either as part of the TARGIT trial or in an off-trial setting. If consent to trial entry and randomisation have not been obtained previously, they can be finalised at this point. The clinical oncologist must then complete the radiotherapy prescription card, which will be a permanent record of the patient's radiotherapy treatment.

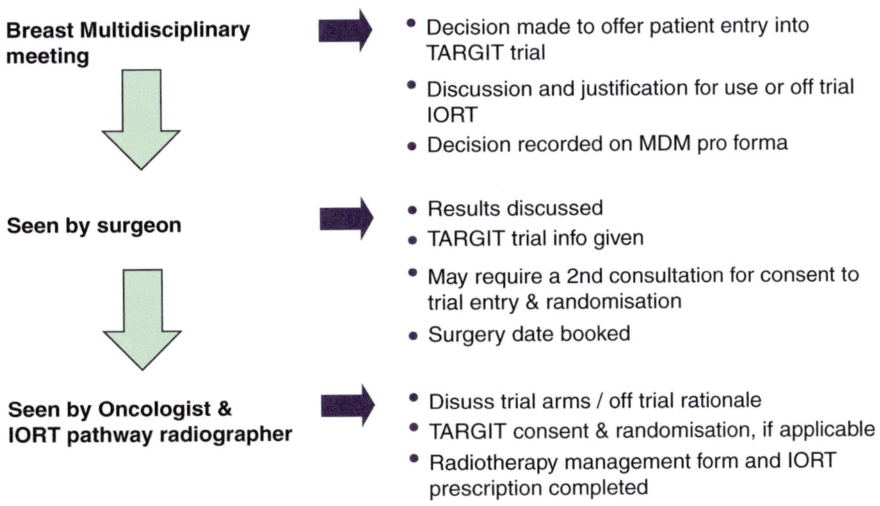

Fig. 18.3 The patient pathway

- Toxicity
- RTOG or LENT SOMA or other
- Fibrosis, telangiectasia, oedema, retraction, ulceration, lymphoedema, hyperpigmentation, pain
- Standardised Photo

- Relapse
- Medical check-up
- Mammography
- Ultrasound

- Quality of Life
- QLQ-C30
- QLQ-BR23

Fig. 18.4 TARGIT A follow-up assessments

18.8 TARGIT-A: Follow-Up Assessments

Follow-up assessments are shown in Fig. 18.4.

References

Anwar IF, Down SK, Rivzi S, Farooq N, Burger A, Morgan A, Hussein MI (2010) Invasive lobular carcinoma of the breast: should this be regarded as a chronic disease? Int J Surg 8:346–352

Hughes KS, Schnaper LA, Berry D, Cirrincione C, McCormick B, Shank B et al (2004) Cancer and Leukemia Group B; Radiation Therapy Oncology Group; Eastern Cooperative Oncology Group. Lumpectomy plus tamoxifen with or without irradiation in women 70 years of age or older with early breast cancer. N Engl J Med 351:971–977

National Institute for Clinical Excellence (2002) Guidance on cancer services: improving outcomes in breast cancer. NICE, London

Njeh CF, Saunders MW, Langton CM (2010) Accelerated partial breast irradiation (APBI): a review of available techniques. Radiat Oncol 5:90

Parkin D, Pisani P, Ferlay J (2008) Global cancer statistics. CA Cancer J Clin. doi:10.3322/canjclin.49.1.33

Polgár C, Van Limbergen E, Pötter R, Kovács G, Polo A, Lyczek J et al (2010) Patient selection for accelerated partial breast irradiation (APBI) after breast-conserving surgery: Recommendations of the Groupe Européen de Curiethérapie-European Society for Therapeutic Radiology and Oncology (GEC-ESTRO) breast cancer working group based on clinical evidence (2009). Radiother Oncol 94:264–273

Smith BD, Arthur DW, Buchholz TA, Haffty BG, Hahn CA, Hardenburgh PH et al (2009) Accelerated partial breast irradiation consensus statement from the American Society for Radiation Oncology (ASTRO). Int J Radiat Oncol Biol Phys 74:987–1001

Vaidya JS, Tobias JS, Baum M, Keshtgar M, Joseph D, Wenz F et al (2004) Intraoperative radiotherapy for breast cancer. Lancet Oncol 5:165–173

Vaidya JS, Joseph DJ, Tobias JS, Bulsara M, Wenz F, Saunders C et al (2010) Targeted intraoperative radiotherapy versus whole breast radiotherapy for breast cancer (TARGIT-A trial): an international, prospective, randomised, non-inferiority phase 3 trial. Lancet 376:91–102

19 Quality Assurance and Training of Targeted Intraoperative Radiotherapy: Establishment of the TARGIT Academy

Mohammed Keshtgar and Frederik Wenz

19.1 Introduction

There is growing interest in accelerated partial breast irradiation, which aims to decrease the volume of breast treated and increase the daily fraction size of radiation. Of the available technologies, only two provide partial breast irradiation in the operating room during surgery, namely use of a mobile linear accelerator (http://www.intraopmedical.com/) and the novel technique of targeted intraoperative radiotherapy (TARGIT) using the INTRABEAM® system (Carl Zeiss Surgical, Oberkochen, Germany).

There has been significant interest in the TARGIT technique since publication of the results of our randomised controlled trial in *The Lancet* (Vaidya et al. 2010), which provided level 1 evidence that, in early breast cancer, a single dose of radiotherapy delivered at the time of surgery using INTRABEAM is safe and that this approach is not inferior to standard whole breast external beam radiotherapy. There is also increasing demand for this innovative technique from patients with early breast cancer due to the advantages already outlined in this textbook.

Although the technique is relatively straightforward, its successful application requires adequate training and attention to detail. The lessons learned from the introduction of new techniques in surgery in the past need to be appreciated, and it is vital that lack of training does not bring this powerful new technique into disrepute.

M. Keshtgar, BSc, FRCSI, FRCS (Gen), PhD (✉)
Division of Surgery and Interventional Sciences, Department of Breast Surgery, University College London Medical School, Royal Free London Foundation NHS Trust, Pond Street, Hampstead NW3 2QG, UK
e-mail: m.keshtgar@ucl.ac.uk

F. Wenz
Department of Radiation Oncology, University Medical Center Mannheim, University of Heidelberg, Theodor-Kutzer-Ufer 1-3, D-68167 Mannheim, Germany
e-mail: frederik.wenz@medma.uni-heidelberg.de, frederik.wenz@umm.de, http://www.umm.de

19.2 TARGIT Academy

We identified the need to establish an academic focal point for this new technology and therefore established the TARGIT Academy in 2010, which is co-directed by Mohammed Keshtgar from the Royal Free and University College London, UK and Frederik Wenz from the University Medical Centre Mannheim and University of Heidelberg. The TARGIT Academy offers high-quality training and the opportunity to establish a broad academic network. The faculty comprises a group of multidisciplinary experts who have been involved with this technology from the outset and have extensive experience in performing the procedure and providing advice in difficult cases.

As targeted intraoperative radiotherapy is an interdisciplinary technique, the TARGIT Academy provides a networking platform which enables interaction and cooperation between surgeons, radiation oncologists, medical physicists and the extended multidisciplinary team.

M. Keshtgar et al. (eds.), *Targeted Intraoperative Radiotherapy in Oncology*,
DOI 10.1007/978-3-642-39821-6_19, © Springer-Verlag Berlin Heidelberg 2014

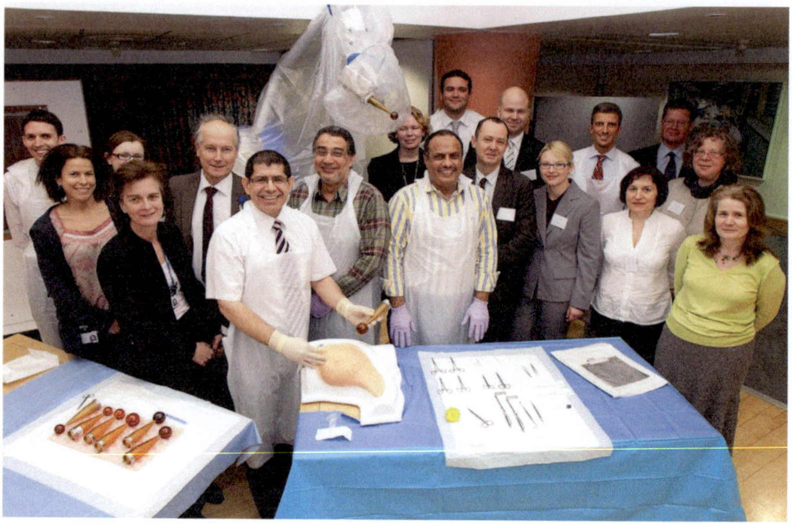

Fig. 19.1 Inauguration of TARGIT Academy at the Royal Free Hospital, London with the faculty from the UCL and University of Mannheim and participants

Use and handling of the intraoperative radiotherapy device, selection of appropriate applicator and adequate placement in the tumour bed are unfamiliar territory for surgeons. Therefore the focus of the Academy is on quality assurance and high standards in clinical education and training. It runs regular training courses in London and Mannheim which are sponsored by the manufacturer of the INTRABEAM system (Carl Zeiss Surgical, Oberkochen, Germany).

As the success of this technique depends on the members of a multidisciplinary team working harmoniously with each other, we encourage the attendance of teams rather than individuals. The first training course of the Academy was launched in February 2011 at the Royal Free Hospital in London (Fig. 19.1). The training involves three phases: theory days plus hands-on experience in a skills laboratory, proctored training and the audit phase.

19.2.1 Theory Days and Hands-on Training

The Academy offers a 2-day extensive training course, run by a multidisciplinary faculty, that provides participants with clinical education and practice, unique first-hand and peer-led training in the proper selection of patients, clinical trial results, information on the safe use of INTRABEAM and precise details on the TARGIT technique. By offering participants a unique first-hand education and intensive hands-on training, the TARGIT Academy accelerates the learning curve to the optimum level within the shortest possible time.

There is also emphasis on the radiobiology and radiation safety aspects of this procedure to ensure that correct guidelines are followed. As the indications for the use of TARGIT are expanding to encompass other tumour sites, these new developments are also covered.

There is also group discussion, troubleshooting and presentations of interesting cases in a mock multidisciplinary meeting setting.

Educational Material. The educational material comprises a full slide set of the training programme along with video recordings of the procedure performed by various surgeons in different settings. A comprehensive reference list with copies of the abstracts from all related publications is also provided.

Development of the TARGIT Training Simulator. As we believe that surgeons and the interdisciplinary team should be equipped with all the appropriate practical skills required to perform the procedure, we have designed and built a

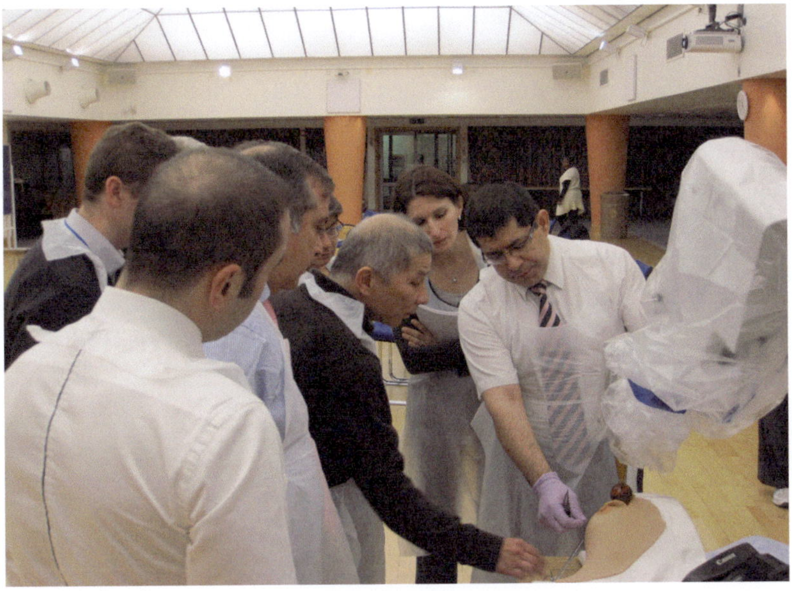

Fig. 19.2 Hans-on Training in progress on a simulator using Intrabeam

model that can be used for training all aspects of this technology.

The training simulator is realistic anatomically and is constructed from hot-melt thermoplastic polymer material with similar physical characteristics and radiation attenuation qualities to the breast. It allows accurate demonstration of the technical aspects of TARGIT. Simulated tumours of different sizes and locations are implanted within the model to mirror a real-life experience as closely as possible.

Participants have an opportunity to practice the implementation of the entire treatment workflow on this specially designed training simulator (Fig. 19.2). There is also in-depth demonstration of the practical aspects based on review of the recorded operative procedure.

19.2.2 Proctored Training

The Academy also facilitates proctored training for TARGIT-naïve centres that have recently acquired the equipment. This is done by an experienced trainer and provides an opportunity for the extended multidisciplinary team, including the operating theatre staff, to familiarise themselves with the technical aspects of the procedure. In order to ensure that an adequate number of trainers are available, a "training the trainer" programme is being designed.

19.2.3 Audit Phase

Centres that intend to join the international randomised trial need to complete an audit phase in which five TARGIT procedures are successfully performed and the relevant proformas sent to the trial steering group for review and approval. This ensures uniformity of practice within the participating centres in the trial.

19.3 TARGIT Academy Website

We are in the process of launching a website (www.targitacademy.com) which members of the Academy will be able to access. On this basis it is intended to develop focus groups that can stay in touch and deal with queries from centres all over the world. All the educational materials and latest developments regarding TARGIT will be posted on the website for access by INTRABEAM users.

19.4 Concluding Remarks

There has been significant interest in the TARGIT technique since the publication of the randomised controlled trial confirming its safety and efficacy. It is essential that as new centres take up this innovative technology worldwide, there is an appropriate training programme in place, and adequate quality assurance, to ensure that this powerful technology is implemented appropriately. We believe that establishment of the TARGIT Academy will go a long way in achieving this objective. The Academy provides at least eight courses a year, split between London and Mannheim.

Reference

Vaidya JS, Joseph DJ, Tobias JS, Bulsara M, Wenz F, Saunders C et al (2010) Targeted intraoperative radiotherapy versus whole breast radiotherapy for breast cancer (TARGIT-A trial): an international, prospective, randomised, non-inferiority phase 3 trial. Lancet 376:91–102

20 Health Economics of TARGIT

Chris Brew-Graves, Stephen Morris, and Michael Alvarado

20.1 What Is Health Economics?

Savedoff (2004) states, "Forty years ago, Kenneth Arrow published "uncertainty and the welfare economics of medical care" in the American Economic Review. This paper become not only one of the most widely cited articles in the field of health economics – indeed, it marked the creation of the discipline."

Health economics can be defined as the application of the theories, tools and concepts of economics as a discipline to the topics of health and health care. Since economics as a science is concerned with the allocation of scarce resources, health economics is concerned with issues relating to the allocation of scarce resources to improve health. This includes resource allocation both between sectors of the economy and the healthcare system and to different activities and individuals within the health case system. Health economics is therefore a broad subject and studies in health economics can, amongst other things, be concerned with economic aspects of health promotion and prevention, the supply and demand of health care, health insurance, regulation of markets for health manpower, cost and benefits of medical research and economic evaluation of health care.

Due to the constant introduction of new treatment alternatives and scarce resources within the health care system, it has become increasingly important to evaluate whether new treatment options achieve health improvements at a reasonable cost. This has led to the emergence of economic evaluation of drugs and other healthcare interventions as one of the major fields of health economics. An economic evaluation is a key part of a more general health technology assessment (HTA) undertaken to gain information for decisions about new as well as established medical technologies. Appleby (2012) shows that, in the past 30 years, total national expenditures on healthcare as a percentage of gross domestic product (GDP) have increased. In the UK this figure rose from 3.9 % in 1960 to 9.4 % in 2010, in Germany it rose from 6.0 % in 1970 to 11.6 % in 2010 and in the USA it rose from 5.1 % in 1960 to 17.6 % in 2010.

20.2 What Are Costs?

A cost can be defined as the value of the resource in its best alternative use of the resource (Lidgren 2007). This is referred to as the opportunity cost. Estimating costs in an economic evaluation involves four steps:

1. All relevant resources are identified and quantified into physical units, such as out-patient visits and number of fractions of radiotherapy.

C. Brew-Graves (✉)
Division of Surgery and Intervention Science, Department of Surgery, University College London, London, UK

S. Morris • M. Alvarado
Division of Surgical Oncology, Department of Surgery, University of California, San Francisco, CA, USA

M. Keshtgar et al. (eds.), *Targeted Intraoperative Radiotherapy in Oncology*,
DOI 10.1007/978-3-642-39821-6_20,

2. The physical unit must be valued, which means assigning a unit cost. According to economic theory, a resource should be priced based on its opportunity cost. However, in practice, the market price of the unit, or its NHS reference price, or HRG tariff, is often used.
3. Multiplication of quantities used by their unit costs.
4. Sum across all cost components

Cost can be split into three categories:

(a) *Direct cost*: borne by the health care system, community and family in directly addressing the problem.
(b) *Indirect cost*: mainly productivity losses caused by the problem or disease, borne by the individual, family, society or employer.
(c) *Intangible cost*: usually the costs of pain, grief and suffering and loss of leisure time. The cost of a life is usually included in case of death.

20.3 Effectiveness

The quality-adjusted life year (QALY) is a measure of disease burden, including both the quality and the quantity of life lived. It is used in assessing the value for money of a medical intervention. The QALY model requires utility-independent, risk-neutral and constant proportional trade-off behaviour.

The QALY is based on the number of years of life that would be added by the intervention. Each year in perfect health is assigned the value of 1.0 down to a value of 0.0 for death. If the extra years will not be lived in full health, for example if the patient is unable to carry out self-care or usual activities, then the extra life years are given a value between 0 and 1 to account for this.

20.3.1 Measuring QALYs

The EQ-5D is a generic (standardised), widely used, well-validated instrument for use as a measure of health outcome, commonly employed in cost-effectiveness analyses. Applicable to a wide range of health conditions and treatments, the EQ-5D health questionnaire provides a simple descriptive profile and a single index value for health status (www.euroqol.org). The instrument contains questions in five domains: mobility, self-care, usual activities, pain/discomfort and anxiety/depression. Response options for each item include:

1. No problems
2. Slight problems
3. Moderate problems or symptoms
4. Severe problems or symptoms
5. Unable to do or extreme symptoms

Patients choose the response that best describes their current experience in each domain, thereby aligning themselves with 1 of 3,125 possible health states (plus two extra for unconscious and dead), making a total of 3,127.

20.4 Perspective

The term "perspective" is used to define the categories of costs to be included in an economic evaluation. Various perspectives may be employed; within the UK context these are:

1. The patient
2. The hospital
3. The Primary Care Trust (PCT)
4. The NHS
5. Society at large (societal)

The "NHS perspective" would imply that only costs to the NHS are to be included whereas the term "societal perspective" implies that all categories of cost should be included (i.e. irrespective of whose responsibility it is to pay the costs). The National Institute for Health and Care Excellence (NICE)'s perspective for the Reference Case used within the Technology Appraisal Programme is "the costs to the NHS and Personal Social Services". This means that only the costs that fall within the remit of these two organisations should be included in Reference Case analyses.

20.5 Economic Evaluation

Economic evaluation is a structured approach to help decision makers to choose between alternative ways of using resources (Morris and Parkin 2009).

The different types of economic evaluation all measure cost in a similar way based on opportunity costs and are therefore usually distinguished by how the consequences of the compared alternatives are measured. Economic evaluations (Table 20.1) are usually divided into four categories (Drummond et al. 2005):

1. Cost minimisation analysis
2. Cost effectiveness
3. Cost utility
4. Cost-benefit analysis.

Other economic evaluations include cost consequences and budgetary analysis/impact. Simoens (Simoens 2009) explains budgetary analysis succinctly: "In addition to information about the efficiency of a new health technology, regulatory agencies in an increasing number of countries now require data about the budgetary impact of the technology on national, regional or local budgets. Whereas an economic evaluation allows decision makers to assess the efficiency of a health technology, a budget impact analysis examines the financial impact of the adoption and diffusion of the technology within a particular setting. Thus, a budget impact analysis considers the affordability of a technology. Specifically, a budget impact analysis explores how a change in the current mix of treatment strategies by the introduction of a new technology will impact spending on a disease."

The most frequently economic analysis used is, however, cost effectiveness. Cost-effectiveness analyses compare the economic and financial impacts of various therapies to determine which treatment option represents the best value for money spent (Foster et al. 2011). An intervention usually is considered cost-effective if its ratio of incremental cost to incremental benefit, often measured in terms of QALYs (i.e. the incremental cost-effectiveness ratio, or ICER), falls under the well-established acceptability thresholds or within the range of other therapies for which payers have demonstrated a willingness to pay.

20.6 Incremental Cost-Effectiveness Ratios

A cost-effectiveness ratio (CER) is the cost per unit of output or effect, and the implication is that the lower the CER, the better. The *incremental* cost-effectiveness ratio is a ratio which specifically compares alternatives which both require

Table 20.1 Summary of economic evaluations

Method	How are benefits measured?	How are results expressed?	What is the decision making rule?
Cost minimisation analysis	Proven equal	In monetary value	Choose that which costs least
Cost benefit analysis	In monetary value	Net present value (NPV) in £ Benefit cost (B:C) ratio	NPV >0 B:C ratio >1
Cost-effectiveness analysis	Natural units, e.g. pain-free days, life years gained	Incremental cost-effectiveness ratio (ICER) = Δ costs/Δ outcome	The option with the lowest ICER is best value for money
Cost consequences analysis	In a variety of different natural units	CERs for each alternative measure of effectiveness	The option with the lowest CER is the best value for money
Cost utility analysis	Utility, commonly measured in terms of quality-adjusted life years (QALYs)	Cost effectiveness ratio = Δ costs/Δ QALYs	The option with the lowest ICER is best value for money

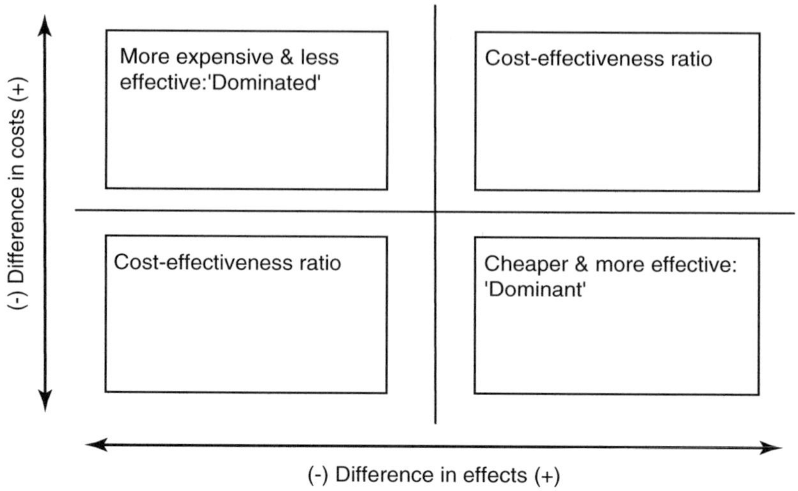

Fig. 20.1 Basic model for health economics

some input, because the costs and effects are incremental to the best alternative:

$$\text{ICER} = \frac{(C_A - C_B)}{(E_A - E_B)}$$

where C denotes cost and E, effectiveness (Fig. 20.1).

The NICE guidelines 2008 (National Institute for Health and Clinical Excellence 2008) consider cost-effectiveness as well as clinical effectiveness. To achieve cost-effectiveness, a new technology should generate more health gain to NHS patients than it displaces as a result of any additional costs imposed on the system (opportunity cost). This trade-off is assessed by comparing the incremental cost per quality-adjusted life year (QALY) gained against the cost-effectiveness threshold. In doing this, NICE is concerned with making decisions which are consistent with maximising population health gains subject to the NHS budget constraint. NICE's perspective for the Reference Case used within the Technology Appraisals Programme is the cost to the NHS and Personal Social Services (PSS); this means that only the costs that fall within the remit of these two organisations should be included in Reference Case analyses.

NICE defines the reference case thus: "The Institute has to make decisions across different technologies and disease areas. It is, therefore, crucial that analyses of clinical and cost effectiveness undertaken to inform the appraisal adopt a consistent approach. To allow this, the Institute has defined a 'reference case' that specifies the methods considered by the Institute to be appropriate for the Appraisal Committee's purpose and consistent with an NHS objective of maximising health gain from limited resources. Submissions to the Institute should include an analysis of results generated using these reference case methods. This does not preclude additional analyses being presented when one or more aspects of methods differ from the reference case. However, these must be justified and clearly distinguished from the reference case." (See (National Institute for Health and Care Excellence 2013) re the NICE 2013 guidance on the reference case.)

Drummond et al. (2005) provide clear guidelines on how to carry out a robust economic analysis. In summary, they state that the analysis should cover:

1. A clear definition of all relevant treatments
2. Definition of the analysis perspective
3. Proper identification, measurement and valuation of costs and outcomes
4. Incorporation of sensitivity analysis when appropriate
5. Adjustment for the differential timing of costs and benefits

20.7 Modelling-Based Economic Evaluation

Economic evaluations often use data from one or several clinical trials, epidemiological studies and databases. Models provide the framework to bring all these data together.

Clinical trials are usually conducted for a limited period of time, yet the real interest may be in examining the costs and benefits over a longer period. Trials often employ intermediate health outcomes whereas economists want to focus on "final" outcomes such as life expectancy; consequently, some form of modelling may be required to extrapolate beyond the end point of the clinical trial and to adjust or supplement the original data. Modelling therefore can be seen as a pragmatic response to the problem of limited time horizons. Data will be required to populate the model.

20.8 Decision Tree Models

A decision tree is a representation of sequential decisions and events with uncertain outcomes (Fig. 20.2). The model structure defines available options for each decision and the possible outcome for each event. By assigning probabilities and values to the different outcomes, the expected value of each outcome can be calculated and the optimal strategy can be identified. Decision tree models are most appropriate for short-term analyses or other situations where the numbers of possible outcomes are limited. Decision tree data can be fed into Markov models to assess long-term or lifetime outcomes.

20.9 Markov Models

Markov models are often used in economic evaluations to model diseases that are recursive and chronic in nature. A Markov model describes the disease process as a series of discrete mutually exclusive and collectively exhaustive health states, meaning that the patient can exist in only one health state at a time and that the patient must be in one of the health states. Transition from one state to another occurs in defined recurring intervals of equal length (Markov cycles) and is governed by transition probabilities that determine the speed at which patients move between states.

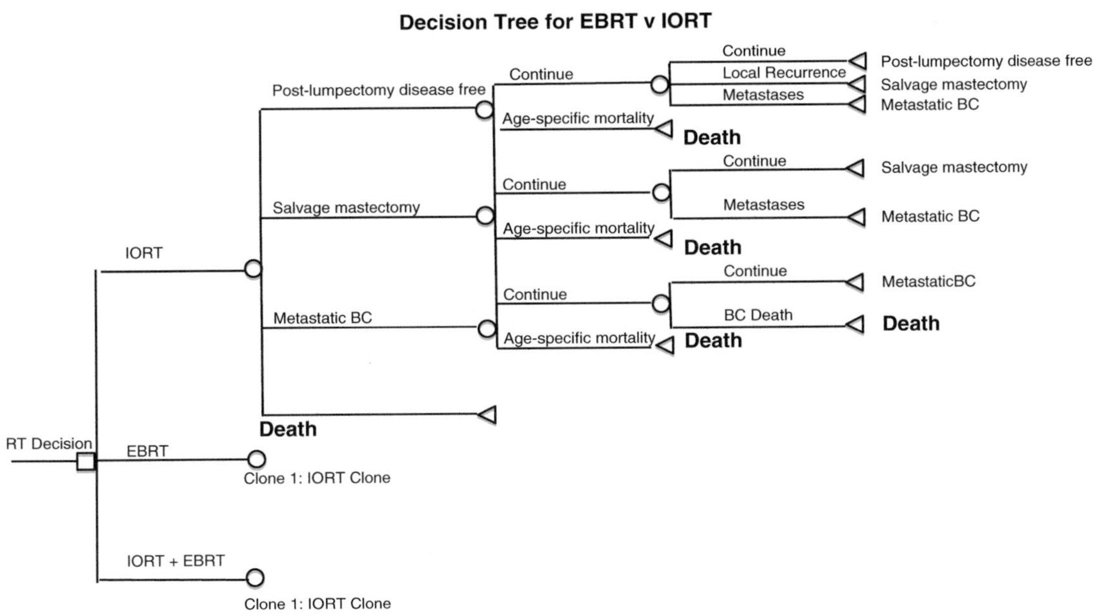

Fig. 20.2 EBRT vs IORT decision tree

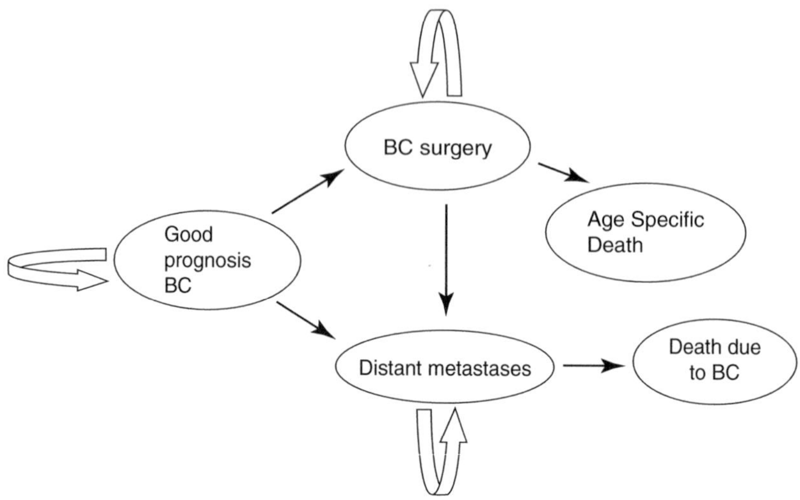

Fig. 20.3 Markov model (From Alvarado et al. 2011)

Heath states from which it is impossible to leave, e.g. death, are described as absorbing states. A Markov model is evaluated by moving a simulated cohort of patients through the model, where fractions of the cohort move to different states in each cycle based on transition probabilities in the model. Each state is typically assigned a cost and an outcome such as QALYs. Moving patients through the model, with a proportion spending time in each state, generates an estimate of mean costs and mean survival. The results obtained when running the model using costs, health effects and transition probabilities associated with different interventions can then be compared, and the incremental costs and effects for the simulated interventions can be calculated (Fig. 20.3).

20.10 TARGIT-A: A Case Study (UK Approach)

20.10.1 Which Evaluation Would You Carry Out?

TARGIT-A is a phase III randomised controlled trial comparing external beam radiotherapy (EBRT) with intraoperative radiotherapy (IORT). EBRT is the current standard of care and IORT is a novel partial breast radiation treatment. Recently published data from Vaidya et al. (2010) show early confirmation of non-inferiority of IORT with respect to local recurrences. Based on these findings, it is appropriate to carry out a cost minimisation analysis of IORT compared with EBRT for early stage breast cancer.

The results of clinical trials cannot be known in advance. No prospective economic evaluation starts out as a cost minimisation analysis; only when the health outcomes generated are demonstrated to be "identical or similar" can a cost minimisation analysis be carried out. In the aforementioned report, clinical effectiveness proved to be equivalent in both arms (at 4 years local recurrences in IORT arm numbered six and in the EBRT arm, five); cost could now be seen as the main decision driver. Steps in the evaluation are described below:

1. *Identify all costs*

   External beam radiotherapy (EBRT):

   Calculate all costs pertaining to the linear accelerator (Linac):

   - Cost of purchasing the equipment
   - Costs of running it, staff and consumables
   - Servicing and maintenance annual costs.

   Important note: As Linacs are used for the treatment of various types of cancer, one must first establish the time/cost associated with breast cancer only; for the purposes of this exercise one cannot use all Linac costs as this would be incorrect.

   What is the planned life span of this equipment?

Table 20.2 Cost allocation

Item	EBRT (£)	IORT (£)
Capital costs	–	
Equipment (INTRABEAM with a 10-year life span)	1,000,000	526,246
Service agreement and maintenance charges/annum	100,000	42,000
Consumables		
Drapes/box of 5	–	102
Applicators each (100 sterilisations)	–	3,052
Radiation shields/box of 10	–	725
5 % of patients require immobilisation shells for PETG each	350	
New breast boards per annum	5,000	
Vac bags for patient positioning for 30 % of patients	1,000	
Hospital costs		
Cost per case – Radiation Physics	–	300
Theatre – per patient (additional cost for IORT treatment)	–	800
CT planning scan 30 min × 2 radiologists, 2.5 h virtual simulation × 1 radiologist, treatment time 20 min per patient × 2 radiologists + 1 h × 2 radiologists' input time (pretreatment) = 19.5 h radiology time for 23 fractions	975	

Divide the costs over the life span, for example 10 years.

Intraoperative radiotherapy (IORT):

This intervention is fairly new and therefore no NHS reference cost data are available. Obtain the costs of:

- Purchasing the equipment
- Running it, recommended staffing, consumables
- Annual servicing and maintenance

What is the life span of the INTRABEAM? (Divide the costs over this period, for example 10 years).

Note that the life spans of the equipment may vary.

Prices used are 2011 prices. The cost allocation table (Table 20.2) shows total costs incurred by site.

Table 20.3 Resource allocation

	EBRT (£)	IORT (£)
Per patient cost		
Capital cost		
Equipment (INTRABEAM with a 10-year life span)	14	527
Service agreement and maintenance charges/annum	1	420
Consumables		
Drapes/box of 5		21
Applicators each (100 sterilisations)		31
Radiation shields/box of 10		73
5 % of patients require immobilisation shells for PETG each	1	
New breast boards per annum	11	
Vac bags for patient positioning for 30 % of patients	1	
Hospital costs		
Cost per case – Radiation Physics		300
Theatre – per patient (additional cost for IORT treatment)		800
CT planning scan 30 min × 2 radiologists, 2.5 h virtual simulation × 1 radiologist, treatment time 20 min per patient × 2 radiologists + 1 h × 2 radiologists' input time (pretreatment) = 19.5 h radiology time for 23 fractions	975	
HRG code		
Cost per patient borne by the hospital	200/ fraction	2,172.00
N.B. consider that approximately 7,000 fractions are deployed per Linac per annum, and that one-third of the work load is breast		

Based on the cost allocation table, a per patient cost for a single dose of EBRT and IORT can be calculated, as shown in the resource table (Table 20.3).

2. *Calculate a unit cost for each unit*

   Price per fraction of EBRT works out as £200.00

   Price per dose of IORT treatment works out as £2,172.00

3. *Calculate quantities used per patient and then multiply by unit costs, giving the cost per patient for each treatment*

Cost per IORT treatment	=£2,172.00
Cost of EBRT for 15 fractions	=£3,000.00
Cost of EBRT for 20 fractions	=£4,000.00
Cost of EBRT for 25 fractions	=£5,000.00
Cost of EBRT for 30 fractions	=£6,000.00

20.10.2 Budgetary Analysis/Impact

Cancer Research UK (CRUK) states that 47,700 women were diagnosed with breast cancer in 2008; approximately 60 % of these women were treated by conservative surgery.

If these patients were to be given IORT at the aforementioned cost of £2,172 per patient (approximated to **£**2,175):
= 2,175 × (60% of 47,700) = **£**62,248,500.00

If 15% of these patients go on to have 20 fractions of EBRT:
= (200 × 20) × (15% of (60% of 47,700))
= **£**17,172,000.00

The cost of IORT would then
= **£**62,248,500.00 + **£**17,172,000.00
= £79,420,500.00

By contrast, the cost of 20 fractions of EBRT at **£**200 per fraction (**£**4,000 per patient)
= 4000 × (60% of 47,700) = £114,480,000.00

Cost of EBRT alone less IORT + 15% EBRT = £35,059,500.00 (saved) based on 2008 incidence figures, and 2011 costs

The NHS could thus potentially save 35 million pounds per annum, for equivalent outcomes in local recurrences.

NICE states clearly how economic appraisals that they approve should be set out. They require the appraisal to have an NHS and PSS perspective; both costs and effectiveness need to be discounted at 3.5 % and their threshold for willingness to pay is £20,000/QALY (Devlin and Parkin 2004) except in exceptional circumstances, e.g. rare diseases, orphaned drugs and end of life therapies.

The calculations above are "per protocol calculations". More in-depth work needs to be carried out, using trial data, to calculate cost of complications in each arm, and compare these.

To provide a full health economics evaluation on targeted IORT, it would be useful to consider other perspectives, for example, the NHS perspective in its totality or the patient perspective, in a separate analysis (in the latter case, evaluating costs incurred by the patient and then comparing those of the EBRT patient with those of the IORT patient). Possibly one could also consider a societal perspective: this evaluation would explore all costs borne by the NHS, Works and Pensions, Health Insurance institutions, the Primary Care Trust and the patient.

Currently QALY data on breast cancer patients treated with whole breast radiotherapy need refreshing; data from the Hayman et al. 1998 study (1998) are now out of date.

In line with the recommendations made by Drummond et al. (2005), the value of these analyses can further be enhanced by including:

- A full sensitivity analysis
- Use of discounting methods

References

Alvarado MD, Mohan AJ, Esserman LJ, Ozanne E (2011) Cost-effectiveness of intraoperative radiation therapy for breast conservation. Breast 20:S62–3

Appleby J (2012) Rises in healthcare spending: will it end? BMJ 345:e7127. doi:10.1136/bmj.e7127

Devlin N, Parkin D (2004) Does NICE have a cost effectiveness threshold and what other factors influence its decisions? Health Econ 13:437–52

Drummond MF, Sculpher MJ, Torrance GW, O'Brien BJ, Stoddart GL (2005) Methods for the economic evaluation of healthcare programmes, 3rd edn. Oxford Medical Publications, New York

Foster TS, Miller JD, Boyle ME, Blieden MB, Gidwani R, Russell MW (2011) The economic burden of metastatic breast cancer: A systematic review of literature from developed countries. Cancer Treat Rev 37:405–15

Hayman JA, Hillner BE, Harris JR, Weeks JC (1998) Cost-effectiveness of routine radiation therapy following conservative surgery for early-stage breast cancer. J Clin Oncol 16:1022–9

Lidgren M (2007) Health economics of breast cancer (thesis). Department of Learning, Informatics, Management and Ethics, Medical Management Centre, Karolinska Institute, Stockholm, Sweden, 2007. Available at http://publications.ki.se/jspui/handle/10616/39580

Morris S, Devlin N, Parkin D (2009) Economic Analysis in Health Care, John Wiley & Sons, UK

National Institute for Health and Care Excellence (2013) Guide to the methods of technology appraisal, 2013. Available at http://publications.nice.org.uk/guide-to-the-methods-of-technology-appraisal-2013-pmg9/the-reference-case

National Institute for Health and Clinical Excellence (2008) Guide to the methods of technology appraisal, 2008. Available at http://www.nice.org.uk/media/B52/A7/TAMethodsGuideUpdatedJune2008.pdf

Savedorf WD (2004) Kenneth arrow and the birth of health economics. Bull WHO 82(2):139–140

Simoens S (2009) Health economic assessment: a methodological primer. Int J Environ Res Public Health 6:2950–66

Vaidya JS, Joseph DJ, Tobias JS, Bulsara M, Wenz F, Saunders C et al (2010) Targeted intraoperative radiotherapy versus whole breast radiotherapy for breast cancer (TARGIT-A trial): an international, prospective, randomised, non-inferiority phase 3 trial. Lancet 376:91–102

Index

M. Keshtgar et al. (eds.), *Targeted Intraoperative Radiotherapy in Oncology*,
DOI 10.1007/978-3-642-39821-6, © Springer-Verlag Berlin Heidelberg 2014

MIX
Papier aus verantwortungsvollen Quellen
Paper from responsible sources
FSC® C105338

If you have any concerns about our products,
you can contact us on
ProductSafety@springernature.com

In case Publisher is established outside the EU,
the EU authorized representative is:
Springer Nature Customer Service Center GmbH
Europaplatz 3, 69115 Heidelberg, Germany

Printed by Libri Plureos GmbH
in Hamburg, Germany